Respiratory Medicine

Series Editor:
Sharon I.S. Rounds

More information about this series at http://www.springer.com/series/7665

Nicholas S. Ward • Mitchell M. Levy

Editors

Sepsis

Definitions, Pathophysiology
and the Challenge of Bedside Management

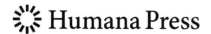 Humana Press

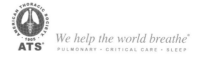 We help the world breathe®
PULMONARY · CRITICAL CARE · SLEEP

Editors
Nicholas S. Ward
Division of Pulmonary Critical Care,
   and Sleep Medicine
Alpert/Brown Medical School
Providence, RI, USA

Mitchell M. Levy
Division of Pulmonary Critical Care,
   and Sleep Medicine
Alpert/Brown Medical School
Providence, RI, USA

ISSN 2197-7372   ISSN 2197-7380   (electronic)
Respiratory Medicine
ISBN 978-3-319-83950-9   ISBN 978-3-319-48470-9   (eBook)
DOI 10.1007/978-3-319-48470-9

Printed on acid-free paper

This Humana Press imprint is published by Springer Nature
The registered company is Springer International Publishing AG
The registered company address is: Gewerbestrasse 11, 6330 Cham, Switzerland

Preface

Sepsis is a disease syndrome that is difficult to understand as well as to treat and has plagued mankind for thousands of years. In this textbook, the editors and authors sought to assemble relatively brief but detailed compilations of what is the state of the science on a variety of key topics. We have chosen topics that range from molecular biology to clinical practice. It is our hope that this text can be used by bench scientists and clinicians alike as a reference to aid in their work. Clinicians can learn more about the biology behind the disease they treat and scientists can gain deeper understanding into how the disease they study plays out in intensive care unit. Together the clinical and scientific elements of this text will hopefully make a reference that is of great value. We have picked as authors those who we feel are leaders in the field they have written about and thus can provide vast experience as well as data from years of study and practice.

Providence, RI, USA   Nicholas S. Ward, MD, FCCM
Providence, RI, USA   Mitchell M. Levy, MD, FCCM

Contents

Contributors

Charles Adams, MD Department of Surgery, Alpert/Brown Medical School, Providence, RI, USA

Brian J. Anderson, MD, MSCE Pulmonary, Allergy and Critical Care Division, Perelman School of Medicine at the University of Pennsylvania, Philadelphia, PA, USA

MaryEllen Antkowiak, MD Division of Pulmonary and Critical Care Medicine, University of Vermont College of Medicine, Burlington, VT, USA

Alfred Ayala, PhD Division of Surgical Research, Department of Surgery, Rhode Island Hospital, Providence, RI, USA

Debasree Banerjee, MD Division of Pulmonary, Critical Care, and Sleep Medicine, Alpert/Brown Medical School, Providence, RI, USA

William Bender Pulmonary, Critical Care and Sleep Medicine, Bellevue Hospital/ NYU School of Medicine, New York, NY, USA

Jason D. Christie Division of Pulmonary, Allergy, and Critical Care Medicine, Perelman School of Medicine, University of Pennsylvania, Philadelphia, PA, USA

Tristen T. Chun, MD Division of Surgical Research, Department of Surgery, Rhode Island Hospital, Providence, RI, USA

Douglas R. Closser, MD Division of Pulmonary, Critical Care, and Sleep Medicine, The Ohio State University Wexner Medical Center, Columbus, OH, USA

Michael Connolly, MD Department of Surgery, Alpert/Brown Medical School, Providence, RI, USA

Elliott D. Crouser, MD Division of Pulmonary, Critical Care, and Sleep Medicine, The Ohio State University Wexner Medical Center, Columbus, OH, USA

Nicholas Csikesz Alpert Medical School of Brown University, Rhode Island Hospital, Providence, RI, USA

Laura Evans Pulmonary, Critical Care and Sleep Medicine, Bellevue Hospital/NYU School of Medicine, New York, NY, USA

Mathew C. Exline, MD Division of Pulmonary, Critical Care, and Sleep Medicine, The Ohio State University Wexner Medical Center, Columbus, OH, USA

Hernando Gomez, MD The Center for Critical Care Nephrology, University of Pittsburgh, Pittsburgh, PA, USA

The CRISMA Center, Department of Critical Care Medicine, University of Pittsburgh, Pittsburgh, PA, USA

Daithi S. Heffernan, MD, FACS, AFRCSI Division of Surgical Research, Department of Surgery, Rhode Island Hospital/Brown University, Providence, RI, USA

Andre C. Kalil, MD Infectious Disease Division, Department of Internal Medicine, University of Nebraska Medical Center, Omaha, NE, USA

John A. Kellum, MD The Center for Critical Care Nephrology, University of Pittsburgh, Pittsburgh, PA, USA

The CRISMA Center, Department of Critical Care Medicine, University of Pittsburgh, Pittsburgh, PA, USA

Mitchell M. Levy, MD, FCCM Division of Pulmonary, Critical Care, and Sleep Medicine, Alpert/Brown Medical School, Providence, RI, USA

Greg S. Martin, MD, MSc Division of Pulmonary, Allergy, and Critical Care Medicine, Emory University School of Medicine, Atlanta, GA, USA

Nuala J. Meyer Division of Pulmonary Allergy, and Critical Care Medicine, Perelman School of Medicine, University of Pennsylvania, Philadelphia, PA, USA

Mark E. Mikkelsen, MD, MSCE Pulmonary, Allergy and Critical Care Division, Perelman School of Medicine at the University of Pennsylvania, Philadelphia, PA, USA

Lucas Mikulic, MD Division of Pulmonary and Critical Care Medicine, University of Vermont College of Medicine, Burlington, VT, USA

Raghavan Murugan, MD The Center for Critical Care Nephrology, University of Pittsburgh, Pittsburgh, PA, USA

The CRISMA Center, Department of Critical Care Medicine, University of Pittsburgh, Pittsburgh, PA, USA

Steven M. Opal, MD Infectious Disease Division, Memorial Hospital of RI, Alpert Medical School of Brown University, Pawtucket, RI, USA

Brittany A. Potz Division of Surgical Research, Department of Surgery, Rhode Island Hospital, Providence, RI, USA

John P. Reilly Division of Pulmonary, Allergy, and Critical Care Medicine, Perelman School of Medicine, University of Pennsylvania, Philadelphia, PA, USA

Bashar Staitieh, MD Division of Pulmonary, Allergy, and Critical Care Medicine, Emory University School of Medicine, Atlanta, GA, USA

Benjamin T. Suratt, MD Division of Pulmonary and Critical Care Medicine, University of Vermont College of Medicine, Burlington, VT, USA

Jean-Louis Vincent, MD Department of Intensive Care, Erasme Hospital, Université Libre de Bruxelles, Brussels, Belgium

Nicholas S. Ward Division of Pulmonary, Critical Care, and Sleep Medicine, Alpert/Brown Medical School, Providence, RI, USA

Whitney A. Young Division of Surgical Research, Department of Surgery, Rhode Island Hospital, Providence, RI, USA

Alex Zarbock Department of Anesthesiology, Intensive Care and Pain Medicine, University of Münster, Münster, Germany

Part I

Chapter 1
Introduction

Mitchell M. Levy and Nicholas S. Ward

Sepsis is a disease that has been known and studied for over 2000 years and yet there is still so much of it we do not understand. Our ignorance is not for lack of effort, however. In just the year 2015, PUBMED listed over 1400 articles published with sepsis as a major topic. The journey to understand sepsis over the years has been a microcosm of our progress all fields of medicine. It began as a common disease with varying outward manifestations and has progressed to become understood as problem that encompasses organs, cells, organelles, cytokines, molecules, and genetics of every part of the body. No longer just a clinical puzzle, it is now studied and discussed in papers ranging from molecular biology, to health services research and it remains a serious concern for practitioners of all branches of medicine.

The word "sepsis," was first used by Hippocrates and derived from the Greek word for "rot" to describe generally the decay or organic matter. Hippocrates went on to associate this sepsis with the human colon and recognized that this process had the ability to release toxins deadly to man. There are descriptions of the clinical entity "sepsis" from Ancient Egypt dating back to 3000 BCE that reflect an understanding similar to ours today of a local insult or injury that results in systemic complications (e.g., a flesh wound resulting in fever). Roman physicians expanded on these ideas, hypothesizing the existence of spontaneously generated invisible creatures in swamps whose emission of putrid fumes ("miasma") caused human disease. As a result, they focused on water purification and the elimination of swamps [1].

In the seventeenth century, Leeuwenhoek's invention of the microscope led to the discovery of "animalcules," the first description of directly observed bacteria,

M.M. Levy, MD, FCCM (✉) • N.S. Ward
Division of Pulmonary, Critical Care, and Sleep Medicine, Alpert/Brown Medical School, Providence, RI, USA
e-mail: mitchell_levy@brown.edu; nward@lifespan.org

© Springer International Publishing AG 2017　　　　　　　　　　　　　　　　3
N.S. Ward, M.M. Levy (eds.), *Sepsis*, Respiratory Medicine,
DOI 10.1007/978-3-319-48470-9_1

and paved the way for the development of germ theory and more targeted public health initiatives. The next 100 years saw discoveries by Koch, Semmelweis, Pasteur, and Lister create not only more understanding of infectious sepsis but real-world methods for preventing it. Ignaz Semmelweis, through his pioneering study of hand washing and puerperal sepsis, gave us one of the first highly effective ways to prevent the disease and Lister followed by advancing these ideas to aseptic surgical techniques. Tragically, Semmelweis was mocked for his research and likely died from staphylococcal sepsis while in an insane asylum.

In the ensuing centuries, the understanding of sepsis showed an increasingly complex disease syndrome triggered by infections with bacteria. For most of this time, sepsis therapy focused heavily on the rapid and effective treatment of infections and the advent of antibiotics was groundbreaking in our ability to save patients with this disease. Indeed, it was thought that antibiotics could possibly eliminate sepsis as a deadly illness. What was found instead was that even when infections are properly diagnosed and treated, patients with sepsis will frequently go on to have organ dysfunction and death.

In the latter half of the twentieth century, this led to the realization that the source of injury in sepsis may not be solely the bacteria. Pioneering researchers such as Roger Bone and many others helped us to realize that it was the body's response to the infection that was causing most of the injury and organ dysfunction. Bone went on to discover (along with others) that this over exuberant pro-inflammatory response often coexisted with an exuberant anti-inflammatory response that limited self injury but opened the door to more infections.

Restoring hemodynamic normalcy to patients with sepsis has been subject of focus for many years as well. However, unlike other forms of shock, restoration of hemodynamics in septic patients does not always prevent or repair organ dysfunction. It has now become clear that even though sepsis appears to exert much of its injury through shock, the true mechanisms of injury are far more complex than just insufficient oxygen delivery. As described in several chapters of this book, sepsis causes dysfunction to occur not just at the organ level but at the cellular and molecular levels. Problems with cell membranes, mitochondria, the coagulation system, and pathologic amplification of inflammatory cascades are now being recognized and the key factors leading to hemodynamic problems and organ dysfunction. These discoveries represent paradigm changing moments in the history of sepsis. Few if any of our current therapies are able to address these problems in a direct fashion.

As the twenty-first century arrived new areas have become important in our understanding and treatment of sepsis. Genetic analysis has shown the ways in which predisposition to severe sepsis may differ among people and this information may help guide both prevention and treatment in years to come. Therapeutically, various other research groups have shown that by bundling well-established existing therapies and practices as part of a comprehensive targeted strategy, sepsis mortality can be reduced. Multi-professional groups such as the Surviving Sepsis Campaign have used data from all corners of research to put together new definitions and treatment strategies, and help guide further research by analyzing where deficiencies lay.

It is our hope that the chapters of this textbook can be used to give researchers and clinicians alike a broad understanding of multiple elements of sepsis while also giving detailed descriptions of the most current evidence on mechanisms, diagnosis, and treatments. The book is organized into four sections. The first is meant to give a perspective the history and impact of sepsis on mankind with sections on epidemiology and definitions. The second section discusses the known mechanisms of sepsis at the molecular, genetic, and cellular levels. The third section details what is known about organ failure in sepsis with specific chapters discussing some of the most important organs such as the lung, kidneys, and coagulation system. The final section of the book discusses key topics in the treatment of the disease such as bundled therapies, source control, and hemodynamic support.

It is a certainty that our understanding of sepsis will continue to grow in the years to come. New technologies will aid this endeavor and enable progress to deeper levels of understanding that are necessary to make new and effective therapies. As these new discoveries coalesce, we will undoubtedly see very different sepsis therapies in the years to come that push beyond antibiotics and vasopressors. It is clear to anyone who studies or treats patients with the disease that we have far to go in eliminating a condition that has threatened lives for millennia.

References

1. Funk DJ, Parrillo JE, Kumar A. Sepsis and septic shock: a history. Crit Care Clin. 2009;25: 83–101. viii

Chapter 2
Sepsis Definitions

Debasree Banerjee and Mitchell M. Levy

Introduction

Sepsis is the tenth leading cause of death in the United States [1]. Mortality in the United States from sepsis is more than the total number of deaths caused by prostate cancer, breast cancer, and AIDS combined [2]. It causes more hospitalizations than acute myocardial infarction and has become a leading cause of hospital expenditure [3, 4]. Ninety percent of physicians feel that sepsis is a "significant financial burden on the health care system in their country" [5]. The Center for Disease Control and Prevention cite an aging population, chronic illness, invasive procedures, immuno-suppressive drugs, chemotherapy, organ transplantation, antibiotic resistance, and increased awareness as causes for the increase in number of reported cases of sepsis each year in the United States. Despite the significance held by this disease in medicine it has been subject to many varying definitions over the years. The ongoing changes in the "definition" of sepsis reflect both a new emphasis on precision, needed for research, and an ever-expanding knowledge of its pathophysiology.

History of the Definition of Sepsis

Origins of the Definition of Sepsis

The word "sepsis" was first used over 2000 years ago [σηψις] in ancient Greek literature, referenced by Homer, Hippocrates, Aristotle, Plutarch, and Galen to describe decay of organic material [6]. In its earliest derivation in 1989, Roger Bone

D. Banerjee, MD (✉) • M.M. Levy, MD, FCCM
Division of Pulmonary, Critical Care, and Sleep Medicine, Alpert/Brown Medical School, Providence, RI, USA
e-mail: banerjed19@gmail.com; Mitchell.levy@brown.edu

© Springer International Publishing AG 2017
N.S. Ward, M.M. Levy (eds.), *Sepsis*, Respiratory Medicine,
DOI 10.1007/978-3-319-48470-9_2

and his colleagues introduced the concept of the "sepsis syndrome" which is the foundation of our systemic inflammatory response syndrome (SIRS) criteria [7]. The sepsis syndrome was first described by Bone in his post hoc analysis of the Methylprednisolone Severe Sepsis Study Group in 1989 where he defined it as "a systemic response to a suspected or documented infection and at least one organ dysfunction" [7]. It consisted of hypothermia or hyperthermia, tachycardia, tachypnea, infection, and end organ dysfunction from hypoperfusion.

1991 International Consensus Conference

Current use of the terminology "sepsis" was born out of the 1991 International Consensus Conference: Distinctions in the Definition of Severe Sepsis (hosted by the Society of Critical Care Medicine, European Society of Intensive Care Medicine, the American College of Chest Physicians, the American Thoracic Society and Surgical Infection Society) [8]. Bone's work formed the basis of the first official definition for sepsis as stipulated by the International Sepsis Definition Conference. Lynn ascribes the philosophy of parsimony of the twentieth century as being one of the more influential factors in the creation of the definition [9]. This definition adopted both threshold decision making and consensus theories. The former enables clinicians at the bedside to ascertain a reasonable pretest probability for the pathology based on clinical and supporting diagnostics such as easy-to-obtain vital signs, while the latter utilizes expert opinion [10]. The goals of this conference were twofold: to allow early bedside detection of disease and subsequent therapeutic intervention and also to standardize research protocols [11]. More modern definitions of sepsis had been based on the central concept of SIRS, a term that describes both a complex immune cascade in response to infection or injury and is also used to delineate the clinical characteristics associated with that response. The clinical use of the term SIRS describes derangements in respiratory rate, heart rate, temperature, and white blood cell count. Meeting two of the four following criteria satisfies the requirement for SIRS: respiratory rate >20 breaths per min or a $PaCo2$ <32 mmHg, heart rate >90 beats per minute, temperature >38 °C or <36 °C, and white blood cell count >12,000/mm^3 or <4000/mm^3 or >10% bandemia [8]. Guidelines stated that sepsis is SIRS with suspected or proven infection, while severe sepsis describes patients who fulfill the criteria for sepsis and in addition have organ dysfunction [12]. In its most severe manifestation, septic shock is defined as "acute circulatory failure characterized by persistent arterial hypotension [including systolic <90 mmHg, mean arterial pressure <65 mmHg, or a drop in systolic blood pressure of >40 mmHg from baseline after adequate fluid resuscitation] unexplained by other causes" [11].

2001 International Consensus Conference

In the interim between 1991 and 2001 when the professional societies decided to revisit the definition, the SIRS criteria were widely used in research protocols [11, 13]. SIRS was acknowledged as a "systemic activation of the innate immune response, regardless of the cause" and therefore not specific to sepsis [11]. This prompted the professional societies consensus statement of 2001 to reject the use of the term SIRS in favor of the "signs and symptoms of sepsis" [11]. This would allow for early intervention as "findings indicative of early organ dysfunction may be the first symptoms noted by clinicians when making [the] assessment [for sepsis]" [11].

It was the goal of this committee to "provide a conceptual and practical framework to define the systemic inflammatory response to infection, which is a progressive injurious process that falls under the generalized term 'sepsis' and includes sepsis-associated organ dysfunction" [11]. The use of multiple organ dysfunction syndrome defined by deranged organ function such that the body cannot heal without intervention has become commonplace in critical care literature and is the basis for the use of the SOFA [12, 14].

The revision in 2001 sought to improve the definition by including clinical symptoms and physical exam findings such as altered mental status, oliguria, decreased capillary refill, and hyperglycemia without known diabetes [11] (Fig. 2.1). The use

Infection[a]
Documented or suspected *and* some of the following[b]:

General parameters
Fever (core temperature >38.3°C)
Hypothermia (core temperature <36°C
Heart rate >90 bpm or >2 SD above the normal value for age
Tachypnea: >30 bpm
Altered mental status
Significant edema or positive fluid balance (>20 ml/kg over 24 h)
Hyperglycemia (plasma glucose >110 mg/dl or 7.7 mM/l) in the absence of diabetes

Inflammatory parameters
Leukocytosis (white blood cell count >12,000/μl)
Leukopenia (white blood cell count <4,000/μl)
Normal white blood cell count with >10% immature forms
Plasma C reactive protein >2 SD above the normal value
Plasma procalcitonin >2 SD above the normal value

Hemodynamic parameters
Arterial hypotension[b] (systolic blood pressure <90 mmHg, mean arterial pressure <70,
   or a systolic blood pressure decrease >40 mmHg in adults or <2 SD below normal for age)
Mixed venous oxygen saturation >70%[b]
Cardiac index >3.5 l min⁻¹ m⁻²[c,d]

Organ dysfunction parameters
Arterial hypoxemia (PaO₂/FIO2 <300)
Acute oliguria (urine output <0.5 ml kg⁻¹ h⁻¹ or 45 mM/l for at least 2 h)
Creatinine increase ≥0.5 mg/dl
Coagulation abnormalities (international normalized ratio >1.5 or activated partial
   thromboplastin time >60 s)
Ileus (absent bowel sounds)
Thrombocytopenia (platelet count <100,000/μl)
Hyperbilirubinemia (plasma total bilirubin >4 mg/dl or 70 mmol/l)

Tissue perfusion parameters
Hyperlactatemia (>3 mmol/l)
Decreased capillary refill or mottling

[a] Defined as a pathological process induced by a micro-organism
[b] Values above 70% are normal in children (normally 75–80%) and should therefore not be used as a sign of sepsis in newborns or children
[c] Values of 3.5–5.5 are normal in children and should therefore not be used as a sign of sepsis in newborns or children
[d] Diagnostic criteria for sepsis in the pediatric population is signs and symptoms of inflammation plus infection with hyper- or hypothermia (rectal temperature >38.5°C or <35°C), tachycardia (may be absent in hypothermic patients) and at least one of the following indications of altered organ function: altered mental status, hypoxemia, elevated serum lactate level, and bounding pulses

Fig. 2.1 Diagnostic criteria for sepsis; adapted from Levy, ICM, 2003;29:530–538

of clinician judgment may seem nebulous but at least one study demonstrated good inter-operator agreement between clinicians for identifying an infectious source in septic patients in the intensive care unit (ICU), though the clinical decision-making process becomes more complex and concordance diminishes as subsets of infections are studied [15, 16]. The authors explain that the thresholds chosen for their criteria were selected to reflect the "'reality' for bedside physicians" [11]. The word "some" is used purposefully to credit physician experience and detection of protean and subtle clinical changes in a patient. This aim was specifically prioritized over using a more clear-cut checklist for purposes of research enrollment [11]. This flexibility while reflecting a more accurate real-life scenario does not allow for easy standardization of the definition.

2010 Merinoff Symposium

Despite the further clarifications crafted at these conferences, it was felt that the definitions did not adequately capture the underlying complex molecular processes that drove the sepsis syndrome. The 2001 meeting had been notable for giving more weight to the host response of severe sepsis rather than the virulence of the specific microbe. This was a well-known concept dating back to William Osler who said "except on few occasions, the patient appears to die from the body's response to infection rather than from [the infection itself]" [17]. However, these earlier definitions still did not address how infection differs from sterile inflammation as seen in severe burns and pancreatitis [18]. It is thought that on a molecular level, the inflammatory cascade triggered by trauma for example is similar to that caused by pathogens in regards to leading to cell death [19]. In 2010, the first meeting of the Global Sepsis Alliance with representatives from various national governments and media was held at the Merinoff symposium to create a "public definition" and a "molecular definition" of sepsis that focuses on the deranged host response to the microbial insult [20]. The results were the following:

1. *Definition of sepsis*: Sepsis is a life-threatening condition that arises when the body's response to an infection injures its own tissues and organs. Sepsis leads to shock, multiple organ failure, and death, especially if not recognized early and treated promptly [20].
2. *Molecular definition of sepsis:* Host-derived molecules and foreign products of infection converge on molecular mechanisms that cause unbalanced activation of innate immunity. Foreign and endogenous molecules interact with pathogen recognition receptors expressed on or in cells of the immune system. Activation of pathogen recognition receptors culminates in the release of immune mediators that produce the clinical signs and symptoms of sepsis [20].

2016 The Third International Consensus Definitions for Sepsis and Septic Shock (Sepsis-3)

The most recent definition of sepsis stems from a 2016 task force which resulted in a change in terminology [21]. Simple infection with signs and symptoms of the inflammatory response but without organ dysfunction, formerly defined as sepsis, is now defined as *infection*. *Sepsis* is now defined as infection with evidence of organ dysfunction (as evidenced by Sequential Organ Failure Assessment [SOFA] score > 2). Previously, this was the definition of *Severe Sepsis*, a term that will no longer be used. This change was instituted primarily because the field was already using sepsis to imply a patient deteriorating with infection and organ dysfunction, leading to considerable confusion between the terms sepsis and severe sepsis. The definition of *Septic Shock* refers to patients with infection who also have hypotension (MAP < 65 mmHg or systolic < 90 mmHg) and are receiving vasopressors and with a lactate > 2 mmol/L.

Difficulties in Defining Sepsis

Shortcomings of the SIRS Criteria

The SIRS criteria are useful because they can facilitate enrollment for research purposes and have been adopted for identification of potentially septic patients but their utility is limited by the lack of specificity. Up to 90% of patients admitted to the ICU fit the criteria for SIRS [22]. In an editorial by Vincent et al., the authors point out fundamental limitations in the current definition of sepsis (SIRS criteria with infection), including, that while all patients with sepsis have a known or presumed infection, not all infected patients have a clinically appreciable physiologic response that can be characterized as a syndrome thus making it challenging to create a practical clinical definition of sepsis [23, 24].

Another concern regarding SIRS criteria is their utility in patients who were already thought to have an acute injury or infection [25]. Gaieski and Goyal thus contend that this method does not properly ascertain the ability of this tool to discriminate undifferentiated patients for early intervention [25]. SIRS does however, have the ability to capture a very high percentage of people with sepsis as studied by Rangel-Frausto, who looked at the spectrum of SIRS/septic shock in the general hospital admissions of an academic center and found 68% fit SIRS criteria, 26% developing sepsis, 18% severe sepsis, and 4% septic shock with an inversely proportionate rate of mortality [26]. Reflecting these beliefs, the 2001 consensus meeting concluded that SIRS captured too broad a population and as such, additional signs and symptoms were proposed to the description and definition of sepsis. Only recently has the field begun to move away from the use of SIRS, propelled by the 2016 consensus definition.

Staging of Sepsis

Another problem with trying to define sepsis comes from the observation that sepsis appears to have stages that can differ significantly in terms of clinical features and immune system characteristics. In general, these stages can be thought of as initiation, amplification, and resolution of the response but as time goes on, it appears even these subcategories may be too general. The 2001 consensus statement acknowledged potential limitations to the definition including the inability to stage or prognosticate the host response to infection [11]. The authors acknowledged the overly sensitive nature of SIRS and proposed PIRO—a hypothetical model for staging sepsis using premorbid conditions (P), the causative infection (I), host response (R), and the severity of organ dysfunction (O) [11]. The PIRO model is a system that allows staging of sepsis to risk stratify patients for illness and also for potential response to therapy [11] (Fig. 2.2). Follow-up studies seem to validate the use of PIRO to risk stratify patients with suspected infection [27].

Similar to oncologic staging, PIRO staging factors criteria such as variable genetic susceptibility to illnesses. It was proposed that this model could also describe the host response to infection [11], for example, a genetic polymorphism that causes a more aggressive inflammatory response to an invading organism [11]. Additionally, early detection of a pathogen through sensitive assays of microbial genomics or transcriptomics would allow further characterization of the host response to infection. Although several studies validate PIRO, it remains to be seen whether this system is robust enough for consistent application in the future. The PIRO system is further limited by the lack of specific genotypic targets that can

Domain	Present	Future	Rationale
Predisposition	Premorbid illness with reduced probability of short tem survival. Cultural or religious beliefs, age, gender	Genetic polymorphisms in components of inflammatory response (e.g., Toll-like receptor, tumor necrosis factor, interleukin 1, CD14); enhanced understanding of specific interactions between pathogens and host diseases	At the present, premorbid factors impact on the potential attributable morbidity and mortality of an acute insult; deleterious consequences of insult depend heavily on genetic predisposition (future)
Insult (infection)	Culture and sensitivity of infecting pathogens; detection of disease amenable to source control	Assay of microbial products (lipopolysaccharide, mannan, bacterial DNA); gene transcript profiles	Specific therapies directed against inciting insult require demonstration and characterization of that insult
Response	SIRS, other signs of sepsis, shock, C-reactive protein	Nonspecific markers of activated inflammation (e.g., procalcitonin or interleukin 6) or impaired host responsiveness (e.g., HLA-DR); specific detection of target of therapy (e.g., protein C, tumor necrosis factor, platelet-activating factor)	Both mortality risk and potential to respond to therapy vary with nonspecific measures of disease severity (e.g., shock); specific mediator-targeted therapy is predicated on presence and activity of mediator
Organ dysfunction	Organ dysfunction as number of failing organs or composite score (e.g.,multiple-organ dysfunction syndrome, logistic organ dysfunction system, Sequential Organ Failure Assessment, Pediatric Multiple Organ Dysfunction, Pediatric Logistic Organ Dysfunction)	Dynamic measures of cellular response to insult – apoptosis, cytopathic hypoxia, cell stress	Response to preemptive therapy (e.g., targeting micro-organism or early mediator) not possible if damage already present; therapies targeting the injurious cellular process require that it be present

Fig. 2.2 PIRO system for staging sepsis; adapted from Levy, ICM, 2003;29:530–538, CCM, 31(4):1250–1256, April 2003

be analyzed quickly and are of phenotypic significance. Once this technology is accessible to the majority of physicians, it could allow for tailored therapy and prognosticating ability.

Problems with in Early Stage Sepsis

Ideally, the criteria by which to recognize a patient suffering from a complex process such as sepsis should be one that is easily memorized, tabulated, and reproducible. The invariable difficulties with recognizing patients early in the disease course for quickly evolving and devastating disease processes such as pulmonary embolism, acute coronary syndrome, and cerebrovascular accidents, for example, have led to evidence-based protocols to allow early intervention when possible. Unfortunately, the dynamic host-pathogen interaction that produces sepsis has not lent itself to methodology with enough sensitivity and specificity to identify high-risk patients without a high false-negative rate or alarm fatigue.

Currently, the focus on the early identification of septic patients includes the use of electronic warning scores that can tabulate patient risk based on data available in the patient chart [28]. Various systems for using the electronic patient record have been studied to identify patients at risk for deterioration. The 2009 Joint Commission stipulated a goal to improve the identification and response to sick ward patients [29]. To implement these medical emergency teams, critical care outreach teams, and rapid response systems to manage sick patients with infectious complications, there needs to be a sensitive method for defining sepsis. This would allow crisis detection of new physiologic deterioration in patients at risk of harm who requires urgent response of a predetermined fashion, whether it is personnel, equipment, or knowledge to then correct the imbalance in needs and care [30, 31].

These warning alert systems have evolved from single parameter tracking and triggering that showed low sensitivity and specificity to multiple parameter system such as the Patient at Risk score, to aggregate weighted systems that take into account the degree of derangement as exemplified by the Modified Early Warning Score (MEWS), which has improved sensitivity and specificity [32]. The MEWS is based on vital signs and documentation of effect of end organ damage in the form of altered consciousness and urine output. There is significant overlap between these chosen variables and those outlined by the professional societies as part of the accepted sepsis criteria.

Adoption of the Term "Septic" in Medical Culture

Another barrier to effective use of sepsis definitions is the common use of the word sepsis or septic by physicians to describe patients who appear very ill and are usually suffering from infection with end organ damage or shock. Patients who simply have at least two of four SIRS criteria in addition to a suspected or proven infection usually are admitted to the general wards and not often described as "septic" despite having fit the clinical definition prior to 2016. The colloquial use of the descriptor "septic" in medical culture is acknowledged in the 2001 guidelines [11]. Other challenges in identifying an effective term include the diverse physiologic responses to infection among individuals and lack of specific biomarkers.

Defining Sepsis Through Clinical or Administrative Data

Reporting of sepsis worldwide and nationally relies on proper documentation. These data help determine epidemiology and trends for incidence, prevalence, mortality, and specific infectious processes that have clinical and research-based public health implications. Governing bodies such as the New York State Department of Health has passed legislation, requiring hospitals to implement guideline-based treatment of sepsis. In addition, this protocol requires that institutions use administrative data to report back to the state department of health regarding their adherence and risk-stratified mortality rates. The Centers for Medicare and Medicaid Services (CMS) has adopted the use of claims based data to ascertain hospital case mix index and other indicators for reimbursement. CMS has required public reporting of hospital outcomes as they relate to medical infections since 2003, when they implemented the Hospital Inpatient Quality Reporting (Hospital IQR) program, as part of Section 501(b) of the Medicare Prescription Drug, Improvement, and Modernization Act. Since that time, more outcome measures on admission diagnoses coding such as pneumonia have been evaluated as part of hospital compensation. The gradual conversion of documentation to electronic medical records has made administrative data use possible by searching diagnosis codes.

Coding

The accurate applicability of data gathered through the use of electronic medical records relies heavily on physician documentation and understanding of coding. Little formal training is done on proper coding and emphasis is placed for billing purposes. Several studies including a recent systematic review have shown that ICD codes are less accurate at capturing sepsis than are reference standards such as documentation in notes [33, 34]. In this era of access to vast stores of data, much important information can be gathered from administrative data, but this is ultimately limited by the accuracy of coding. Coding also has implications for reimbursement and coders, trained to comb charts and ascribe proper codes for billing may lack the perspective that accurate coding provides for research and epidemiologic purposes [35]. The particular instrument used to abstract data should be matched to the outcome being evaluated as different tools have lesser or greater sensitivity to capture the population of interest and will capture a sample of mixed purity. Accurate estimation of sepsis incidence will be important for resource allocation and public reporting [36].

Criteria

Given the previously mentioned limitations of using billing data to identify sepsis patients, there have been efforts to use other forms of data from the medical record. The methods have sought to use existing medical data or specific data input from the physician or nurse providers [33]. There have been few validated methods of medical record data extraction for estimating the incidence of sepsis. Even among these protocols there is great variation in estimates, as wide as threefold [36]. Over the last two decades, several groups have attempted to identify accurate instruments for utilizing administrative data, specifically the *International Classification of Disease 9* (ICD9). We anticipate that future studies will incorporate ICD10.

Angus Criteria

One of the first protocols using administrative data, the Angus criteria, was validated by comparing a nurse-driven identification of a population of patients with the clinical syndrome of sepsis [3]. The algorithm for the Angus criteria first looks to identify patients coded for severe sepsis or septic shock. If patients do not have this code, all discharge diagnoses are reviewed for an infection code, if present then procedure codes/diagnoses codes are checked for organ dysfunction codes. Upon clinical review, the false-positive charts were most commonly found to have a different etiology of the organ dysfunction than sepsis.

Iwashyna et al. conducted a single center validation of the Angus implementation [37] (Fig. 2.3). This group looked at all patients admitted to the general medical wards from 2009 to 2010, reviewed by three internal medicine hospitalists by a

	True Positives (n = 60)	False Positives (n = 32)
Cardiovascular	27.6%	20.0%
95% CI	8.6%, 46.4%	0.8%, 39.3%
Neurological	26.4%	37.9%
95% CI	0.2%, 52.7%	0.0%, 87.4%
Hematologic	11.9%	18.0%
95% CI	0.0%, 27.2%	0.2%, 35.8%
Hepatic	0.8%	2.0%
95% CI	0.0%, 2.5%	0.0%, 6.4%
Renal	82.6%	32.1%
95% CI	71.4%, 93.8%	4.0%, 60.1%
Respiratory	9.9%	0.0%
95% CI	2.5%, 17.3%	0.0%, 10.9%

These values incorporate sampling weights.
CI indicates confidence interval.

Fig. 2.3 Prevalence of organ dysfunction by ICD9 among true positive and false-positive hospitalizations meeting the Angus criteria; adapted from Iwashyna et al., Med Care. 2014 Jun;52(6):e39–43

structured instrument (gold standard was clinical judgment from chart review of randomly selected positive and negatively screened cases) [37]. This revealed over 3000 patients who met the criteria (13.5% of cases sampled) [37]. After review, the Angus was found to have a positive predictive value of approximately 70%, negative predictive value of 91.5%, with a sensitivity of 50% and specificity of 96% [37]. This captured mostly patients with severe sepsis but not exclusively and thus the authors point out that its limitations should be noted, especially for the purposes of use in research [37].

Martin Criteria

A model created by Martin et al. sorts patients either by codes for septicemia, septicemic, bacteremia, disseminated fungal infection, disseminated candida infection or disseminated fungal endocarditis in addition to an organ dysfunction code or an explicit diagnosis: severe sepsis or septic shock [37]. The Martin implementation had a positive predictive value of 97.6% with a sensitivity of 16% [37]. The drawbacks to this instrument include the less formal use by physicians of the term "septicemic" (not requiring microbiologic data which is in discordance with the American Medical Association definition 2009 coding guidelines) [37]. Also, when it is used properly, it will miss immunologic and coagulopathic organ dysfunction caused by culture negative infection [37].

In this study, three trained hospitalists reviewed the charts sampled. This approach allowed for a more thorough study but highlights the lack of inter-operator agreement in chart review even for clinical judgment of sepsis, which was used as the gold standard for determination. Using the explicit criteria for diagnosis, there is a positive predictive value of 100% though sensitivity drops to less than 10% [37]. The authors point out that this is also limited to a single center and may vary across institutions [37].

Comparison of Different Methods

The variability in cohorts identified by different methodologies for data abstraction has been seen not only in the United States but globally, as reported by Wilhelms et al. [38]. A retrospective study looking at data from 1987 to 2005 using both the Angus and Martin implementation yielded widely different patient groups (with a small percentage only [16.3%] being captured by both tools) [38]. It should be noted that Sweden did not have a specific code for severe sepsis at the time of this study. In addition, this study included data prior to the consensus statement from 1991 defining sepsis. Despite these limitations, there was a rising trend for capture of sepsis coding irrespective of methodology used [38]. Practices surrounding sepsis vary geographically as assessed by a survey-based study that demonstrated

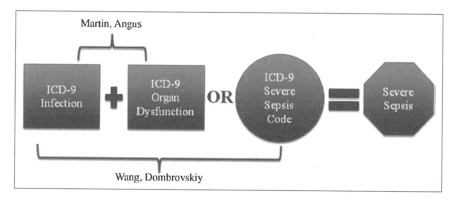

Fig. 2.4 Comparison of ICD classification systems; adapted from Gaieski et al. CCM 2013; 41:1167–74

different mortality based on place of admission to the ICU and different compliance with the sepsis bundle which may affect coding [39].

Comparing four methods head to head, Gaieski found that annual incidence of sepsis calculations varied up to 350%, with ab ate values ranging from 300 per 100,000 to 1031 per 100,000 [36, 40, 41] (Fig. 2.4). This study was conducted over a 6 year period from 2004 to 2009 and there was an annual increase in incidence in sepsis independent of the method used [36]. ICD9 codes for sepsis, severe sepsis, and septic shock were not implemented until 2002, and data extractions using these terms were not examined until more recently. The divergence in estimates for the incidence of sepsis may be attributed to the increase in ICD9 codes for sepsis, which doubled during that period [36].

This group performed a retrospective cohort study using the nationwide inpatient sample (NIS) which is a public database sponsored by the Agency for Healthcare Research and Quality. In 2009, 44 states participated, capturing over 1000 hospitals and eight million admissions and is thought to represent one-fifth of the national sample [36]. The four techniques used were Angus, Martin, Wang, and Dombrovskiy, the former two using ICD9 codes for infection and organ dysfunction to identify severe sepsis and the latter pair using either infection plus organ dysfunction or a specific severe sepsis code. Gaeiski mentions that there is more variability in the ability to capture infection with the ICD9 which includes over 1000 codes infection versus organ dysfunction that only encompasses 13 by comparison [36].

Annual growth was estimated by comparing 2009 data to 2004 data and assuming proportional increase. The average age of septic patients was similar among the four tools, while Angus and Wang captured more females, Wang and Dombrovskiy captured patients with longer average length of stay and number of organ dysfunctions. In this study period, approximately 40 million patients were found, thought to represent 20% of the national average [36]. Mortality estimates were described by total number of deaths and also case fatality rate and it was found that overall mortality increased, however case fatality rate decreased over 6 years [36]. This is in part due

Code Abstraction Method	Sensitivity to Identify Severe Sepsis Cases (n = 1735)[a]	95% Confidence Interval
1. Severe sepsis (ICD–9-specific coding method, 995.92)	20.5%	18.6% to 22.4%
2. Combining end-organ dysfunction and infection codes (the Angus coding method)	47.2%	44.8% to 49.5%
Code Abstraction Method	Sensitivity to Identify Septic Shock Cases (n = 321)[a]	95% Confidence Interval
1. Severe sepsis (ICD–9-specific coding method, 995.92)	49.5%s	44.0% to 55.0%
2. Septic shock (ICD–9-specific coding method, 785.52)	42.4%	37.0% to 47.8%
3. Combining end-organ dysfunction and infection codes (the Angus coding method)	75.1%	70.4% to 79.8%

ICD-9 = *International Classification of Diseases*, 9th Revision.
[a]Cases of septic shock (n = 321) were encompassed within the severe sepsis (n = 1735) population.
Categorical data are presented as proportions.

Fig. 2.5 Sensitivities of two difference code abstraction methods for identifying cases of severe sepsis and septic shock determined by patient-level data; adapted from Whittaker SA et al., Crit Care Med. 2013;41(4):945–53

to improved interventions for sepsis such as early identification, fluid resuscitation, and timely administration of antibiotics despite a rise in the number of patients suffering from sepsis.

Overall, although Angus and Wang may be more sensitive and therefore identify patients with lower severity of illness, Dombrovskiy and Martin are less sensitive but capture more severely ill patients [36]. Only a small percentage of patients identified with the four instruments were assigned a specific sepsis code [36]. It was also found that of those patients with septic shock only half also were coded for severe sepsis [36]. This implies that the singular use of either the severe sepsis or septic shock code could greatly underestimate the incidence of both. Of those with specific sepsis coding, more were likely to have had higher severity of illness and identified with Dombrovskiy and Martin than with Angus and Wang [36]. A similar study in Sweden by Wilhelms found a large variation in capture based on which methodology was used for data abstraction [38]. It is important to note, however, in Gaeiski's study, organ dysfunction and mortality could not be attributed specifically to sepsis as individual charts were not made available to the authors [36].

Whittaker et al. looked to study the sensitivity of various methods and assess whether patient outcome differed among variable coding [35] (Fig. 2.5). This retrospective cohort focused on ED admissions and validated coding through chart review. It was found that age, gender, and race did not affect specific coding for sepsis [35]. Of 1735 patients admitted with severe sepsis or septic shock, only 21.5% received a corresponding ICD9 code from 2005 to 2009 [35]. Similar to prior studies, the Angus classification was more sensitive than specific diagnostic coding for severe sepsis and septic shock and that there was no added benefit to using a combined approach [35]. Of those admitted directly to the ICU, 36% received the specific ICD9 code versus 6% of ward patients who fulfilled the criteria [35]. In addition, lower presenting systolic blood pressure, higher serum lactate measurements, higher Acute Physiology and Chronic Health Evaluation (APACHE-II) scores all correlated with proper coding [35].

Trends in Mortality and Disability in Sepsis

Given what appears to be a decline in mortality in sepsis, the impetus for accurately identifying hospitalized patients and therefore tracking trends in sepsis include redistribution of funds to disease states that are emerging public health issues or with increasing mortality and morbidity [42]. In addition, this further informs the accurate measurement of quality improvement and therapeutic intervention outcomes (accurately identifying secular trends in sepsis mortality) [42] (Fig. 2.6).

In an editorial by Iwashyna and Angus, the authors discuss the role of the Will Rogers effect as initially published by Feinstein et al. that describes the role of increased awareness and testing as well as the inclusion of less sick patients into the category of severe sepsis, which might then give the appearance of increased incidence and improved mortality [43]. Feinstein and colleagues described this phenomenon as it relates to lead time bias for cancer diagnosis and prognosis but is applicable to sepsis as pointed out by Iwashyna and Angus, who also suggest that increased awareness may influence changes in practice, not only in terms of coding, but for increasing admission to ICUs [44]. This may account for the observation that the initial estimate of 750,000 of sepsis present in 1996 has increased through the years to upward of three million [3, 36].

A meta-analysis to estimate the mortality trends in severe sepsis by Stevenson et al. compared clinical trial data from usual care group in multicenter sepsis trials searched on MEDLINE from 1991 to 2009 and data extraction from NIS samples

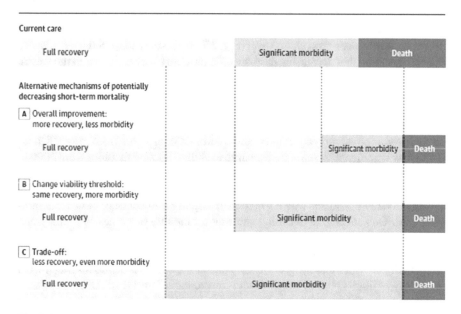

Fig. 2.6 Potential mechanisms of decreasing short-term mortality among patients across a distribution of illness severity; adapted from Iwashyna TJ, Angus DC. JAMA. 2014;311(13):1295–7

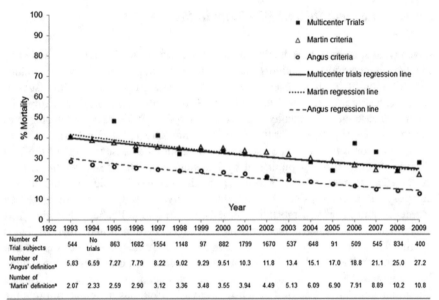

Number of Trial subjects	544	No trials	863	1682	1554	1148	97	882	1799	1670	537	648	91	509	545	834	400
Number of 'Angus' definition[a]	5.83	6.59	7.27	7.79	8.22	9.02	9.29	9.51	10.3	11.8	13.4	15.1	17.0	18.8	21.1	25.0	27.2
Number of 'Martin' definition[a]	2.07	2.33	2.59	2.90	3.12	3.36	3.48	3.55	3.94	4.49	5.13	6.09	6.90	7.91	8.89	10.2	10.8

[a] Survey-weighted number of patients identified each year through specified administrative data algorithm, x 10⁵

Fig. 2.7 Mortality trends in severe sepsis using martin and Angus criteria; adapted from Stevenson et al., Crit Care Med. 2014 Mar;42(3):625–31

from 1993 to 2009, using both Angus and Martin definitions showed a similar trend in decrease in case-specific mortality from sepsis in both arms (with a sample size of 14,418, adjusted for case mix index among institutions, stratified by severity of illness by several scoring systems) [42] (Fig. 2.7). This study was conducted because of the suggestion that decreasing case-specific mortality was attributed to the way in which ICD9 coding was utilized. Coding of less severe cases of sepsis would result in spurious decline in case fatality rate [42, 45–47]. Increase in coding for sepsis might in part be financially driven [36]. Another phenomenon to explain this trend is discharge from hospital to acute care prior to hospital death (increased survival to discharge without significant improvement in functional status from prior). Kumar et al. show significant increase in discharge to skilled nursing facilities from 2000 to 2007, using the Martin classification of severe sepsis on the NIS cohort. Interestingly, they also note the increase in practice of appropriate transition to comfort care in certain critically ill patients which would then magnify the decline of in-hospital mortality [48]. One concern about using short-term mortality outcomes as primary end points to critical care literature is the effect of discharging increasingly debilitated patients to long-term care facilities. Iwashyna and Angus describe the "mortality/morbidity trade off" when choosing a "viability threshold," which is defined as the "degree of severity of illness beyond which death is unavoidable" [44] (Fig. 2.8).

These estimates are subject to inaccuracies related to the way in which the data is abstracted. Kaukonen and coauthors worked to eliminate some inflation bias by using a bedside nurse to score and identify severe sepsis after the initial abstraction

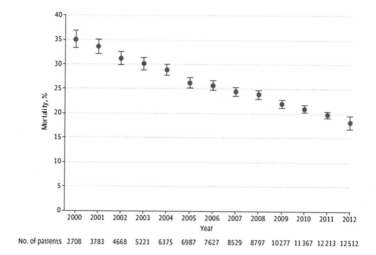

Fig. 2.8 Mean annual mortality in patients with severe sepsis; adapted from Kaukonen KM et al., JAMA. 2014;311(13):1308–16

through administrative claims to capture the patients admitted to the ICU with infection [49]. The authors account for secular change in trends of mortality by comparing death in sepsis to critically ill patients as a whole and also by adjusting for death by the APACHE III score [49].

Future Directions

In daily practice, clinicians often use the word "septic" to describe a patient who appears toxic and by strict definition usually qualifies as having severe sepsis as evidenced by organ dysfunction usually among the neurologic, cardiovascular, pulmonary, renal, and hepatic or coagulation systems. The 2001 review cited the European Society of Intensive Care Medicine/Society of Critical Care Medicine survey that demonstrated that 67% of physicians were concerned about not having a common definition of sepsis and 17% of those interviewed provided a unified definition of sepsis despite the consensus statement produced in 1991 [5]. Gaieski and Goyal proposed biomarker use, genetic profiling, and/or severity scores with bacterial assays to bolster our diagnostic ability [25]. The hope is to put sepsis diagnosis more in line with diseases such as acute myocardial infarction for which there is a serum marker for testing [11]. Unfortunately, to date, no single or panel of biomarkers has been shown to have the balance of sensitivity and specificity to be clinically useful. The current sepsis definition may cause a high false-positive rate; however, we must decide as physicians whether a life-threatening illness is better served by a simplified over-sensitive diagnostic tool or the one that may have a higher positive predictive value for serious illness but may not capture a sizeable portion of patients with the potential to become more ill and who may benefit from early intervention.

Conclusions

As outlined in this chapter, there are various methods for defining sepsis and estimating the incidence and trends in mortality from administrative data. With the advent of the electronic medical record, vast amounts of data can be sorted to provide statistics on large samples. Using administrative datasets for determination of sepsis incidence and prevalence has significant flaws, which leads to great variability and ultimately, inaccuracy in the estimate of sepsis. Earlier studies quoted a mortality rate between 28% and 50% [50]. The true estimate of sepsis-related mortality is now in flux as the traditionally accepted values may be imprecise from variations in coding, inclusion criteria for randomized, controlled trials, and other factors.

Even with the recent revision of sepsis definitions, the ability for clinicians to identify patients with sepsis early remains a significant challenge. Twenty five years after the first publication establishing sepsis definitions the field still lacks proven, objective tools for diagnosing sepsis. For now, clinicians caring for patients with sepsis must wait and hope that, similar to the fields of cardiology and oncology, further research will provide the objective means necessary for early, accurate diagnosis and treatment.

References

1. Murphy SL, Xu J, Kochanek KD. Deaths: final data for 2010. Natl Vital Stat Rep. 2013;61(4):1–117.
2. National Institute of General Medical Sciences. Sepsis Fact Sheet. 2014.
3. Angus DC, Linde-Zwirble WT, Lidicker J, Clermont G, Carcillo J, Pinsky MR. Epidemiology of severe sepsis in the United States: analysis of incidence, outcome, and associated costs of care. Crit Care Med. 2001;29(7):1303–10.
4. Elixhauser A, Friedman B, Stranges E. Septicemia in U.S. Hospitals, 2009: Statistical Brief #122. Healthcare Cost and Utilization Project (HCUP) Statistical Briefs. Rockville, MD: Agency for Health Care Policy and Research (US); 2006.
5. Poeze M, Ramsay G, Gerlach H, Rubulotta F, Levy M. An international sepsis survey: a study of doctors' knowledge and perception about sepsis. Crit Care. 2004;8(6):R409–13.
6. Geroulanos S, Douka ET. Historical perspective of the word "sepsis". Intensive Care Med. 2006;32(12):2077.
7. Bone RC, Fisher Jr CJ, Clemmer TP, Slotman GJ, Metz CA, Balk RA. Sepsis syndrome: a valid clinical entity. Methylprednisolone Severe Sepsis Study Group. Crit Care Med. 1989;17(5):389–93.
8. American College of Chest Physicians/Society of Critical Care Medicine Consensus Conference: definitions for sepsis and organ failure and guidelines for the use of innovative therapies in sepsis. Crit Care Med. 1992;20(6):864–74.
9. Lynn LA. The diagnosis of sepsis revisited—a challenge for young medical scientists in the 21st century. Patient Saf Surg. 2014;8(1):1.
10. Pauker SG, Kassirer JP. The threshold approach to clinical decision making. N Engl J Med. 1980;302(20):1109–17.
11. Levy MM, Fink MP, Marshall JC, Abraham E, Angus D, Cook D, et al. 2001 SCCM/ESICM/ ACCP/ATS/SIS international sepsis definitions conference. Intensive Care Med. 2003;29(4):530–8.

12. Bone RC, Balk RA, Cerra FB, Dellinger RP, Fein AM, Knaus WA, et al. Definitions for sepsis and organ failure and guidelines for the use of innovative therapies in sepsis. The ACCP/SCCM Consensus Conference Committee. American College of Chest Physicians/Society of Critical Care Medicine. Chest. 1992;101(6):1644–55.
13. Veloso T, Neves A, Vincent JL. Are the concepts of SIRS and MODS useful in sepsis? New York: Elsevier; 2009.
14. Vincent JL, de Mendonca A, Cantraine F, Moreno R, Takala J, Suter PM, et al. Use of the SOFA score to assess the incidence of organ dysfunction/failure in intensive care units: results of a multicenter, prospective study. Working group on "sepsis-related problems" of the European Society of Intensive Care Medicine. Crit Care Med. 1998;26(11):1793–800.
15. Mikkelsen ME, Gaieski DF. Classifying infections in the ICU: seeking certainty in an uncertain environment. Crit Care Med. 2013;41(10):2452–3.
16. Klein Klouwenberg PM, Ong DS, Bos LD, de Beer FM, van Hooijdonk RT, Huson MA, et al. Interobserver agreement of Centers for Disease Control and Prevention criteria for classifying infections in critically ill patients. Crit Care Med. 2013;41(10):2373–8.
17. W.O. The Evolution of Modern Medicine. 1904.
18. Vincent JL, Opal SM, Marshall JC, Tracey KJ. Sepsis definitions: time for change. Lancet. 2013;381(9868):774–5.
19. Andersson U, Tracey KJ. HMGB1 is a therapeutic target for sterile inflammation and infection. Annu Rev Immunol. 2011;29:139–62.
20. Czura CJ. "Merinoff symposium 2010: sepsis"—speaking with one voice. Mol Med. 2011;17(1–2):2–3.
21. Singer M, Deutschman CS, Seymour CW, Shankar-Hari M, Annane D, Bauer M, et al. The third international consensus definitions for sepsis and septic shock (sepsis-3). JAMA. 2016;315(8):801–10.
22. Sprung CL, Sakr Y, Vincent JL, Le Gall JR, Reinhart K, Ranieri VM, et al. An evaluation of systemic inflammatory response syndrome signs in the Sepsis Occurrence in Acutely Ill Patients (SOAP) study. Intensive Care Med. 2006;32(3):421–7.
23. Vincent JL. Dear SIRS, I'm sorry to say that I don't like you. Crit Care Med. 1997;25(2):372–4.
24. Kaukonen KM, Bailey M, Pilcher D, Cooper DJ, Bellomo R. Systemic inflammatory response syndrome criteria in defining severe sepsis. N Engl J Med. 2015;372(17):1629–38.
25. Gaieski DF, Goyal M. What is sepsis? What is severe sepsis? What is septic shock? Searching for objective definitions among the winds of doctrines and wild theories. Expert Rev Anti Infect Ther. 2013;11(9):867–71.
26. Rangel-Frausto MS, Pittet D, Costigan M, Hwang T, Davis CS, Wenzel RP. The natural history of the systemic inflammatory response syndrome (SIRS). A prospective study. JAMA. 1995;273(2):117–23.
27. Howell MD, Talmor D, Schuetz P, Hunziker S, Jones AE, Shapiro NI. Proof of principle: the predisposition, infection, response, organ failure sepsis staging system. Crit Care Med. 2011;39(2):322–7.
28. Huh JW, Lim CM, Koh Y, Lee J, Jung YK, Seo HS, et al. Activation of a medical emergency team using an electronic medical recording-based screening system. Crit Care Med. 2014;42(4):801–8.
29. Jones L, King L, Wilson C. A literature review: factors that impact on nurses' effective use of the Medical Emergency Team (MET). J Clin Nurs. 2009;18(24):3379–90.
30. McCurdy MT, Wood SL. Rapid response systems: identification and management of the "pre-arrest state". Emerg Med Clin North Am. 2012;30(1):141–52.
31. Devita MA, Bellomo R, Hillman K, Kellum J, Rotondi A, Teres D, et al. Findings of the first consensus conference on medical emergency teams. Crit Care Med. 2006;34(9):2463–78.
32. Churpek MM, Yuen TC, Huber MT, Park SY, Hall JB, Edelson DP. Predicting cardiac arrest on the wards: a nested case-control study. Chest. 2012;141(5):1170–6.
33. Wei WQ, Teixeira PL, Mo H, Cronin RM, Warner JL, Denny JC. Combining billing codes, clinical notes, and medications from electronic health records provides superior phenotyping performance. J Am Med Inform Assoc. 2015.

34. Jolley RJ, Sawka KJ, Yergens DW, Quan H, Jette N, Doig CJ. Validity of administrative data in recording sepsis: a systematic review. Crit Care. 2015;19:139.
35. Whittaker SA, Mikkelsen ME, Gaieski DF, Koshy S, Kean C, Fuchs BD. Severe sepsis cohorts derived from claims-based strategies appear to be biased toward a more severely ill patient population. Crit Care Med. 2013;41(4):945–53.
36. Gaieski DF, Edwards JM, Kallan MJ, Carr BG. Benchmarking the incidence and mortality of severe sepsis in the United States. Crit Care Med. 2013;41(5):1167–74.
37. Iwashyna TJ, Odden A, Rohde J, Bonham C, Kuhn L, Malani P, et al. Identifying patients with severe sepsis using administrative claims: patient-level validation of the angus implementation of the international consensus conference definition of severe sepsis. Med Care. 2014;52(6):e39–43.
38. Wilhelms SB, Huss FR, Granath G, Sjoberg F. Assessment of incidence of severe sepsis in Sweden using different ways of abstracting International Classification of Diseases codes: difficulties with methods and interpretation of results. Crit Care Med. 2010;38(6):1442–9.
39. Levy MM, Artigas A, Phillips GS, Rhodes A, Beale R, Osborn T, et al. Outcomes of the Surviving Sepsis Campaign in intensive care units in the USA and Europe: a prospective cohort study. Lancet Infect Dis. 2012;12(12):919–24.
40. Dombrovskiy VY, Martin AA, Sunderram J, Paz HL. Rapid increase in hospitalization and mortality rates for severe sepsis in the United States: a trend analysis from 1993 to 2003. Crit Care Med. 2007;35(5):1244–50.
41. Wang HE, Shapiro NI, Angus DC, Yealy DM. National estimates of severe sepsis in United States emergency departments. Crit Care Med. 2007;35(8):1928–36.
42. Stevenson EK, Rubenstein AR, Radin GT, Wiener RS, Walkey AJ. Two decades of mortality trends among patients with severe sepsis: a comparative meta-analysis. Crit Care Med. 2014;42(3):625–31.
43. Feinstein AR, Sosin DM, Wells CK. The Will Rogers phenomenon. Stage migration and new diagnostic techniques as a source of misleading statistics for survival in cancer. N Engl J Med. 1985;312(25):1604–8.
44. Iwashyna TJ, Angus DC. Declining case fatality rates for severe sepsis: good data bring good news with ambiguous implications. JAMA. 2014;311(13):1295–7.
45. Lagu T, Rothberg MB, Shieh MS, Pekow PS, Steingrub JS, Lindenauer PK. Hospitalizations, costs, and outcomes of severe sepsis in the United States 2003 to 2007. Crit Care Med. 2012;40(3):754–61.
46. Lindenauer PK, Lagu T, Shieh MS, Pekow PS, Rothberg MB. Association of diagnostic coding with trends in hospitalizations and mortality of patients with pneumonia, 2003–2009. JAMA. 2012;307(13):1405–13.
47. Hall WB, Willis LE, Medvedev S, Carson SS. The implications of long-term acute care hospital transfer practices for measures of in-hospital mortality and length of stay. Am J Respir Crit Care Med. 2012;185(1):53–7.
48. Kumar G, Kumar N, Taneja A, Kaleekal T, Tarima S, McGinley E, et al. Nationwide trends of severe sepsis in the 21st century (2000–2007). Chest. 2011;140(5):1223–31.
49. Kaukonen KM, Bailey M, Suzuki S, Pilcher D, Bellomo R. Mortality related to severe sepsis and septic shock among critically ill patients in Australia and New Zealand, 2000–2012. JAMA. 2014;311(13):1308–16.
50. Wood KA, Angus DC. Pharmacoeconomic implications of new therapies in sepsis. Pharmacoeconomics. 2004;22(14):895–906.

Chapter 3
Epidemiology of Sepsis: Current Data and Predictions for the Future

Bashar Staitieh and Greg S. Martin

Introduction

The history of sepsis is deeply intertwined with advancements in the study of infectious diseases. As far back as Hippocrates (circa 400 BCE), sepsis has been understood to be a destructive process that brings with it the release of systemic toxins, but it was not until the discovery of microorganisms and the consequent recognition of their relationship to infectious pathology that the study of sepsis as a field came into its own. Modern discussions of sepsis have focused on the importance of early recognition and treatment of the disease. In this chapter, we will focus on the epidemiology of sepsis in the light of its changing patterns over time across the globe.

Incidence and Outcome of Sepsis

The consensus definition of sepsis has enabled investigators to study the incidence of the disease through time in different settings. Surveys have been conducted in many, if not most, developed and undeveloped nations and offer a few general points to review before delving into specific cohorts (Table 3.1). First, the incidence of sepsis alone in hospitalized patients may not be as important or easy to quantify as the number of patients who progress to severe sepsis and septic shock (particularly those requiring ICU admission). Many patients requiring hospital admission will meet criteria for the systemic inflammatory response syndrome (SIRS, detailed elsewhere in this volume) and many will have at the very least a suspected infection and will thus qualify for sepsis under traditional definitions. Clearly, if sepsis

B. Staitieh, MD • G.S. Martin, MD, MSc (✉)
Division of Pulmonary, Allergy, and Critical Care Medicine, Emory University
School of Medicine, 615 Michael Street, Suite 205, Atlanta, GA 30322, USA
e-mail: bashar.staitieh@emory.edu; greg.martin@emory.edu

© Springer International Publishing AG 2017
N.S. Ward, M.M. Levy (eds.), *Sepsis*, Respiratory Medicine,
DOI 10.1007/978-3-319-48470-9_3

Table 3.1 Key studies of the epidemiology of sepsis

Authors	Methodology	Study period	Selected key findings
Rangel-Frausto et al. [1]	Prospective cohort of patients meeting SIRS criteria in study ICUs and wards in a single academic center	1992–1993	Evolution of SIRS to sepsis in 26%, to severe sepsis in 18%, and septic shock in 4%
Angus et al. [3]	Observational cohort study of patients (hospital-wide) meeting criteria for severe sepsis using state hospital discharge records linked with population data	1995	Severe sepsis incidence of ~2.3/100 hospital discharges, mortality rate of ~29%, estimated annual cost of $16.7 billion
Brun-Buisson et al. (for French ICU group) [22]	Two-month prospective survey of all patients admitted to 170 French ICUs meeting criteria for severe sepsis and septic shock	1994	Severe sepsis in 6.3/100 ICU admissions, ~60% 28 days mortality
Martin et al. [7]	Retrospective cohort study of all hospitalized patients diagnosed with sepsis (per ICD-9-CM codes) using the National Hospital Discharge Survey	1979–2000	Increasing rates of sepsis leading to increasing absolute mortality (with decrease in mortality rate)
Padkin et al. [41]	A retrospective observational cohort study of prospectively-collected data from 91 ICUs in England, Northern Ireland, and Wales. Examined patients meeting criteria for severe sepsis within the first day of their ICU stay	1995–2000	27.1% of patients met criteria for severe sepsis, with mortality rates of 35% during ICU stay and 47% during hospital stay
Vincent et al. (for EPIC II group) [4]	One-day prospective, point-prevalence study of adult patients from 1265 ICUs from 75 countries.	May 8, 2007	51% of ICU patients infected, hospital mortality rate 33% versus 15% in uninfected patients

represents a clinically relevant spectrum of disease from infection to organ dysfunction to shock, then identifying and naming each stage of the disease is important. To that end, a study by Rangel-Frausto in 1995 evaluated the incidence of SIRS and the natural history of the syndrome [1]. The authors found that approximately 68% of patients admitted to their survey units (both wards and ICU) met criteria for SIRS, with 26% of that group developing sepsis, 18% developing severe sepsis, and 4% developing septic shock. Furthermore, large studies of administrative data sets that rely on coding for surrogates of sepsis (e.g., bacteremia) may underreport the true prevalence. The setting of the cohort is also of paramount importance: one would expect to see a high percentage of patients with sepsis in general medical wards or trauma ICUs of large urban hospitals, and would expect to see far fewer in smaller community facilities. One notable attempt to study the epidemiology of sepsis specifically in an academic setting was undertaken by Sands et al. in 1997 [2]. In a study of eight academic medical centers in a prospective observational trial, the authors found an incidence of sepsis of 2.0 cases per 100 hospital admissions, septic shock in 25% at onset of sepsis, and an overall mortality rate of 34% at 28 days.

Given the inherent difficulties in studying SIRS and sepsis in isolation, far more attention has been paid to patients meeting criteria for severe sepsis and septic shock, a fact that reflects both the incredible amount of resources required to care for these patients, as well as their high risk of death and other complications. A study by Angus et al. in 2001 [3] linked discharge records to U.S. Census data and estimated the incidence of severe sepsis in the United States at 300 cases per 100,000 people (studies of cohorts outside the United States have often found a lower incidence, as discussed below). Over 50% of patients in the cohort who developed severe sepsis required ICU services during the course of their hospital admissions. Several studies have attempted to ascertain the prevalence of sepsis within intensive care units generally. A seminal example of this effort was published in 2009 by Vincent, who led a team of investigators in studying the prevalence of sepsis on 1 day across almost 1300 ICUs in 75 countries, encompassing almost 14,000 patients in the EPIC II trial [4]. In that study, around 70% of patients were infected on arrival to the ICU and infection independently increased the risk of mortality twofold both in the ICU and in-hospital.

Also of note is a recent study by Whittaker et al. [5] that examined the trajectory and outcomes of patients admitted through the emergency department to a non-ICU setting. They found that approximately 45% of patients with severe sepsis were admitted to a non-ICU setting between 2005 and 2009 (with the rate increasing over time) and that 12.5% eventually required transfer to an ICU, particularly oncology patients and patients with markers of higher illness severity on presentation. Another recent study by Rohde et al. [6] examined the rates of recognition of sepsis as well as the predominant organ dysfunctions outside the ICU. Using a random sampling of patients from one tertiary care academic center, the authors found that severe sepsis was documented appropriately in only 47% of cases and that cardiovascular (hypotension) and renal dysfunction were the most common end-organ manifestations in patients admitted to non-ICU settings (66% and 64% of patients, respectively). The authors conclude that severe sepsis on the wards is both poorly documented and that the epidemiology is potentially different from what has been seen previously in the ICU setting.

In terms of incidence over time, Martin et al. found an increase in both sepsis and sepsis-related deaths over the past two decades in the United States using data collected from the National Hospital Discharge Survey between 1979 and 2000 in a study published in 2003 [7]. The incidence increased by approximately 13.7% per year over the 22 year span studied. Importantly, although the overall mortality rate declined over time (from 27.8% to 17.9%), the rising incidence resulted in an increase in number of deaths overall (from 21.9 deaths/100,000 people in 1979 to 43.9/100,000 in 2000). More recently, another study of sepsis trends in the United States by Kumar et al. in 2011 found similar results using the Healthcare Costs and Utilization Project's Nationwide Inpatient Sample, with the number of severe sepsis hospitalizations increasing from 143/100,000 persons in 2000 to 343 in 2007 [8]. Mortality rate decreased from 39% to 27% and hospital length-of-stay decreased from 17.3 days to 14.9. Many other studies from across the world (some discussed below) have found similar evidence of increasing incidence of sepsis over time as mortality rates continue to decrease. Many explanations have been offered for these findings, notably the increasing use of immunosuppressive medications for organ transplantation and chemotherapy, as well as changes in coding rates of organ dysfunction over time. In any case, these trends are expected to continue for the foreseeable future, particularly in industrialized nations.

While administrative databases do carry the caveats described above, one recent study by Stevenson et al. compared data from the "usual care" arms of severe sepsis clinical trials to data from administrative data sets from 1991 to 2009 and found similar mortality rates between the two groups, suggesting that administrative data may be appropriate for use in monitoring mortality trends over time [9]. Despite that, wide variability exists depending on the method used to study the incidence of sepsis, as shown in a study by Gaieski et al. published in 2013 [10]. The authors studied the period between 2004 and 2009 using several different methods, including ICD-9 codes as well as methods published by Angus [3], Martin [7], Wang [11], and Dombrovskiy [12]. Angus et al. [3] used hospital discharge records from seven states and ICD-9-CM codes for infection and organ dysfunction. Martin et al. [7] made use of the National Hospital Discharge Survey, a database containing the records of a representative sample of hospitals across the United States, and used ICD-9-CM codes for infection and organ dysfunction. Wang et al. [11] based their study on the Compressed Mortality File, a database that contains demographic data and causes for all deaths in the United States, and identified cases based on ICD-10 codes for infection and severe sepsis. The study by Dombrovskiy et al. [12] used the Nationwide Inpatient Sample, a database sponsored by the Agency for Healthcare Research and Quality, along with ICD-9-CM codes for infection and severe sepsis. The incidence of sepsis varied markedly (up to 3.5-fold) depending on the method used, with almost 300 cases/100,000 population using the methods of Dombrovskiy, and 1031 cases/100,000 population using the methods of Wang. Rates of severe sepsis were closer between methods (approximately 13.0–13.3%), but in-hospital mortality rates showed a wider range (14.7% using the method of Wang et al. and 29.9% using the method of Dombrovskiy et al.). In addition, Gaieski et al. noted an increase in the use of sepsis ICD-9 codes by more than double over the 6 year period between 2004 and 2009. Additionally, as billing codes and quality improvement data are increasingly used to identify sepsis, septic shock, and its mortality, incentives to record or not record these data increase.

An attempt to validate the use of administrative data in epidemiologic studies of sepsis was published by Iwashyna et al. [13]. The authors used the "Angus" implementation to identify cases of severe sepsis and septic shock (cases with ICD9 codes for severe sepsis and septic shock or codes for infection and associated organ dysfunction are termed "Angus-positive," cases without such codes are termed "Angus-negative") and compared the results to the gold-standard of direct physician review of cases. They found that the Angus method had a positive predictive value of 70.7% and a negative predictive value of 91.5% when compared to direct physician review. Sensitivity was 50.4% and specificity was 96.3%. The authors conclude that

Angus implementation is a reasonable but imperfect method for identifying patients with severe sepsis.

The improvement in mortality rates over time may be due in part to the development of bundled care plans for septic patients. As shown by Barochia et al. in a study published in 2010 that analyzed the use of bundle (i.e., protocolized) care versus non-protocolized care found a consistent benefit to protocolized care ($I^2 = 0\%$, $p = 0.87$) in decreases of time to antibiotics and increases in appropriateness of antibiotics ($p \leq 0.0002$ for both factors) [14]. A more recent study by Miller et al. in 2013 found a decrease in mortality in patients whose care complied with specific sepsis care bundle components: inotropes, red cell transfusions, glucocorticoids, and lung protective ventilation after adjusting for severity of illness [15]. They noted an improvement in all-or-none bundle compliance over time (from 4.9% in 2004 to 73.4% in 2010) and a concomitant improvement in mortality during the study period (from 21.2% in 2004 to 8.7% in 2010).

Another interesting effort to address the changing patterns of sepsis was published by Gaieski et al. [16]. The authors examined the effects of severe sepsis case volume on inpatient mortality and found an inverse relationship, with mortality varying from 18.9% in lower volume centers (<50 cases/year) to 10.4% in higher volume centers (>500 cases/year) over the period between 2004 and 2010 in a nationally representative sample of hospital admissions.

Another recent study that examined the effect of sepsis admissions on overall hospital mortality was published by Liu et al. in 2014 [17]. The study examined two complementary inpatient cohorts, Kaiser Permanente Northern California and the Nationwide Inpatient Sample using both explicit ICD9 codes for sepsis and implicit codes (infection with associated organ dysfunction). Overall, the researchers found that sepsis contributed to one in every two to three deaths, again highlighting both the common and deadly nature of the disease.

Global Cohorts

Outside the United States, several other cohorts deserve mention. A study by Harrison et al. in 2006 of the epidemiology of severe sepsis in the United Kingdom using the Intensive Care National Audit and Research Centre Case Mix Programme Database found a rate of 27% of ICU admissions with severe sepsis (up from 23.6% in 1996 to 28.7% in 2004) [18]. As was seen in the United States, mortality rate decreased (from 48.3% in 1996 to 44.7% in 2004) but absolute number of deaths increased due to the higher incidence (from 9000 to 14,000 over the same period). In 2004, van Gestel et al. examined the point prevalence of severe sepsis in the Netherlands across 47 ICUs and found that it accounted for around 0.6% of hospital admissions and 11% of ICU admissions [19]. Another point prevalence study of severe sepsis in ICUs in Australia and New Zealand found an incidence of around 12% of ICU admissions and around .08% of the population [20]. A more recent study of 171 ICUs in Australia and New Zealand found a decrease in mortality due to severe sepsis with and without shock in the period between 2000 and 2012 [21]. A French cohort studied by the EPISEPSIS group in 1995 had a prevalence of severe sepsis of 6.5% in ICUs [22], up to almost 15% when the group published findings on a similar cohort in 2004 [23]. An observational cohort of Emergency Department admissions to a University hospital in the West Indies published by Edwards et al. in 2013 found a rate of approximately 1.3% of patients with sepsis, 15.4% of whom had either severe sepsis or septic shock [24]. Overall mortality was 25%, despite a lack of protocols for early goal-directed therapy. One notable study to examine total hospital incidence of [23] sepsis in a prospective cohort in Spain was published by Esteban et al. in 2007. The incidence relative to total hospital admissions was 4.4% and only 32% of patients with severe sepsis were cared for in an ICU [25].

The reasons for such heterogeneity in sepsis incidence around the world are myriad and have been discussed in several recent papers. Adhikari et al., in a study on the global burden of critical illness published in 2010, detailed how different countries have wide ranges of ICU bed availability (e.g., 30.5 beds/100,000 people in the United States versus 8.6/100,000 in the United Kingdom) [26]. Countries with lower numbers of ICU beds will likely admit only the sickest patients, while countries with higher numbers will tend to accept patients who are not as critically ill. As a result, those with fewer ICU beds will tend to under-report the total prevalence of the disease [27]. Other complicating factors include the variety of hospital sizes within a country, the variety of definitions for what constitutes an ICU, and the problematic nature of risk-adjustment models in this setting [28].

The Cost of Sepsis

Many studies have evaluated the costs of caring for sepsis. A report by the Healthcare Costs and Utilization Project found that sepsis resulted in the highest aggregate costs of any hospital diagnosis in 2009 at 15.4 billion U.S. dollars [29]. The average cost per stay was approximately $18,000 and costs grew at an average annual rate of 11.3%. Sepsis ranked highest among the top three most expensive diagnoses (the others being osteoarthritis and coronary atherosclerosis), with the rate of increase in costs outpacing hospital spending by two to three times. A European trial by Brun-Buisson et al. in 2003 found the total cost of sepsis care to be around Euro 26,000 for sepsis (~USD 36,000), Euro 35,185 (~USD 48,000) for severe sepsis, and Euro 27,083 (~USD 37,000) for septic shock [30]. Importantly, the authors found a significant difference in cost depending on the route of acquisition of sepsis, with ICU-acquired infections approximately 2.5 times as costly as other cases. A UK group found a similar effect, with cost of care rising significantly in patients who acquired sepsis after their second day in the ICU (up to a high of around $18,000 in total costs) [31]. A study of German ICUs published in 2007 estimated that care of the individual sepsis patient accounted for around Euro 1100 ± 400 per day (roughly USD 1500) [32]. It should again be noted that countries with more

ICU beds will tend to admit patients who are on the average less ill than patients in countries with fewer beds and that the cost of care in ICUs is significantly higher than on the wards.

The costs of postoperative sepsis were evaluated in a study by Vaughan-Sarrazin et al. published in 2011 in a cohort of patients treated at 118 Veterans Affairs hospitals in the United States [33]. In the cohort, 564 out of a total of 13,878 patients undergoing general surgery developed sepsis (a rate of 4.1%). Average cost for patients who did not develop sepsis was $24,923 and average cost for patients who did develop sepsis was $88,747, 3.6 times higher. With those data in mind, the authors conclude that a strong financial incentive exists to prevent the development of sepsis (in addition to implications for patient care well-being).

Long-Term Outcomes

It should be noted that many, if not most, studies of the sepsis spectrum report 30-day and/or 90-day mortality. Emerging data suggests that even longer time points may yield important data. A systematic review of long-term mortality and quality of life (>3 months) in sepsis by Winters et al. in 2010 found ongoing mortality beyond short-term end points and consistent impairment in quality of life as well [34]. The authors suggest that longer-term endpoints may paint a more accurate picture of the natural history of the disease and the interventions we use to mitigate it. A study by Iwashyna et al. also published in 2010 supports that conclusion, finding an odds ratio of 3.34 for moderate to severe cognitive impairment among survivors of severe sepsis in a cohort drawn from the Health and Retirement study (mean age 76.9 years old) [35]. The authors also found a high rate of functional impairment among survivors, with a mean increase of 1.57 limitations among those who had no limitations prior to their hospital stay for severe sepsis. Another study by Iwashyna et al. in 2012 of a large Medicare cohort also found that a large portion of survivors suffered from functional disability (almost 480,000 out of the 640,000 patients studied) and moderate to severe cognitive impairment (around 106,000 patients) [36]. There was little change in sepsis mortality, however, from 73.5% to 71.3% over the span of 1996 to 2008. Another study by Storgaard et al. in 2013 found a mortality rate of 33% for severe sepsis and septic shock at 30 days and a hazard ratio of 2.7 in the next 1 year and a ratio of 2.3 over the next 3 years, again pointing to a significant long-term impact of the disease [37]. A more recent study of healthcare utilization in survivors of severe sepsis that made use of Medicare claims found a higher rate of post-discharge mortality in sepsis versus non-sepsis admissions in the year after admission (44.2% versus 31.4%), as well as a steeper decline in days spent at home (−38.6 days), and a greater increase in the proportion of days spent alive in a facility (5.4%) [38]. Another recent study by Liu et al. [39] examined patient-level factors contributing to readmissions and healthcare utilization after sepsis. They found that healthcare utilization increased threefold after admission for sepsis and that most factors leading to increased utilization were present prior to initial sepsis admission (e.g., comorbid disease burden and high pre-sepsis healthcare utilization).

Demographic and Genetic Factors

Gender

A number of demographic factors have been found to affect a person's risk of developing sepsis. In the previously mentioned EPISEPSIS study, men were more likely to develop sepsis by a ratio of almost 2:1 with an average age of around 65 [22]. Although the authors saw no difference in mortality between men and women, survivors tended to be younger than non-survivors (61 versus 70 years, $p < .001$). After adjusting for sex in the population-at-large, Martin et al. showed a significantly higher risk of sepsis in men as well, with a relative risk of 1.28. In addition, sepsis developed later in life for women than men (62.1 versus 56.9 years), and the age of the overall population increased over the duration of the study (from 57.4 in the period between 1979 and 1984 to 60.8 years of age in the period between 1995 and 2000) [40]. A study by Padkin et al. of ICUs in the United Kingdom found an increased rate of sepsis in men (54% of patients admitted to the ICU) and the median age was 65 years [41]. A multicenter Italian study published in 2013 also found an increased risk of sepsis in men (63.5% of patients admitted to ICUs with severe sepsis), but interestingly found an increase in mortality among women with severe sepsis (OR 2.33) despite similar rates of overall ICU mortality between men and women [42]. The increased mortality in women may be explained at least partially by experimental evidence that women demonstrate more robust inflammatory responses to LPS than men [43]. Interestingly, an Austrian study of resource utilization by men and women in the ICU found that, despite more severe illness among women, men accounted for much greater levels of resource utilization and a higher number of invasive procedures, neither of which translated into improvement in mortality rate [44]. Both age and gender might be mitigated as risk factors by a study of comorbid conditions (discussed below), but the fact remains that both factors correlate well with the risk of sepsis in many different populations.

Race

The contribution of race to sepsis risk has been difficult to tease out, likely due to the myriad variables complicating the equation. Race itself is a difficult concept to study, owing to its changing definition over time. In addition, what was once considered a biological category influenced by genetics and ancestry is now thought to be primarily a social construction of culture, class, and environment. Given the complex nature of the terminology itself, it becomes difficult to study the epidemiology of a particular disease within a specific racial group (as opposed to a particular ethnic group, for example). That said, comorbid conditions such as end-stage renal disease are more prevalent in certain ethnic groups than others, and competing demographic factors such as socio-economic status (SES) certainly play an important role in the overall burden of disease in a particular community (due to access to healthcare, etc.). For the purposes of this review, we will use the terminology adhered to by the authors of the individual studies we discuss. In most larger cohorts, whites have significantly lower rates of sepsis. In the cohort of Martin et al., blacks and other non-whites had a relative risk of approximately 2.0 for the development of sepsis. Blacks had the highest mortality rate from sepsis (23.3%) and developed sepsis at the youngest ages (47.4 years on average). In a study by Mayr et al. of seven US states and infection-related Emergency Department visits, black patients had a 67% higher risk of severe sepsis when compared to white patients and an 80% higher mortality rate. The authors also found an increased rate of infection in black patients (47.3 versus 34.0 per 1000 population) and an increased risk of associated organ dysfunction (OR 1.29), both of which help to explain the racial disparities [45]. Barnato et al. found similar disparities in studying a cohort of six hospital referral areas in the United States using data from the US Census that showed an incidence of severe sepsis of 6.08/1000 population in black patients (versus 4.06 and 3.58/1000 for Hispanics and whites, respectively) [46]. After adjusting for SES, black patients still had an adjusted rate ratio of 1.44 for the development of severe sepsis. In addition, blacks had a higher case fatality rate than Hispanics and whites (with rates of 32.1%, 30.4%, and 29.3% respectively). Slightly conflicting data were found by Dombrovskiy et al. in a study of a New Jersey database published in 2008 [47]. In that cohort, black and white patients had similar case fatality rates from severe sepsis, but black patients were of significantly lower age (61.6 versus 72.8 years), at significantly higher risk of comorbidities such as HIV and diabetes, and were at much higher risk of poor health care coverage (3.96 times white patients). Taken together, it is likely that black patients do indeed have a greater predisposition to severe sepsis, but it is as yet unclear whether that predisposition results from specific genetic factors, environmental factors, or comorbid conditions. In terms of the level of care provided to patients of different races within the same hospital, a study by Mayr et al. found no differences between the care received by blacks and whites for pneumonia, but did note that hospitals that served primarily black patients were less likely to provide timely antibiotics (OR .84) [48].

Interestingly, a study by Mendu et al. found improved survival in all-cause critical illness among patients in Boston, Massachusetts who did not speak English as their primary language (30-day odds ratio 0.69) [49]. The effect was not confounded by indicators of severity of disease, specific language spoken, and neighborhood poverty index (a proxy for SES). While the authors did not report the specific difference in mortality rate for sepsis alone, they did note that controlling for sepsis as an admitting diagnosis did not alter their primary conclusions.

Socioeconomic Status

In terms of SES itself, many studies have noted the relationship between SES and access to ICU care, as well as overall intensity of care. A systematic review by Fowler et al. noted that patients without health insurance are less likely to receive critical care services (odds ratio 0.56) and may experience worse clinical outcomes [50].

A Danish cohort studied by Koch et al. in 2013 found a strong association between bacteremia and 30-day mortality (crude hazard ratio 1.38 between low and high levels of education and 1.58 between low versus high income tertile) [51]. Substance abuse rates, social support, pre-existing comorbidities, location of acquisition of infection, and infectious agent were all significantly different between SES groups. Correcting for those differences attenuated much of the difference in mortality between SES groups (adjusted hazard ratio 1.15 between low and high levels of education and 1.29 between low versus high income tertile).

A multicenter observational study by Mendu et al. [52] of almost 15,000 critically ill patients examined the relationship between neighborhood poverty rate and the development of bloodstream infections. After multivariate analysis, neighborhood poverty rates in the two highest quintiles (20–40% and >40%) were strongly associated with an increased risk for bloodstream infection (26% and 49%, respectively) relative to the lowest quintile (neighborhood poverty rate < 5%).

Biological Factors

Genetics also play a significant role in the development of sepsis and susceptibility to infections and are discussed fully in a separate chapter. A study by Sørenson et al. published in 1998 looked at genetic susceptibilities to a range of diseases by following a cohort of children in Denmark adopted between 1924 and 1926 [53]. Environmental factors seemed to play a role in the development of cancers and vascular disease (odds ratio 5.16 and 3.02, respectively, for death of adoptee when an adoptive parent died of one of those diseases), and genetic factors played a role in cardio/cerebrovascular disease (OR 4.52) and infections (OR 5.81) when the authors studied the frequency of adoptee death when the biologic parents died of one of the above. More recently, Henckaerts et al. reviewed the DNA of 774 MICU patients and found that polymorphisms in NOD2 and TLR4 (both important for innate immunity) were associated with an increased risk of bacteremia and increased in-hospital mortality (OR 4.26 and 2.27, respectively) [54]. Another study of genetics in critically ill patients by Sutherland et al. found a significantly increased risk of infection in patients with single nucleotide polymorphisms of CD14, mannose-binding lectin, and TLR2 [55]. A polymorphism of Mal, an adaptor protein downstream of TLR2 and TLR4, was found by Kohr and colleagues to provide protection against bacteremia and certain specific infectious pathogens [56]. A study by Agnese et al. found a significantly increased risk of gram-negative infections in ICU patients with specific TLR4 polymorphisms (79% versus 17%, $p > .004$) [57]. While mutations in the pathways listed above have been well studied in the literature, it is important to note that not every study evaluating them has shown consistent results. In addition, a great many other genetic pathways are under investigation, more fully detailed in a recent review by Waterer et al. [58]. Genetic polymorphisms have not yet cracked the code for vulnerability to sepsis, but they hold out the promise of a more specific biomarker in the near future.

Comorbidities

Many diseases predispose patients to the development of sepsis, but a few specific entities deserve special attention for their significant effects on overall rates and outcomes. In particular, malignancy, HIV infection, obesity, and diabetes mellitus all appear to increase susceptibility to infection.

Malignancy

Malignancy, particularly hematologic malignancy, seems to be the most significant risk factor. A cohort study by Williams et al. in 2004 found, in a survey of hospital data from six states in 1999, around 30,000 cases of severe sepsis out of a total of around 606,000 total cancer cases (a rate of around 5%) [59]. Nationally, they estimated around 126,000 cancer patients would develop sepsis (around 16 cases per 1000 cancer patients). The relative risk of hospitalization for severe sepsis in patients with cancer was approximately 3.96, with a mortality rate of 8.5%, and a cost of 3.4 billion dollars annually. Analysis of the National Hospital Discharge Survey in 2006 by Danai et al. found even more dramatic results, with 1465 cases per 100,000 cancer patients, and a relative risk of 9.77 compared to patients without underlying malignancy [60]. When the data were analyzed in terms of race, they found that blacks and other non-white races had a higher incidence of sepsis relative to whites (with relative risks of 1.28 and 1.47, respectively). Male cancer patients were more likely to develop sepsis than female cancer patients with a relative risk of 1.98. In addition, multivariate analysis found that the presence of cancer independently increased the risk of death from sepsis with an adjusted odds ratio of 1.98. In terms of specific cancer types, pancreatic cancer caused the greatest increase in the risk of sepsis (with 14,468 cases/100,000 patients), followed by multiple myeloma, leukemia, lung cancer, and lymphoma.

HIV

Despite the great advances made in the treatment of HIV with anti-retroviral therapies, patients with HIV continue to be at increased risk of developing sepsis. A study by Greenberg et al. found that 13.7% of ICU patients were HIV seropositive. Of that group, the majority of their acute infections were nosocomial (112 out of a total of 194 infections) [61]. The inpatient mortality rate was 42% for HIV patients with severe sepsis in the ICU. Interestingly, in a multivariate regression model, markers associated with HIV were not independently predictive of hospital mortality (e.g., CD4 count, use of HAART), but APACHE II score was (OR 1.12). A cohort of patients studied by Coquet et al. found an increase in annual admissions of HIV patients to the ICU from 1996 to 2005, but a steady decrease in ICU and 90-day mortality between 1996 and 1997 and between 2004 and 2005 from 25% and 37.5%, respectively, to 8.6% [62]. Severe sepsis was among the strongest predictors of mortality in HIV patients admitted to the ICU (behind specific organ failures and coma) with an OR of 3.67. Those data were corroborated by another study by Japiassú et al. of 88 HIV-infected patients admitted to the ICU of an infectious diseases research center [63]. The rate of severe sepsis in that population was 50% and severe sepsis was the strongest independent predictor of mortality, both 28-day (OR 3.13) and 6-month (OR 3.35). Respiratory infections accounted for the majority of cases of severe sepsis, as discussed further below.

Obesity

Obesity, defined as a body-mass index (BMI) ≥ 30 kg/m^2, is a tremendous public health problem throughout the developed world. According to a recent systematic review of the 2013 Global Burden of Disease Study, the proportion of adults with a BMI of 25 kg/m^2 or higher increased from 28.8% to 36.9% between 1980 and 2013 in men and 29.8% to 38.0% in women [64]. The proportion of obese children and adolescents in developed countries also increased substantially. In addition to the well-established cardiovascular risks of obesity, patients are also at increased risk of a range of other diseases, including malignancies of multiple types. Obese patients also appear to be at significantly increased risk for infection. While the mechanism of susceptibility is not fully understood, adipose tissue does appear to contribute actively to inflammation, with both leptin and adiponectin playing important roles in the balance of immune functions. A retrospective study by Yaegashi et al. in 2004 of obese medical ICU patients found that morbid obesity (BMI ≥ 40 kg/m^2) increases the risk of sepsis from 6.1% to 26.7% over obese patients [65]. A matched cohort study published the same year by Bercault et al. found similar results, with mechanically ventilated obese patients being significantly more likely to acquire a diagnosis of septic shock during their ICU than their non-obese counterparts (8% versus 3%, $p < 0.05$) [66]. In a more recent population-based cohort study by Wang et al., the morbidly obese were more likely than the non-obese to develop sepsis (HR 1.57) [67]. They also found increased waist circumference (>102 cm in men and >88 cm in women) to be a better predictor for the risk of sepsis than BMI (HR 1.34).

Interestingly, a large multinational cohort study by Arabi et al. published in 2013 found that obese patients had a lower mortality rate due to sepsis than non-obese patients (OR 0.80 for obese patients, 0.61 for morbidly obese patients), but that the association between obesity and survival disappeared when they controlled for variations in sepsis management [68]. Specifically, obese patients seem to receive less intravenous fluid per kilogram and lower antibiotic doses per kilogram than the non-obese. A recent retrospective cohort study by Gaulton et al. corroborated those data, finding no difference between mortality rates in the obese and non-obese due to sepsis. Another recent study by Prescott et al. again found that obesity conferred a protective effect against mortality at 1 year (OR 0.59 for obese patients and 0.46 for morbidly obese patients) [69].

Diabetes

Diabetes mellitus (DM), defined as a fasting glucose ≥126 mg/dL, a 2-h glucose of ≥200 mg/dL after a 75 g oral glucose challenge test, and/or a hemoglobin A1c level of ≥6.5, carries with it an increased risk of infection and sepsis. In a prospective cohort study published in 2005, Muller et al. found a higher risk of lower respiratory tract infection (OR for patients with type I DM of 1.42 and for type 2 DM of 1.32) and urinary tract infection (DM1 OR 1.96 and DM2 OR 1.24) as well as increased risks of both mucus membrane and skin infections [70]. The incidence rate for sepsis in diabetes patients in the cohort of Danai et al. mentioned above was found to be 700.8/100,000 [60] and Stegenga et al. found that 22.7% of all septic patients were diabetic in a retrospective analysis of a clinical trial [71]. That cohort also showed no increase in the mortality rate of sepsis in patients with underlying diabetes. Other studies have found conflicting data, however [72], and the true impact of sepsis on diabetic patients is as yet unclear.

Etiology and Source of Infection

In the cohort of Martin et al., gram-negative organisms dominated as the primary etiology of sepsis between 1979 and 1987 [7]. After that period, gram-positive organisms became the dominant bacteria. By 2000, gram-positive organisms accounted for 52.1% of infections, gram negatives for 37.6%, and fungi for 4.6%. Polymicrobial and anerobic organisms accounted for the rest of the infections in the cohort. Overall, the rate of gram-positive infections increased by the highest relative amount, an average of 26.3% per year in the period studied. In addition, the rate of fungal infections increased 207%, from 5321 cases in 1979 to 16,042 in 2000. The shift in etiologic agent may be due to increases in invasive procedures and hospital infection rates. In contrast, the EPIC II point prevalence study found a higher prevalence of gram-negative infections than gram positive (62% versus 47%, with the overlap representing polymicrobial infections) [4]. An etiologic agent was isolated in 70% of the total cohort. *Staphylococcus aureus* alone accounted for 20.5% of total infections and *Pseudomonas* accounted for around 20%. Several agents were independently associated with hospital mortality in multivariate logistic regression analysis: *Enterococcus*, *Pseudomonas*, and *Acinetobacter* [4]. A recent study by Ani et al. [73] that made use of the Nationwide Inpatient Sample database found that between 1999 and 2008, the most common causes of severe sepsis were gram-negative organisms, particularly *Escherichia coli*, but that *S. aureus* had the highest mortality hazard ratio (1.38).

In most cohorts, the lungs are the most common site of infection leading to sepsis. In the EPIC II cohort, the lungs accounted for approximately 64% of the total infections, followed by abdominal (20%), bloodstream (15%), and renal/GU infections (14%). The first EPISEPSIS cohort found similar numbers, with respiratory infections responsible for more cases of severe sepsis than any other site (41%) [22]. In the cohort published by Angus et al. in 2001, respiratory infections accounted for 45.8% of all severe sepsis, with bacteremia of unspecified site causing the highest relative mortality (41.2%) [3]. The cohort of community-acquired sepsis published by Storgaard found that urinary infections accounted for the highest percentage (36%) [37]; the discrepancy may be due to the selection of community-acquired sepsis in particular, as the weight of evidence strongly supports the notion that respiratory infections are the most common cause of sepsis by a wide margin.

A retrospective observational study of Canadian hospitals and ICUs by Leligdowicz published in 2014 found an association between the etiologic agent and the mortality rate [74]. With around 70% culture positivity in the cohort overall, gram positives were the most common etiologic agent (34.2% versus 25.7% gram negatives). As in prior cohorts, the lung was the most common site of infection for the development of sepsis. After adjusting for a number of factors known to affect mortality in sepsis, disseminated infections and intra-abdominal infections accounted for the highest risk of mortality by source.

An interesting attempt to find the underlying connection between organism, site of infection, and mortality rate was published in 2004 by Cohen et al. In a meta-analysis of 510 articles encompassing over 55,000 patients with microbiologic confirmation of infection, the authors demonstrated the importance of stratifying clinical trials not just by source of infection and etiologic agent, but also by the interaction between the two. They note, for example, that catheter-related bloodstream infection due to coagulase negative *Staphylococcus* is a wholly different process than the same site of infection due to *Candida* [75].

Conclusions

Sepsis has been recognized as a severe inflammatory response to infection since the days of the Ancient Greeks. Through the work of pioneering scientists and physicians, the connection between causative agents and the response of the host came to the fore. More recent advances in epidemiology have led to an understanding of sepsis as a common disease with potentially catastrophic complications. Consensus definitions have allowed sepsis to be studied as a global problem, with coordinated networks analyzing trends in incidence and outcome and giving insights into demographic trends and comorbidities associated with the development of the disease. Persons of non-white races appear more vulnerable to the disease, as do patients with underlying malignancy, HIV, obesity, or diabetes. Despite improvements in sepsis care, the rising incidence of the disease has resulted in an increase in mortality in the last few decades. Respiratory infections remain the primary source of infection, and gram-positive organisms appear to be eclipsing gram-negatives as the primary etiologic agents driving the disease.

Advances in epidemiology have greatly improved our ability to understand who is most vulnerable to the continuum of sepsis. These advances will point the way toward ever more sophisticated mechanistic questions regarding the development of the disease process. As our understanding of the disease improves and our treatments become more targeted, these epidemiologic tools will help us understand the effect of our interventions on the overall incidence and mortality of sepsis. The recent increase in the number of sepsis cases has shown no sign of abating, and we have every reason to expect the trend to continue into the future. We expect that mortality rate will continue to decline, though, as advances in medical knowledge enter the clinical arena. Concomitant advances in other fields will undoubtedly change the spectrum of infectious source and agent, but coordinated networks will balance those shifts by offering a greater understanding of the dynamics of the disease across the world.

References

1. Rangel-Frausto MS, Pittet D, Costigan M, Hwang T, Davis CS, Wenzel RP. The natural history of the systemic inflammatory response syndrome (SIRS). A prospective study. JAMA. 1995;273(2):117–23.
2. Sands KE, Bates DW, Lanken PN, Graman PS, Hibberd PL, Kahn KL, et al. Epidemiology of sepsis syndrome in 8 academic medical centers. JAMA. 1997;278(3):234–40.
3. Angus DC, Linde-Zwirble WT, Lidicker J, Clermont G, Carcillo J, Pinsky MR. Epidemiology of severe sepsis in the United States: analysis of incidence, outcome, and associated costs of care. Crit Care Med. 2001;29(7):1303–10.
4. Vincent JL, Rello J, Marshall J, Silva E, Anzueto A, Martin CD, et al. International study of the prevalence and outcomes of infection in intensive care units. JAMA. 2009;302(21):2323–9.
5. Whittaker SA, Fuchs BD, Gaieski DF, Christie JD, Goyal M, Meyer NJ, et al. Epidemiology and outcomes in patients with severe sepsis admitted to the hospital wards. J Crit Care. 2014;30(1):78–84. Epub 2014 Jul 22
6. Rohde JM, Odden AJ, Bonham C, Kuhn L, Malani PN, Chen LM, et al. The epidemiology of acute organ system dysfunction from severe sepsis outside of the intensive care unit. J Hosp Med. 2013;8(5):243–7.
7. Martin GS, Mannino DM, Eaton S, Moss M. The epidemiology of sepsis in the United States from 1979 through 2000. N Engl J Med. 2003;348(16):1546–54.
8. Kumar G, Kumar N, Taneja A, Kaleekal T, Tarima S, McGinley E, et al. Nationwide trends of severe sepsis in the 21st century (2000–2007). Chest. 2011;140(5):1223–31.
9. Stevenson EK, Rubenstein AR, Radin GT, Wiener RS, Walkey AJ. Two decades of mortality trends among patients with severe sepsis: a comparative meta-analysis. Crit Care Med. 2014;42(3):625–31.
10. Gaieski DF, Edwards JM, Kallan MJ, Carr BG. Benchmarking the incidence and mortality of severe sepsis in the United States. Crit Care Med. 2013;41(5):1167–74.
11. Wang HE, Devereaux RS, Yealy DM, Safford MM, Howard G. National variation in United States sepsis mortality: a descriptive study. Int J Health Geogr. 2010;9:9.
12. Dombrovskiy VY, Martin AA, Sunderram J, Paz HL. Rapid increase in hospitalization and mortality rates for severe sepsis in the United States: a trend analysis from 1993 to 2003. Crit Care Med. 2007;35(5):1244–50.

13. Iwashyna TJ, Odden A, Rohde J, Bonham C, Kuhn L, Malani P, et al. Identifying patients with severe sepsis using administrative claims: patient-level validation of the angus implementation of the international consensus conference definition of severe sepsis. Med Care. 2014;52(6):e39–43.

14. Barochia AV, Cui X, Vitberg D, Suffredini AF, O'Grady NP, Banks SM, et al. Bundled care for septic shock: an analysis of clinical trials. Crit Care Med. 2010;38(2):668–78.

15. Miller 3rd RR, Dong L, Nelson NC, Brown SM, Kuttler KG, Probst DR, et al. Multicenter implementation of a severe sepsis and septic shock treatment bundle. Am J Respir Crit Care Med. 2013;188(1):77–82.

16. Gaieski DF, Edwards JM, Kallan MJ, Mikkelsen ME, Goyal M, Carr BG. The relationship between hospital volume and mortality in severe sepsis. Am J Respir Crit Care Med. 2014;190(6):665–74.

17. Liu V, Escobar GJ, Greene JD, Soule J, Whippy A, Angus DC, et al. Hospital deaths in patients with sepsis from 2 independent cohorts. JAMA. 2014;312(1):90–2.

18. Harrison DA, Welch CA, Eddleston JM. The epidemiology of severe sepsis in England, Wales and Northern Ireland, 1996 to 2004: secondary analysis of a high quality clinical database, the ICNARC Case Mix Programme Database. Crit Care. 2006;10(2):R42.

19. van Gestel A, Bakker J, Veraart CP, van Hout BA. Prevalence and incidence of severe sepsis in Dutch intensive care units. Crit Care. 2004;8(4):R153–62.

20. Finfer S, Bellomo R, Lipman J, French C, Dobb G, Myburgh J. Adult-population incidence of severe sepsis in Australian and New Zealand intensive care units. Intensive Care Med. 2004;30(4):589–96.

21. Kaukonen KM, Bailey M, Suzuki S, Pilcher D, Bellomo R. Mortality related to severe sepsis and septic shock among critically ill patients in Australia and New Zealand, 2000–2012. JAMA. 2014;311(13):1308–16.

22. Brun-Buisson C, Doyon F, Carlet J, Dellamonica P, Gouin F, Lepoutre A, et al. Incidence, risk factors, and outcome of severe sepsis and septic shock in adults. A multicenter prospective study in intensive care units. French ICU Group for Severe Sepsis. JAMA. 1995;274(12):968–74.

23. Brun-Buisson C, Meshaka P, Pinton P, Vallet B. EPISEPSIS: a reappraisal of the epidemiology and outcome of severe sepsis in French intensive care units. Intensive Care Med. 2004;30(4):580–8.

24. Edwards R, Hutson R, Johnson J, Sherwin R, Gordon-Strachan G, Frankson M, et al. Severe sepsis in the emergency department—an observational cohort study from the university hospital of the West Indies. West Indian Med J. 2013;62(3):224–9.

25. Esteban A, Frutos-Vivar F, Ferguson ND, Penuelas O, Lorente JA, Gordo F, et al. Sepsis incidence and outcome: contrasting the intensive care unit with the hospital ward. Crit Care Med. 2007;35(5):1284–9.

26. Adhikari NK, Fowler RA, Bhagwanjee S, Rubenfeld GD. Critical care and the global burden of critical illness in adults. Lancet. 2010;376(9749):1339–46.

27. Linde-Zwirble WT, Angus DC. Severe sepsis epidemiology: sampling, selection, and society. Crit Care. 2004;8(4):222–6.

28. Angus DC, Sirio CA, Clermont G, Bion J. International comparisons of critical care outcome and resource consumption. Crit Care Clin. 1997;13(2):389–407.

29. Wier LM, Pfuntner A, Maeda J, Stranges E, Ryan K, Jagadish P, et al. HCUP facts and figures: statistics on hospital-based care in the United States, 2009. Rockville, MD: Agency for Healthcare Research and Quality; 2011.

30. Brun-Buisson C, Roudot-Thoraval F, Girou E, Grenier-Sennelier C, Durand-Zaleski I. The costs of septic syndromes in the intensive care unit and influence of hospital-acquired sepsis. Intensive Care Med. 2003;29(9):1464–71.

31. Edbrooke DL, Hibbert CL, Kingsley JM, Smith S, Bright NM, Quinn JM. The patient-related costs of care for sepsis patients in a United Kingdom adult general intensive care unit. Crit Care Med. 1999;27(9):1760–7.

32. Moerer O, Plock E, Mgbor U, Schmid A, Schneider H, Wischnewsky MB, et al. A German national prevalence study on the cost of intensive care: an evaluation from 51 intensive care units. Crit Care. 2007;11(3):R69.

33. Vaughan-Sarrazin MS, Bayman L, Cullen JJ. Costs of postoperative sepsis: the business case for quality improvement to reduce postoperative sepsis in veterans affairs hospitals. Arch Surg. 2011;146(8):944–51.
34. Winters BD, Eberlein M, Leung J, Needham DM, Pronovost PJ, Sevransky JE. Long-term mortality and quality of life in sepsis: a systematic review. Crit Care Med. 2010;38(5):1276–83.
35. Iwashyna TJ, Ely EW, Smith DM, Langa KM. Long-term cognitive impairment and functional disability among survivors of severe sepsis. JAMA. 2010;304(16):1787–94.
36. Iwashyna TJ, Cooke CR, Wunsch H, Kahn JM. Population burden of long-term survivorship after severe sepsis in older Americans. J Am Geriatr Soc. 2012;60(6):1070–7.
37. Storgaard M, Hallas J, Gahrn-Hansen B, Pedersen SS, Pedersen C, Lassen AT. Short- and long-term mortality in patients with community-acquired severe sepsis and septic shock. Scand J Infect Dis. 2013;45(8):577–83.
38. Prescott HC, Langa KM, Liu V, Escobar GJ, Iwashyna TJ. Increased 1-year healthcare use in survivors of severe sepsis. Am J Respir Crit Care Med. 2014;190(1):62–9.
39. Liu V, Lei X, Prescott HC, Kipnis P, Iwashyna TJ, Escobar GJ. Hospital readmission and healthcare utilization following sepsis in community settings. J Hosp Med. 2014;9(8):502–7.
40. Martin GS, Mannino DM, Moss M. The effect of age on the development and outcome of adult sepsis. Crit Care Med. 2006;34(1):15–21.
41. Padkin A, Goldfrad C, Brady AR, Young D, Black N, Rowan K. Epidemiology of severe sepsis occurring in the first 24 hrs in intensive care units in England, Wales, and Northern Ireland. Crit Care Med. 2003;31(9):2332–8.
42. Sakr Y, Elia C, Mascia L, Barberis B, Cardellino S, Livigni S, et al. The influence of gender on the epidemiology of and outcome from severe sepsis. Crit Care. 2013;17(2):R50.
43. van Eijk LT, Dorresteijn MJ, Smits P, van der Hoeven JG, Netea MG, Pickkers P. Gender differences in the innate immune response and vascular reactivity following the administration of endotoxin to human volunteers. Crit Care Med. 2007;35(6):1464–9.
44. Valentin A, Jordan B, Lang T, Hiesmayr M, Metnitz PG. Gender-related differences in intensive care: a multiple-center cohort study of therapeutic interventions and outcome in critically ill patients. Crit Care Med. 2003;31(7):1901–7.
45. Mayr FB, Yende S, Linde-Zwirble WT, Peck-Palmer OM, Barnato AE, Weissfeld LA, et al. Infection rate and acute organ dysfunction risk as explanations for racial differences in severe sepsis. JAMA. 2010;303(24):2495–503.
46. Barnato AE, Alexander SL, Linde-Zwirble WT, Angus DC. Racial variation in the incidence, care, and outcomes of severe sepsis: analysis of population, patient, and hospital characteristics. Am J Respir Crit Care Med. 2008;177(3):279–84.
47. Dombrovskiy VY, Martin AA, Sunderram J, Paz HL. Occurrence and outcomes of sepsis: influence of race. Crit Care Med. 2007;35(3):763–8.
48. Mayr FB, Yende S, D'Angelo G, Barnato AE, Kellum JA, Weissfeld L, et al. Do hospitals provide lower quality of care to black patients for pneumonia? Crit Care Med. 2010;38(3):759–65.
49. Mendu ML, Zager S, Moromizato T, McKane CK, Gibbons FK, Christopher KB. The association between primary language spoken and all-cause mortality in critically ill patients. J Crit Care. 2013;28(6):928–34.
50. Fowler RA, Noyahr LA, Thornton JD, Pinto R, Kahn JM, Adhikari NK, et al. An official American Thoracic Society systematic review: the association between health insurance status and access, care delivery, and outcomes for patients who are critically ill. Am J Respir Crit Care Med. 2010;181(9):1003–11.
51. Koch K, Norgaard M, Schonheyder HC, Thomsen RW, Sogaard M. Effect of socioeconomic status on mortality after bacteremia in working-age patients. A Danish population-based cohort study. PLoS One. 2013;8(7):e70082.
52. Mendu ML, Zager S, Gibbons FK, Christopher KB. Relationship between neighborhood poverty rate and bloodstream infections in the critically ill. Crit Care Med. 2012;40(5):1427–36.
53. Sorensen TI, Nielsen GG, Andersen PK, Teasdale TW. Genetic and environmental influences on premature death in adult adoptees. N Engl J Med. 1988;318(12):727–32.

54. Henckaerts L, Nielsen KR, Steffensen R, Van Steen K, Mathieu C, Giulietti A, et al. Polymorphisms in innate immunity genes predispose to bacteremia and death in the medical intensive care unit. Crit Care Med. 2009;37(1):192–201. e1–3

55. Sutherland AM, Walley KR, Russell JA. Polymorphisms in CD14, mannose-binding lectin, and Toll-like receptor-2 are associated with increased prevalence of infection in critically ill adults. Crit Care Med. 2005;33(3):638–44.

56. Khor CC, Chapman SJ, Vannberg FO, Dunne A, Murphy C, Ling EY, et al. A Mal functional variant is associated with protection against invasive pneumococcal disease, bacteremia, malaria and tuberculosis. Nat Genet. 2007;39(4):523–8.

57. Agnese DM, Calvano JE, Hahm SJ, Coyle SM, Corbett SA, Calvano SE, et al. Human toll-like receptor 4 mutations but not CD14 polymorphisms are associated with an increased risk of gram-negative infections. J Infect Dis. 2002;186(10):1522–5.

58. Waterer GW, Bruns AH. Genetic risk of acute pulmonary infections and sepsis. Expert Rev Respir Med. 2010;4(2):229–38.

59. Williams MD, Braun LA, Cooper LM, Johnston J, Weiss RV, Qualy RL, et al. Hospitalized cancer patients with severe sepsis: analysis of incidence, mortality, and associated costs of care. Crit Care. 2004;8(5):R291–8.

60. Danai PA, Moss M, Mannino DM, Martin GS. The epidemiology of sepsis in patients with malignancy. Chest. 2006;129(6):1432–40.

61. Greenberg JA, Lennox JL, Martin GS. Outcomes for critically ill patients with HIV and severe sepsis in the era of highly active antiretroviral therapy. J Crit Care. 2012;27(1):51–7.

62. Coquet I, Pavie J, Palmer P, Barbier F, Legriel S, Mayaux J, et al. Survival trends in critically ill HIV-infected patients in the highly active antiretroviral therapy era. Crit Care. 2010;14(3):R107.

63. Japiassu AM, Amancio RT, Mesquita EC, Medeiros DM, Bernal HB, Nunes EP, et al. Sepsis is a major determinant of outcome in critically ill HIV/AIDS patients. Crit Care. 2010;14(4):R152.

64. Ng M, Fleming T, Robinson M, Thomson B, Graetz N, Margono C, et al. Global, regional, and national prevalence of overweight and obesity in children and adults during 1980–2013: a systematic analysis for the Global Burden of Disease Study 2013. Lancet. 2014 May 28;384(9945):766–81.

65. Yaegashi M, Jean R, Zuriqat M, Noack S, Homel P. Outcome of morbid obesity in the intensive care unit. J Intensive Care Med. 2005;20(3):147–54.

66. Bercault N, Boulain T, Kuteifan K, Wolf M, Runge I, Fleury JC. Obesity-related excess mortality rate in an adult intensive care unit: a risk-adjusted matched cohort study. Crit Care Med. 2004;32(4):998–1003.

67. Wang HE, Griffin R, Judd S, Shapiro NI, Safford MM. Obesity and risk of sepsis: a population-based cohort study. Obesity (Silver Spring). 2013;21(12):E762–9.

68. Arabi YM, Dara SI, Tamim HM, Rishu AH, Bouchama A, Khedr MK, et al. Clinical characteristics, sepsis interventions and outcomes in the obese patients with septic shock: an international multicenter cohort study. Crit Care. 2013;17(2):R72.

69. Prescott HC, Chang VW, O'Brien Jr JM, Langa KM, Iwashyna T. Obesity and 1-year outcomes in older Americans with severe sepsis. Crit Care Med. 2014 Apr 8;42(8):1766–74.

70. Muller LM, Gorter KJ, Hak E, Goudzwaard WL, Schellevis FG, Hoepelman AI, et al. Increased risk of common infections in patients with type 1 and type 2 diabetes mellitus. Clin Infect Dis. 2005;41(3):281–8.

71. Stegenga ME, Vincent JL, Vail GM, Xie J, Haney DJ, Williams MD, et al. Diabetes does not alter mortality or hemostatic and inflammatory responses in patients with severe sepsis. Crit Care Med. 2010;38(2):539–45.

72. Kornum JB, Thomsen RW, Riis A, Lervang HH, Schonheyder HC, Sorensen HT. Type 2 diabetes and pneumonia outcomes: a population-based cohort study. Diabetes Care. 2007;30(9):2251–7.

73. Ani C, Farshidpanah S, Bellinghausen Stewart A, Nguyen HB. Variations in organism-specific severe sepsis mortality in the United States: 1999–2008. Crit Care Med. 2014 Sep 16;43(1):65–77.
74. Leligdowicz A, Dodek PM, Norena M, Wong H, Kumar A. Association between source of infection and hospital mortality in patients who have septic shock. Am J Respir Crit Care Med. 2014;189(10):1204–13.
75. Cohen J, Cristofaro P, Carlet J, Opal S. New method of classifying infections in critically ill patients. Crit Care Med. 2004;32(7):1510–26.

Part II

Chapter 4
Overview of the Molecular Pathways and Mediators of Sepsis

Tristen T. Chun, Brittany A. Potz, Whitney A. Young, and Alfred Ayala

Abbreviations

APC	Antigen presenting cell
ATP	Adenosine triphosphate
CARS	Compensatory anti-inflammatory response syndrome
CAUTI	Catheter-associated urinary tract infections
CLABSI	Central line-associated blood stream infections
DAMP	Danger-associated molecular patterns
DC	Dendritic cell
DIC	Disseminated intravascular coagulation
DNA	Deoxyribonucleic acid
fMLP	Formyl-methionyl-leucyl-phenylalanine

T.T. Chun, MD
Division of Surgical Research, Department of Surgery, Rhode Island Hospital,
593 Eddy Street Aldrich 226, Providence, RI 02903, USA
e-mail: tristen_chun@brown.edu

B.A. Potz, MD
Division of Surgical Research, Department of Surgery, Rhode Island Hospital,
2 Dudley Street MOC 360, Providence, RI 02905, USA
e-mail: brittany_potz@brown.edu

W.A. Young, MD
Division of Surgical Research, Department of Surgery, Rhode Island Hospital,
593 Eddy Street Aldrich 242, Providence, RI 02903, USA
e-mail: wyoung1@lifespan.org

A. Ayala, PhD (✉)
Division of Surgical Research, Department of Surgery, Rhode Island Hospital,
593 Eddy Street Aldrich 227, Providence, RI 02903, USA
e-mail: aayala@lifespan.org

© Springer International Publishing AG 2017
N.S. Ward, M.M. Levy (eds.), *Sepsis*, Respiratory Medicine,
DOI 10.1007/978-3-319-48470-9_4

HDL	High density lipoprotein
HMGB-1	High mobility group box-1
HSP	Heat shock protein
ICU	Intensive care units
IL	Interleukin
iNKT	Invariant natural killer T cell
iPRS	Intracellular patterns recognition systems
LBP	Lipopolysaccharide biding protein
LDL	Low density lipoprotein
LPS	Lipopolysaccharide
LTA	Lipoteichoic acid
MAC	Membrane attack complex
MAPK	Mitogen-activated protein kinase
MARS	Mixed antagonistic response syndrome
MCP	Monocyte chemotactic protein
MHC	Major histocompatibility complex
MIF	Migration inhibitory factor
MMP	Matrix metalloproteinase
MOF	Multiple organ failure
MSOF	Multisystem organ failure
NADPH	Nicotinamide adenine dinucleotide phosphate
NK	Natural killer cell
NKT	Natural killer T cell
NO	Nitric oxide
PAMP	Pathogen-associated molecular patterns
PAR	Protease-activated receptor
PG	Prostaglandin
PRR	Pattern recognition receptors
RA	Receptor antagonist
RIG-I	Retinoic-acid-inducible gene I
RNA	Ribonucleic acid
RNS	Reactive nitrogen species
ROS	Reactive oxygen species
S1P	Sphingosine-1 phosphate
sIL-R	Soluble interleukin receptor
SIRS	Systemic inflammatory response syndrome
TCR	T cell receptor
TGF	Transforming growth factor
TLR	Toll-like receptors
TNF	Tumor necrosis factor
VAP	Ventilator-associated pneumonia
VLDL	Very low density lipoprotein

Background

Sepsis is a common and expensive clinical entity in critically ill patient populations and intensive care units in the United States and around the world. Sepsis is associated with high morbidity and mortality universally due to the lack of treatment available to modulate this inflammatory syndrome aside from supportive care. While supportive care has improved drastically over the last several decades it is estimated that ~750,000 cases of sepsis occur annually in the US resulting in death in 18–44% of cases. The US has spent as much at 17 billion dollars a year on sepsis alone [1–3]. Thus, understanding the molecular pathways and immune dysfunction in sepsis is critically important for both the bedside management of these patients and the scientific community. Such insight into the natural history and the trajectory of sepsis not only should enable a deeper scientific understanding of the molecular pathways that drive this pathological condition but also should direct pharmacological development of new and novel therapies to modulate this morbid syndrome.

In this respect, sepsis is considered a complex clinical syndrome that develops when host response to pathogen and/or injured tissue becomes inappropriately amplified. Dysregulation of this immune response to infection, thus, becomes a harmful host response. This results in disruption of the balance between eliminating invading pathogens and damage to host tissues, organs, and organ systems. Sustained immunosuppression and infection occur with dysregulated immune response to invading pathogens [4, 5].

Systemic Inflammatory Response Syndrome (SIRS) is defined by the presence of two or more of the following criteria: body temperature <36 °C or >38 °C, heart rate >90 beats per minute, respiratory rate > 20 or $PaCO_2$ < 32 mmHg, white blood cell count <4000 cells/mm^3 (4×10^9 cells/L) or >12,000 cells/mm^3 (12×10^9 cells/L), or the presence of greater than 10% immature (band forms) neutrophils [6]. SIRS is a systemic inflammatory condition that can be induced by trauma, stress, or infection. Sepsis exists when two or more SIRS criteria are met in the setting of a known infectious source. When organ dysfunction, hypo-perfusion, and hypotension are evident, severe sepsis is thought to be present [7]. Persistent dysregulation of the immune system and presence of sustained infection can result in multisystem organ failure (MSOF).

Compensatory Anti-inflammatory Response Syndrome (CARS) is a hypo-inflammatory phase that was initially thought to have evolved so as to offset the pro-inflammatory response/SIRS. However, in sepsis, it was initially proposed that when the CARS response predominated over SIRS, there was a state of immune suppression, which predisposed patients to developing/being vulnerable to secondary infection [4, 5]. In Intensive Care Units (ICUs), these secondary infections are often nosocomial infections like catheter-associated urinary tract infections (CAUTI), ventilator-associated pneumonia (VAP) and central line-associated blood stream infections (CLABSI). However, over time it has become apparent that more of a mixed antagonistic response syndrome (MARS) exists in which both aspects of the pro- (SIRS) and anti-inflammatory response (CARS) are concomitantly altered and/or dysregulated (Fig. 4.1).

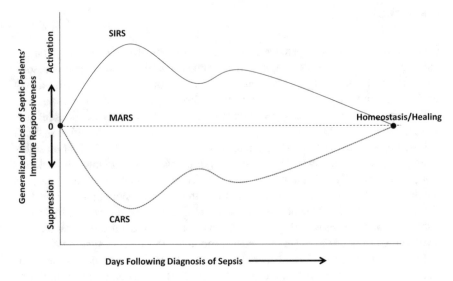

Fig. 4.1 Generalized indices of septic patients' immune responsiveness as a function of time. Both aspects of SIRS and CARS exist to comprise MARS (*SIRS* Systemic Inflammatory Response Syndrome, *CARS* Compensatory Anti-inflammatory Response Syndrome, *MARS* Mixed Antagonistic Response Syndrome)

Introduction to Innate and Adaptive Immune Responses

The *innate* immune system is the first line of host defense against foreign pathogens, and is not specific to any particular antigen. It is older and more primitive than the adaptive immune system and can be found in a wide range of plant and animal species. It is comprised of physical barriers via cells of the epithelium (e.g. the skin and mucosa), chemical barriers (e.g. acids in the stomach) and biological barriers (e.g. normal microflora of the skin and the gastrointestinal tract). In addition, the innate immune system is comprised of various cellular components and molecular factors that are directly or indirectly microbicidal and can regulate the inflammatory response (Fig. 4.2). Examples of these include the complement and coagulation systems, histamines and lipid mediators, cytokines and chemokines and a variety of leukocytes (or white blood cells) that circulate in the peripheral blood. The responses are typically rapid and conserved (or generic) in nature. Unlike the adaptive immunity, the innate immune system is triggered immediately upon challenge by offending pathogens and exhibits no adaptation or memory characteristics to prior known stimuli. Lastly, the innate immune response is believed to be a product of many diverse processes, rather than a single defined physiological system.

Adaptive or acquired immunity is cell mediated. It is an evolutionarily young system, restricted only to vertebrates. Adaptive immunity relies on the function of RAG recombinase genes for somatic recombination of gene segments that code for antigen receptors (i.e., novel immunoglobulin and T cell receptor molecules).

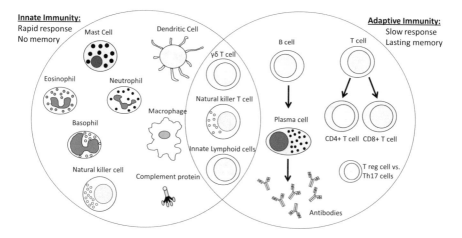

Fig. 4.2 Cellular components of innate and adaptive immunity. γδ T cells and Natural killer T cell have aspects of both innate and adaptive immunity and may serve as an important bridge between the two systems

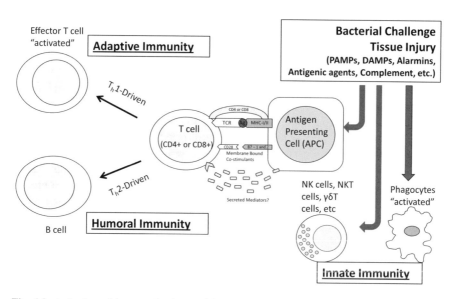

Fig. 4.3 Activation of innate, adaptive, and humoral immunity following bacterial challenge or tissue injury

Once antigen presenting cells (APCs) encounter bacterial or tissue damage-related molecular patterns they present these antigens for immune response (Fig. 4.3). Pathogen-associated molecular patterns (PAMPs) are unique and conserved molecular patterns present in a variety of pathogens (bacterial, fungal, viral, protozoal molecular sequences not found in mammalian cells) (Fig. 4.4). Examples of PAMPs

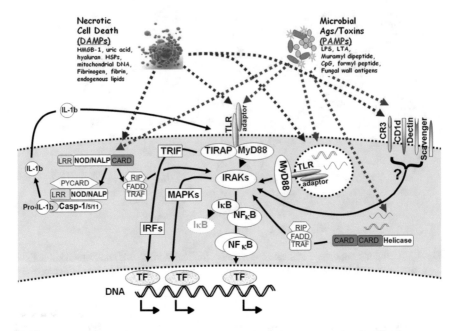

Fig. 4.4 Pathogen-associated molecular patterns (PAMPs) and danger-associated molecular patterns (DAMPs). Subsequent molecular events in response to these stimuli are depicted in this diagram

include endotoxin/lipopolysaccharide (LPS), bacterial deoxyribonucleic acid (DNA), soluble RNA (sRNA), double-stranded RNA (dsRNA), flagellin, peptidoglycan, zymosan and fungal glucans (fungal cell wall components), and glycosylphospho-lipids [8]. Danger-Associated Molecular Patterns (DAMPs) are endogenous cellular components only present or released during necrotic cell injury/death. DAMPs include heat shock proteins, fibrinogen, fibronectin, hyaluran, biglycans, uric acid, high mobility group box-1 (HMGB-1), and mitochondrial components (a source of fMLP) [9, 10]. Pattern recognition receptors (PRR) are the receptors on the surface of immune and non-immune cells that recognize PAMPs and DAMPs.

Innate Immunity

The innate immune response occurs through pattern recognition receptors (PRRs) on the surface of immune cells, which recognize and bind the conserved PAMPs of the invading microorganism or the DAMPs from the injured/dying cells (mentioned earlier) (Fig. 4.5). This triggers complex intracellular signaling cascades that result in gene activation and secretion of a variety of pro-inflammatory mediators. A number of families of surface PRRs have been described, including Toll-like receptors (TLRs), scavenger receptors, formyl peptide receptors, integrin/dectin family members, and mannose receptors.

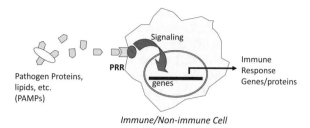

Fig. 4.5 Innate immune response occurs through pattern recognition receptors (PRRs) on the surface of immune and non-immune cells that recognize pathogens (PAMPs, DAMPS, etc.)

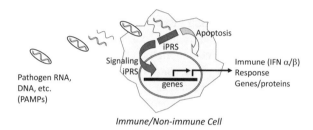

Fig. 4.6 Intracellular patterns recognition systems (iPRSs) also exist to perceive pathogens within intracellular compartments or in the cytosol of immune and non-immune cells

Alternatively, a system of intracellular patterns recognition systems (iPRSs) also appears to exist to perceive invasive intracellular pathogens, e.g., viruses and intracellular bacteria (Fig. 4.6). This system can also respond to the PAMPs and the DAMPs, and, when activated, it leads to the activation of transcription factors that can also upregulate the expression of pro-inflammatory mediators. These iPRSs include protein kinase R, nucleotide-oligomerization domain leucine-rich repeat (NOD-LRR) proteins like inflammasome, cytoplasmic caspase activation, and recruiting domain helicases such as retinoic-acid-inducible gene I (RIG-I)-like helicases. Natural killer and invariant natural killer T cells, gamma-delta T cells and other cytotoxic cells, e.g., innate lymphoid cells, can also become activated and stimulate a nonspecific and rapid immune response to infection (Fig. 4.2). Overtime, the immune system is then able to tolerate self antigens and attack anything that it perceives as foreign, thereby defending the body against invading microorganisms.

Adaptive Immunity

APCs have major histocompatibility complexes which present antigen via CD4 receptors to T cells (CD4$^+$ or CD8$^+$ T cells) (Fig. 4.3). Major histocompatibility complex (MHC) falls into two subtypes, MHC-I and MHC-II. MHCs are a group of cell surface markers on vertebrates that mediate cell–cell interactions with leukocytes and other cells. Each MHC displays an epitope or portion of a protein. This epitope can be foreign such as a particular molecular or protein pattern from a pathogen (nonself) or from within the individual's/host's own molecular and cellular patterns (self). MHC-II are present on APCs like macrophages, B cells, and dendritic cells. An APC ingests an antigen and after processing the antigen displays a portion of it, an epitope, in its MHC-II. MHC-II bind to CD4+ or helper T cells which display both CD4 receptors and T cell receptors (TCR). A naïve helper T cell binds an APC and the TCR comes in contact with the epitope from the APC's MHC-II. Based on the cytokines present and the local tissue environment the naïve T cell (T_0) differentiates into an effector, memory, or regulatory T cell though the process of polarization.

MHC-I on the other hand are present on most all nucleated cells and again through the process of antigen presentation displays epitope, but in this case to cytotoxic (CD8+) T cells that can induce programmed cell death by apoptosis of infected target cells containing (thus the term "cellular immunity") pathogens like viruses and intracellular microbes (mycoplasma, rickettsia). Importantly, for either of these forms of T cell activation to move forward normally membrane bound co-stimulatory, co-inhibitory and/or select secreted factors serve as up or downregulators (act as "check point proteins") of the antigen presentation cell and T cell binding interaction. Once activated, CD4+ and CD8+ T cells stimulate B cells to produce antibodies via a Th-1 response. These antibodies persist in the body and result in long-term "humoral immunity." CD4+ T cell can also act via a Th-2 response to present antigen to T effector cells. (Figs. 4.2 and 4.3). Eventually regulatory T cells (e.g., Th17 and T regulatory subpopulations) coordinate a shift from a Th-1 type response to a Th-2 response allowing for long-term memory of the foreign antigen. Memory enables coordination of an expedited immune response when a given foreign antigen is re-encountered in the future. This memory is the mechanism by which vaccinations work to prevent disease. Introduction of a killed or partial attenuated bacterial or viral pathogen stimulates activation of T cells (CD8+ T cells in a Th-1-dependent fashion resulting in antibody production by B cells). When an antigen is re-encountered antibody production is increased and the clonal population of immunoglobulin stimulates cell-mediated immune response to infection. Through antigen-immunoglobulin binding agglutination, macrophages become primed for phagocytosis and this stimulates the complement pathway to neutralize infection [6, 11–13].

Cells Involved in Immune Response in Sepsis

The innate immune response is mediated by leukocytes (white blood cells) that are initially derived from the bone marrow and/or thymus, circulate in the peripheral blood and home to the site of inflammation early in the course of infection. These include circulating monocytes, tissue macrophages, neutrophils and dendritic cells, natural killer cells, eosinophils, basophils, and mast cells. As described earlier, some of these innate leukocytes have the ability to fight invading pathogens by engulfing and destroying them through a process called phagocytosis (Fig. 4.2). This process is critical in removing cellular debris and creating an optimal environment for tissue repair and healing. Some of these cells are capable of processing the antigens of these pathogens and displaying them on their surfaces, resulting in antigen presentation through the MHC to the TCR on the surface of T-cells (Fig. 4.3). This provides an important link between innate and adaptive immune responses. We will describe some of the leukocytes involved in innate immune response in detail below with a particular focus on cellular and molecular changes that occur in response to sepsis.

Monocytes and Macrophages

Monocytes are large leukocytes that arise from myeloid precursor cells in primary lymphoid organs such as the fetal liver and bone marrow. These cells circulate in the peripheral blood and are recruited into tissues at sites of inflammation, where they differentiate into large phagocytic cells called macrophages. Monocytes and macrophages play an important role in innate immune response through their ability to phagocytose and fight invading pathogens until effective adaptive response can develop. In addition, they have a crucial role in coordinating an inflammatory response, producing a variety of regulatory cytokines and chemokines, such as tumor necrosis factor (TNF)-α, interleukin (IL)-1 and IL-6, and IL-8, as examples, involved in recruiting other cells of innate immune response to the sites of inflammation. Some of the cytokines released are responsible for causing fever upon infection, thus, their effects can be both local and systemic. Monocytes and macrophages have an additional role in adaptive immune response as APCs. They can capture and present these antigens to activated T cells in the lymph nodes. This triggers a cascade of important cellular and molecular events in adaptive immunity. In sepsis, it is known that the oxidative burst capacity in monocytes, which is important in generating reactive oxygen species to fight and destroy pathogens in innate immune response, is significantly attenuated [14]. The production of some inflammatory cytokines in response to select stimuli appears to be affected in sepsis as well. Upon activation with LPS, (a component of bacterial endotoxin that can induce a strong immune response in most eukaryotic species) monocytes appear to have a diminished capacity to release TNF, IL-1α, IL-1β, and IL-6 [14]. However, such production of inflammatory cytokines appears to be unchanged or even enhanced when other stimuli are used or when other cytokines are examined. There is no global decrease in the release of cytokines in sepsis, but rather a specific alteration of cytokine production in response to specific stimuli takes place. Thus, the term "reprogrammation" of monocytes in sepsis may be appropriate [15, 16].

Dendritic Cells

Dendritic cells (DCs) are potent antigen-presenting cells that have been recently found to participate in innate immune response. These cells mostly arise from the bone marrow, but are found in nearly every tissue in the body where they come in contact with invading pathogens. Based on their function and origin, they can be subcategorized into conventional dendritic cells, Langerhans cells, plasmacytoid dendritic cells, and monocyte-derived dendritic cells [17]. During the early phase of infection, immature DCs fight bacterial, viral, and fungal pathogens through secretion of TNF-α and reactive nitrogen intermediates [18]. As DCs functionally mature, they migrate into lymphoid organs to activate T and B lymphocytes to generate adaptive immune response [19]. DCs also stimulate natural killer cells (NKs) in secondary lymphoid organs through various cytokines, which results destruction and elimination of invading pathogens at the site of infection [20]. Therefore, DCs are becoming increasingly recognized as an important bridge between innate and adaptive immune responses. In sepsis, several important alterations to this molecular architecture can result. There is increased apoptosis of both immature and mature DCs. T cell activation and release of certain cytokines by DCs are also impaired, potentially leading to the development of immune suppression in sepsis [21].

Neutrophils

Neutrophils are the most common type of circulating leukocytes in mammals, and they are a key component of innate immune response. Neutrophils arise from myeloid precursor cells in the bone marrow, and are released into the systemic circulation with a short lifespan of 24–48 h. Severe infection or inflammatory response can result in release of immature neutrophils, such as band cells, meta-myelocytes, and myelocytes, from the bone marrow, resulting in an increased number of immature cells in the peripheral blood. This phenomenon is known as the "left shift." Like macrophages, neutrophils can recognize invading pathogens through receptors on their surface and eliminate them through phagocytosis. Neutrophils are also characterized by the presence of cytoplasmic granules that are abundant in proteases and oxidative enzymes. This allows them to penetrate cellular structures and destroy invading microorganisms effectively. These granules can be subdivided into primary, secondary, and tertiary granules (or C particles). Primary granules contain acid hydrolase, myeloperoxidase, elastase, lysozyme, and cathepsins. Secondary granules contain collagenase, alkaline phosphatase, and lactoferin. Tertiary granules contain gelatinase and cathepsins. Once pathogens are phagocytosed by neutrophils, they are secluded in a cytoplasmic vesicle called a phagolysosome, where degradation of the phagocytosed particle occurs through fusion with these cytoplasmic granules. This entire process is enhanced by a variety of cytokines, including TNF-α, IL-1, IL-6, and IL-8, which are implicated in "priming" neutrophils for increased efficacy [22]. The neutrophils' short lifespan outside of the bone marrow is critically important in maintaining a balance between their effectiveness in fighting pathogens and their potential to cause damage to surrounding tissue [23]. The generation of reactive oxygen species and release of proteases from the granules have significant cytotoxic effects and often cause damage to vascular endothelial cells as well as parenchymal cells [24]. In the absence of inflammatory stimuli, however, neutrophils undergo constitutive apoptosis (or programmed cell death). Apoptotic neutrophils have impaired ability to migrate to the site of inflammation and dispense granules to eliminate invading pathogens [25]. This delicate balance between destruction of microorganism and its control through apoptosis is disrupted in sepsis. Neutrophils isolated from septic animal models and patients have been shown to not only display reduced capacity to migrate to the site of inflammation, but also have prolonged survival through delayed apoptosis, potentially contributing to tissue injury and organ dysfunction in sepsis [26, 27].

Natural Killer Cells

Natural killer (NK) cells are another type of granular lymphocytes that have an important role in cell-mediated, cytotoxic innate immunity. These cells arise from common thymic lymphoid progenitor cells and express PRRs and/or a NK-cell receptor complex on their surface that can recognize only a select conserved motif on the surface of a variety of pathogens, including bacteria, viruses as well as certain types of tumor cells. NK cells do not carry antigen-specific recognition molecules, like the T-cell receptor complex of the classical alpha-beta CD4$^+$/CD8$^+$ T cell, on their surface, making them part of the innate immunity system. They are characterized by the presence of cytoplasmic granules containing lytic enzymes, called granzymes, and perforin, which forms pores in the cellular membrane allowing the granzymes to enter the target cells they can kill. This process ultimately leads to apoptosis. Such cytotoxic mechanisms are crucial in fighting off pathogens early in the course of host cell infection, before adaptive immune responses typically develop. NK cells are also an important source of circulating cytokines, such as interferon-γ, IL-12, and IL-6, and are implicated in septic shock [28]. Increased cytotoxic activity has been correlated with severe organ dysfunction and poor outcome in severe sepsis and septic shock [29].

Other Innate Regulatory Cells

Gamma-delta (γδ) T cells are a special subpopulation of T lymphocytes that develop under the influence of other leukocytes in the thymus and in the periphery. Unlike other T lymphocytes that contain TCRs comprised of alpha (α) and beta (β) chains on their surface, γδ T cells, as their name suggests, have TCRs with one γ chain and one δ chain. γδ T cells interact with B cells to develop immunologic memory through TCRs as part of adaptive immunity. However, these cells often do not require formal antigen presentation and processing, and are capable of rapidly responding to a select group of antigens via their PPRs. Thus, γδ T cells are becoming increasingly recognized as an important cellular component of the innate immunity system as well.

Natural killer T (NKT) cells have the properties of both NK cells and T lymphocytes. Unlike other T lymphocytes that express TCRs with variable α and β chains, the majority of NKT cells express TCRs that are extremely limited in diversity. Therefore, these cells are often referred to as invariant NKT (iNKT) cells. NKT cells recognize and respond to cells that contain lipid and glycolipid antigens presented by the MHC I-like molecule named CD1d. NKT cells are activated nonspecifically by cytokines and soluble mediators, and they are often capable of responding to antigens that are ignored by conventional αβ T cells. Therefore, NKT cells are described to straddle the border between innate and adaptive immunity. Upon activation, NKT cells produce both pro- and anti-inflammatory cytokines. In sepsis, NKT cells appear to play a role in controlling immune response with their unique ability to interact with components of the innate and the adaptive immune responses [30].

CD4⁺/CD8⁺ T and B Lymphocyte Cells

B and T lymphocytes comprise approximately 2% of the peripheral blood cells; the vast majority of lymphocytes are localized in hematopoietic tissue and lymphatics. T progenitor cells are derived in the bone marrow, then migrate to the thymus and once maturation occurs are released as mature T cells. Naïve T cells are those located in bone marrow or thymus, once mature T cells are activated through antigen presentation they become effector T cells. CD4⁺ or helper T cells are neither cytotoxic nor phagocytitic, rather they modulate the immune response. CD4⁺ T cells become activated when they encounter a cognate antigen in the context of MHC-II stimulating cytokine release from the CD4⁺ T cell. Antigen presentation can induce two subtypes of immune responses from the CD4⁺ T helper cell. Th-1 type response is generally stimulated by intracellular pathogens like virus and intracellular bacteria. It is defined by interferon-gamma production, which induces macrophages and stimulates B cells to generate oposin and complement (cell-mediated immunity). A Th-2 response is defined by IL-4 production which activates B cells to make neutralizing antibodies (humoral immunity). A Th-2 type response generally occurs with extracellular bacteria, parasites, and toxin.

When intracellular bacteria or viruses replicate in a host cell, the host degrades (processes) the pathogen and displays various protein epitopes in MHC-I. Naïve CD8⁺ T lymphocytes are activated through this process, differentiate and clonally expand. These clones travel systemically to localize to cells in distal tissue sites displaying MHC-I with that same protein epitope. When the protein epitope is encountered, the cytotoxic CD8$^+$ T lymphocytes release perforin and granulysin to create pores in the host cell and induce apoptosis of the infected host cell. This process must be tightly regulated to minimize bystander tissue damage. With the clearance of the infected/target "nonself" antigen$^+$-MHC-I$^+$ cells, most of the effector CD8$^+$ T cells are then cleared by phagocytosis. However, memory of the event is maintained by a few CD8$^+$ that are selectively retained.

B lymphocytes produce antibody or immunoglobulin. Immunoglobulin is a large protein which can be membrane bound or free in circulation which recognizes, binds, and neutralizes antigen. B cells have a B cell receptor, this receptor is limited to recognizing only one antigen. Once the B cell receptor encounters its antigen, the B cell differentiates into a plasma cell that secretes large amounts of immunoglobulin (antigen specific), which in turn binds the antigen, flagging a cell for phagocytosis by macrophages and/or the binding of complement.

Alterations in Sepsis

In sepsis, there is rapid decrease in the circulating lymphocyte population. The magnitude and persistence of lymphopenia correlates with risk of developing nosocomial infection and mortality. Loss of B cells, CD4$^+$ T cells, and dendritic cells has been observed in nonsurvivors of sepsis [31]. Sepsis is also associated with the development of a state of lymphoid anergy, where less interferon-gamma production, as well as, IL-2 and TNF-α production is evident in response to standard lymphoid T-cell receptor-mediated stimuli. Greater anergy correlates with poorer septic outcome. It as also been posited that the shift away from Th-1 response limits the effective host antimicrobial response to infection and hampers bacterial clearance, thus, resulting in persistence of infection [32, 33]. T regulatory cells are a novel subset of CD4$^+$ and CD8$^+$ T cells that exhibit an active suppressive phenotype. They negatively regulate the innate and adaptive immune response. Sepsis is associated with an increased numbers/survival of T-regulatory cells in the peripheral blood and spleen of septic patients/animals. It is unclear if this is protective or deleterious to septic morbidity or mortality.

Inflammatory Cytokines and Chemokines

During the all stages of sepsis, the innate immune system releases large amounts of cytokines, chemokines, complement activation products, coagulation factors, lipid molecules, reactive oxygen species, reactive nitrogen species, antimicrobial peptides, and intracellular defensins, which not only serve to regulate/activate the immune response but also, in systemic excess, serve to drive the "cytokine storm" involved in sepsis. The adaptive immune response is then induced upon interaction with APCs which have ingested the foreign pathogen. These cells then proliferate to generate effectors cells which themselves release certain cytokines [34]. Cytokines and chemokines are small proteins of substantial importance in tissue immunity.

TNF-α and IL-1

After being triggered by a stimulus (i.e., PAMPs and/or DAMPs), macrophages release a number of early proinflammatory mediators including TNF-α, IL-1, IL-6, Interferon-gamma (INF-gamma), IL-8, and monocyte chemotactic protein (MCP-1). Two important pro-inflammatory cytokines produced during the initial and early phase of the septic inflammatory response are TNF-α and IL-1. These cytokines target a broad range of cells including all leukocytes, endothelial cells, epithelial cells, and organ-specific cells such as hepatocytes and fibroblasts. As a result, these cells produce other pro-inflammatory mediators including (1) cytokines (IFN-γ, IL-6, IL-8, IL-12, IL-17, and macrophage migration inhibitory factor (MIF)); (2) chemokines (IL-8, macrophage inflammatory protein (MIP-1, -2), macrophage chemokine protein, thymus activation-regulated chemokine (TARC)); (3) oxidative markers (ROSs, RNSs, and eicosanoids); and (4) proteolytic enzymes [35].

MIF and HMGB-1

Migration Inhibitory Factor (MIF) and High Mobility Group Box (HMGB)-1 are thought to be two central cytokines in critical illness induced by SIRS and sepsis. MIF is a special regulatory cytokine with a unique protein structure and its receptor is distinct from other cytokine receptor families. It is expressed constitutively and stored in intracellular pools. Therefore, it does not require de novo synthesis before secretion. It is produced in a wide spectrum of cells including DCs, monocytes, macrophages, lymphocytes, neutrophils, eosinophils, basophils, mast cells, all non-immune mucosal cell types that are in direct contact with the external environment, and the skin. MIF is also produced in high levels in tissues involved in the stress responses including the hypothalamus-pituitary-adrenal axis [36]. MIF acts as a stress response mediator and pro-inflammatory cytokine upon induction by glucocorticoids, which are produced at high levels in sepsis. MIF sustains the inflammatory response by delaying the removal of activated monocytes/macrophages by apoptosis. This prolongs production of cytokines, nitric oxide (NO), matrix metalloproteinases (MMPs), and prostaglandins (PGs) [4]. HMGB-1 is a non-histone nuclear DNA binding protein which regulates nucleosome structure and gene transcription. It has also recently been identified as a DAMP/alarmin involved as a late mediator in inflammatory sepsis. In sepsis, HMGB-1 is released in large quantities into the extracellular environment, which allows it to act as a mediator of systemic inflammation [4]. It induces DC maturation and migration of immune cells to the site of injury as well as their release of cytokines and other inflammatory mediators.

HMGB-1 also has pro-inflammatory effects on the endothelium, is involved in tissue repair and regeneration, and stimulates angiogenesis [35]. HMGB-1 plasma levels in intensive care patients correlated with the disseminated intravascular coagulation (DIC) score and sepsis-induced multiple organ failure (MOF) [23]. Higher levels of HMGB-1 in plasma have been found in nonsurvivable septic patients [35]. The number of endogenous host cell molecules that serve as endogenous DAMPs and alarmins is growing rapidly. Some other examples include uric acid, hyaluran, heat shock protein (HSP) family members, fibrinogen, fibronectin, and certain endogenous lipids [23].

Future Diagnostic Inflammatory Markers

The use of cytokines as inflammatory markers capable of predicting outcomes in septic patients is still under research/debate and has been difficult as these are shared with a variety of other inflammatory conditions/diseases. Some of the possible candidates are listed below.

Interleukin-6 is a pro inflammatory cytokine produced by lymphocytes, fibroblasts, and monocytes. IL-6 has a variety of broad effects including activation of B and T lymphocytes, proliferative effects and induction of acute phase proteins produced in the liver. It has been suggested that IL-6 concentrations in sepsis is the best marker of the severity and outcome for sepsis [37].

IL-8 is a CXC chemokine that is produced by mononuclear phagocytes, neutrophils, lymphocytes, endothelial cells, epithelial cells and a variety of mesothelial cell types in response to endotoxin, IL-1β, and TNF-α during sepsis. IL-8 chemoattracts and activates neutrophils to the site of tissue damage and inflammation. Neutrophils respond by changing shape, adhering to endothelial cells, and increasing production of ROSs. In septic patients, the plasma concentration on IL-8 has been reported to peak at 3–4 h after the initial diagnosis of severe septic shock and the concentrations of circulating IL-8 appear to correlate with worse outcomes [23].

IL-17A is pro inflammatory cytokine that is produced by Th17 cells (which we briefly mentioned earlier), neutrophils, CD8+ T cells, NK cells, and other T helper and T cell subtypes during sepsis. IL-17A can trigger the production of many cytokines including IL-1β, IL-6 and TNF-α which provides cross talk between lymphocytes and phagocytes. It has been shown the increased IL-17A levels have adverse effects during experimental sepsis and that neutralization of IL-17A markedly improves survival in animals [34].

IL-7 is a hematopoietic growth factor that has recently been shown to have a role in lymphocyte survival and expansion during sepsis. IL-7 is produced by stromal cells in lymphoid tissues. It induces a T cell survival signal through the IL-7R receptor. IL-7 also induces proliferation of naïve CD4+ and CD8+ T cells. It is currently being studied in clinical trials to boost immune effector cell functions in immune-deficient patients [34].

One study found that increased plasma concentrations of pro-inflammatory (IL-6, TNF-α, IL-1β, KC, MIP-2, MCP-1 and eotaxin) and anti-inflammatory (TNF soluble receptors, IL-10, IL-1 receptor antagonist [IL-1RA]) cytokines were observed in early deaths (days 1–5) of septic patients. They found that plasma levels of IL-6, TNF-α, KC, MIP-2, IL-1RA, TNF soluble receptor I and TNF soluble receptor II accurately predicted mortality within 24 h. In contrast, these parameters were not elevated in either the late deaths or survivors. This study suggests that initial inflammatory response correlates to early but not late septic mortality [38].

Anti-Inflammatory Cytokines

During the course of sepsis an anti-inflammatory response develops. This response is made up of anti-inflammatory cytokines and mediators such as IL-10, IL-4, IL-6, IL-13, P10, P75, P55, transforming growth factor-β (TGF-β), IL-1RA, soluble TNF receptors, soluble interleukin receptors (sIL-Rs), glucocorticoids, and eicosanoids. These mediators are released from T regulatory cells, macrophages and PMNs among other cells. Several anti-inflammatory cytokines; however, have both pro- and anti-inflammatory properties depending on the nature of the danger signals, the nature of the target cells and the timing of the exposure. In addition, some pro-inflammatory cytokines may exert anti-inflammatory properties depending on the cell:cell context and/or concentration of the cytokine [35].

IL-10

IL-10 is a potent anti-inflammatory cytokine released during sepsis. It is produced by activated T helper 2 CD4+cells, T regulatory cells, B cells, monocytes, and several other cell types. IL-10 can upregulate other regulatory molecules and/or receptors as well including IL-1RA, CD32, and chemokine receptor 1 (CCR1) and CCR4. During sepsis the expression of IL-10 is prolonged and sustained. Elevations of blood monoctyes IL-10 mRNA expression or plasma IL-10 levels may be of prognostic significance as high IL-10 expression has been found to be associated with worse outcomes in pediatric patients with sepsis [23].

Chemotactic Cytokines

Certain chemotactic cytokines (chemokines) have also been linked to impaired leukocyte responsiveness during sepsis, especially members of the CC chemokine family. In addition to IL-8 discussed earlier; TARC (CCL17) and the macrophage-derived chemokine (MDC/CCL22) are reported to be expressed in high concentrations by alternatively activated macrophages (cells activated by IL-4 and IL-13) and, thus, serve as markers of this alternatively activated phenotype in macrophages [23]. It has also been shown that decreased expression of key activating chemokine receptors by various leukocyte subpopulations in sepsis may lead to impaired chemokine responsiveness in these cells [39].

Complement and Coagulation Cascades

The inflammatory reaction in sepsis activates the complement and coagulation systems which in turn promote inflammation. Complement may be activated through three distinct routes (the classical, lectin and alternative pathways) which all converge at the level of C3 [35]. Complement acts as both a pathogen recognition receptor and an effector. The inflammatory properties of complement during sepsis are divided into three categories: (1) opsonization; which contributes to phagocytosis and subsequent killing of the pathogens via the membrane attack complex; (2) promotion and expansion of the inflammatory cascade; and (3) coordination of inflammatory events by the anaphylatoxins (C3a and C5a). C3a and C5a are anaphylatoxins generated by activation of all three complement pathways. They serve to enhance vascular permeability, smooth muscle contraction and serve as chemo-attractants for leukocytes [35]. The terminal C5b-9 complement complex forms the membrane attack complex (MAC) which is capable of creating a physical pore in the pathogen membrane causing leakage and cell death [35].

Coagulation can be activated by two pathways: the Factor XII-dependent intrinsic pathway and the Tissue Factor (TF)-dependent, extrinsic pathway. These converge at factor X and ultimately result in thrombin formation. The release of thrombin amplifies the production of more pro-inflammatory mediators. Thrombin can cleave C3 and C5 of the complement cascade. C5a, in turn, can amplify the expression of TF. Binding of other coagulation proteases to protease-activated receptors (PARs) is an important mechanism in the modulation of inflammation by coagulation. For example, binding of thrombin and TF-Factor VIIa complex to their respective PARs enhances production of pro-inflammatory cytokines. In addition, TF is also produced directly in response to pro-inflammatory cytokine activation by endothelial and mononuclear cells [23, 35].

The function of the three anticoagulant pathways that prevent systemic activation of coagulation in normal conditions (anti-thrombin, activated protein C, and Tissue factor pathway inhibitor) are impaired during sepsis leading to clinical DIC and severe inflammation [4].

Antimicrobial Peptides

Antimicrobial peptides are defined as ribosomal-derived proteins that have microcidal activity. In sepsis, the cytokines produced by local innate immune cells (macrophages and dendritic cells) can induce the local production of antimicrobial products which are thought to be important in providing host defense at mucosal/epithelial surfaces. Anti-microbial products defend against extracellular bacteria through permeabilization of the bacterial membrane, opsonization, chemokine function, and modulation of cytokine production. Anti-microbial products are also thought to be involved in pathogen recognition, inflammation, pathogen clearance, and resolution of inflammation during sepsis [35].

In humans, two major classes of antimicrobial peptides, defensins and cathelicidin, have been described. HCAP-18/LL-37, the only endogenous human cathelicidin-18 identified, is a major protein of the specific granules in neutrophils. It is also found in monocytes, keratinocytes, and airway epithelia. Defensins make up 30–50% of the granule proteins in human neutrophils and can structurally be defined as α- or β-defensins. Alpha-defensins are mainly produced by neutrophils and intestinal paneth cells whereas β-defensins are primarily expressed by epithelial cells of the skin, urinary tract and tracheobronchial lining. There is constitutive production of β-defensins at sites such as epithelial tissues that are steadily exposed to potentially infectious microbes. Secretion is induced by the contact of cells with microbes and pro-inflammatory mediators [23]. Other defensins include c type lectins, S100 proteins, elastase inhibitors, and regenerating proteins [35].

Lipid Mediators

Adipose tissue has been found to secrete a variety of bioactive substances, adipo-cytokines, which exert protective roles in different organs during the septic inflammatory response. Adiponectine, an adipo-cytokine, has a strong ability to exert several anti-inflammatory responses in macrophages and endothelial cells. It has been shown to inhibit macrophage LPS-induced production of TNF-α, to inhibit HMGB1, and to induce various anti-inflammatory cytokines such as IL-10R and IL-1R antagonists. Visfatin, a pre B cell colony enhancing factor, has been shown to activate human leukocytes to release IL-1β, TNF-β and IL-6 as well as to increase the surface expression of co stimulatory molecules via MAPK pathways [34].

In sepsis, high density lipoprotein (HDL), low density lipoprotein (LDL), and very low density lipoprotein (VLDL) can bind and neutralize the bioactivity of bacterial components such as lipolysaccharide (LPS) and lipoteichoic acid (LTA). During sepsis circulating levels of HDL decline resulting in elevated circulating LPS levels. Native HDL can suppress the inhibitory activity of LPS binding protein (LBP) which may contribute to its pro-inflammatory property by enhancing monocyte responses to LPS [36].

Sphingosine-1 Phosphate (S1P) is a bioactive sphingolipid metabolite that regulates diverse cellular processes, including cell growth, cellular differentiation, lymphocyte trafficking, vascular integrity, and pro inflammatory cytokine production. S1P is formed by phosphorylation of sphingosin in a reaction catalyzed by two isoforms of sphogosine kinase (Sphk1 and Sphk2). Sphk1 is activated by numerous stimuli including LPS and pro-inflammatory cytokines. In sepsis, the pro-inflammatory cytokines promote the formation of S1P, which in turn activates lymphocytes and promotes further cytokine release [34].

Prostanoids and Leukotriene

Prostanoids are a subclass of eicosanoids consisting of the prostaglandins (e.g. PGE2), the thromboxanes (thromboxane A2) and the prostacyclins (PGI2) which have been proven to play a role in the inflammatory reaction in sepsis. Prostaglandins play an active role in inflammation and anaphylactic reactions. Thromboxanes play a role in platelet aggregation and vasoconstriction and prostacyclins play a role in platelet anti-aggregation and vasodilatation. Leukotrienes (LTB4), also a subclass of eicosanoids, serve has inflammatory mediators produced in leukocytes. Leukotrienes use lipid signaling to regulate the immune response. Both leukotrienes and prostanoids are arachidonic metabolites and have been proven to participate in the pathophysiology of shock. It is thought that the circulatory dysfunction associated with shock is a result of unfavorable balance of arachidonic acid metabolites. Prophylactic and post-treatment regimes of nonsteroidal anti-inflammatory agents that block all arachidonic acid cyclo-oxygenation products have been shown to improve survival of and circulatory function in experimental setting of endotoxic shock [40].

Reactive Oxygen Species (ROSs), Reactive Nitrogen Species (RNSs), and Nitric Oxide (NO)

ROSs and RNSs are pivotal to the defense against invading pathogens during sepsis by performing intracellular signaling for several cytokines and growth factors, acting as second messenger for hormones, serving in redox regulation, and participating in intracellular killing of bacterial pathogens in phagocytosis. ROS and RNS also participate in modulation of ion channels, kinases, membrane receptors, apoptosis, transcription factors, and gene expression [36]. Overwhelming production of ROSs and RNSs results in oxidative and nitrosative stress, respectively, key elements in the deleterious process of experimental sepsis. Neutrophils are the major source of ROS and RNS. ROS and RNS are produced via the membrane bound enzyme complex nicotinamide adenine dinucleotide phosphate (NADPH) oxidase. Pro-inflammatory mediators, immune complexes, and bacteria can activate NADPH oxidase to produce ROS and RNS. Excess generation of ROSs and RNSs, in combination with depleted levels of reduced glutathione, an important intramitochondrial antioxidant, have been found to inhibit adenosine triphosphate (ATP) generation. Myeloperoxidases, from neutrophil azurophilic granules, produce hypochlorous acid from hydrogen peroxide and chloride anions. These superoxide free radicals are highly cytotoxic and neutrophils use them to damage and destroy pathogens. During experimental sepsis, superoxide radicals and NO generate peroxynitrite, which causes DNA strand breakage and initiate lipid peroxidation changing the functions of the ion channels, cell signaling proteins, receptors, enzymes, and transcription factors [4, 23].

NO is produced as a pro-inflammatory mediator in response to inflammatory stimuli by a number of cells. NO maintains normal homeostasis by reducing leukocyte adhesion, platelet aggregation, relaxation of vascular smooth muscle and preservation of mucosal integrity. During experimental sepsis, NO is released at high concentrations causing vasodilation, increases in vascular permeability and inhibition of mitochondrial respiration which leads to decreased ATP synthesis and cellular apoptosis [23].

Immune Resolution of Sepsis

After tissue insult by pathogen or tissue damage, the pro-inflammatory state is upregulated. However, for wound healing and recovery to commence the initial pro-inflammatory state must be turned off or downregulated. Downregulation or anti-inflammatory mechanisms of the immune system results in the arrest, quiescence, or cell death by apoptosis of immune cells. Initially, dissipation of inflammatory signals begins the process of downregulation. As pathogen, microbes and necrotic cell debris is removed less inflammatory signal exists. The complement and coagulation cascade are activated by injury and infection. As injury and infection resolve there is lack of danger signals from these cascades decreases immune cell activation.

Active suppression by release of anti-inflammatory mediators also decreases immune cell activation. Some anti-inflammatory mediators are glucocorticoids, catecholamines, prostaglandin-E, nitric oxide, cytokines (IL-1, IL-4, IL-10, IL-13), and TGF-β. These anti-inflammatory mediators act as competitive antagonist of pro-inflammatory ligand and downregulate activating signal transduction. Anti-inflammatory cytokines and TGF-β also actively suppress phagocytic cells and lymphocytes. Once an immune response has been ongoing there is a Th-1 to Th-2 shift in T lymphocyte phenotype. CD4$^+$ and CD8$^+$ T suppressor cells become activated suppressing the immune cell response. Dendritic cells also have immune suppressive functions. Monocytes transition to a late response with a transition to an anti-inflammatory phenotype and produce anti-inflammatory cytokines IL-6, IL-1, IL-10 and PGE$_2$. Activation of co-inhibitory receptors can also block activating signals, leading to T lymphocyte anergy and immune suppression/tolerance. Finally, immune cell response is resolved by induction of apoptosis [41] (Fig. 4.7).

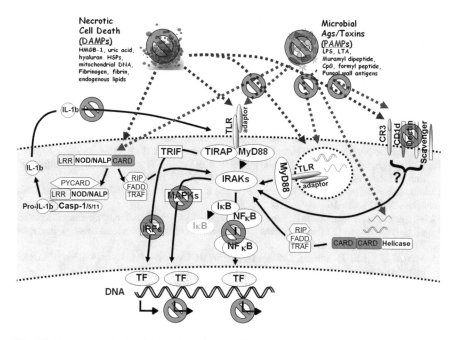

Fig. 4.7 Immune resolution. Molecular pathways affected during immune resolution are depicted in this diagram

Summary

In brief, we have generally (but not exhaustively) overviewed some of the salient immunological pathways/processes that are involved/recruited during the response to the diverse stimuli associated with the response severe injury and/or septic challenge. Hope here being that this provides a framework for understanding/considering the diverse nature of the therapeutic modalities that have been considered and will be proposed for the treatment of the critically ill injured/septic patient.

References

1. Angus DC, Linde-Zwirble WT, Lidicker J, Clermont G, Carcillo J, Pinsky MR. Epidemiology of severe sepsis in the United States: analysis of incidence, outcome, and associated costs of care. Crit Care Med. 2001;29:1303–10.
2. Martin GS, Mannino DM, Eaton S. The epidemiology of sepsis in the United States from 1979 through 2000. N Engl J Med. 2003;16:1546–54.
3. Van Ruler O, Schultz MJ, Reitsma JB. Has mortality from sepsis improved and what to expect from new treatment modalities: review of current insights. Surg Infect (Larchmt). 2009;10:339–48.
4. Cinel I, Opal SM. Molecular biology of inflammation and sepsis. Crit Care Med. 2009;37:291–304.

5. Ward NS, Casserly B, Ayala A. The compensatory anti-inflammatory response syndrome (CARS) in critically ill patients. Clin Chest Med. 2008;29:617–25.
6. Burnet FM. The clonal selection theory of acquired immunity. Nashville, TN: Vanderbilt University Press; 1959.
7. Matzinger P. The Danger Model: a renewed sense of self. Science. 2002;296:301–5.
8. Hemmi H, Akira S. Recognition of pathogen-associated molecular patterns by TLR family. Immunol Lett. 2003;85(2):85–95.
9. Matzinger P. Tolerance, danger, and the extended family. Annu Rev Immunol. 1994;12:991.
10. Matzinger P. Friendly and dangerous signals: is the tissue in control? Nat Immunol. 2007;8:11.
11. Perl M, Chung CS, Garber M, Huang X, Ayala A. Contribution of anti-inflammatory/immune suppressive processes to the pathology of sepsis. Front Biosci. 2006;11:272–99.
12. Mai J, Wang H, Yang XF. Th 17 cells interplay with Foxp3+ Tregs in regulation of inflammation and autoimmunity. Front Biosci. 2010;15:986–1006.
13. Marshall JC, Charbonney E, Gonzalez PD. The immune system in critical illness. Clin Chest Med. 2008;29:605–16.
14. Von Knethen A, Tautenhahn A, Link H, Lindemann D, Brune B. Activation-induced depletion of protein kinase C alpha provokes desensitization of monocytes/macrophages in sepsis. J Immunol. 2005;174:4960–5.
15. Muñoz C, Carlet J, Fitting C, Misset B, Bleriot JP, Cavaillon JM. Dysregulation of in vitro cytokine production by monocytes during sepsis. J Clin Invest. 1991;88:1747–54.
16. Adib-Conquy M, Cavaillon JM. Compensatory anti-inflammatory response syndrome. Thromb Haemost. 2009;101:36–47.
17. Mbongue J, Nicholas D, Firek A, Langridge W. The role of dendritic cells in tissue-specific autoimmunity. J Immunol Res. 2014;857143 doi:10.1155/2014/857143. Epub 2014 Apr 30
18. Serbina NV, Salazar-Mather TP, Biron CA, Kuziel WA, Pamer EG. TNF/iNOS-producing dendritic cells mediate innate immune defense against bacterial infection. Immunity. 2003;19:59–70.
19. Banchereau J, Steinman RM. Dendritic cells and the control of immunity. Nature. 1998;392:245–52.
20. Barreira da Silva R, Münz C. Natural killer cell activation by dendritic cells: balancing inhibitory and activating signals. Cell Mol Life Sci. 2011;68:3505–18.
21. Huang X, Venet F, Chung CS, Lomas-Neira J, Ayala A. Changes in dendritic cell function in the immune response to sepsis. Cell- & tissue-based therapy. Expert Opin Biol Ther. 2007;7:929–38.
22. Klebanoff SJ, Vadas MA, Harlan JM, Sparks LH, Gamble JR, Agosti JM, et al. Stimulation of neutrophils by tumor necrosis factor. J Immunol. 1986;136:4220–5.
23. Thakkar RK, Huang X, Lomas-Neira J, Heffernan D, Ayala A. Sepsis and the immune response. In: Essential immunology for surgeons. Oxford, UK: Oxford University Press; 2011. p. 303–42.
24. Jaeschke H, Smith CW. Mechanisms of neutrophil-induced parenchymal cell injury. J Leukoc Biol. 1997;61:647–53.
25. Luo HR, Loison F. Constitutive neutrophil apoptosis: mechanisms and regulation. Am J Hematol. 2007;83:288–95.
26. Alves-Filho JC, de Freitas A, Spiller F, Souto FO, Cunha FQ. The role of neutrophils in severe sepsis. Shock 2008;Suppl 1;3–9.
27. Jimenez MF, Watson RW, Parodo J, Evans D, Foster D, Steinberg M, et al. Dysregulated expression of neutrophil apoptosis in the systemic inflammatory response syndrome. Arch Surg. 1997;132:1263–70.
28. Goldmann O, Chhatwal GS, Medina E. Contribution of natural killer cells to the pathogenesis of septic shock induced by Streptococcus pyogenes in mice. J Infect Dis. 2005;191:1280–6.
29. Zeerleder S, Hack CE, Caliezi C, van Mierlo G, Eerenberg-Belmer A, Wolbink A, et al. Activated cytotoxic T cells and NK cells in severe sepsis and septic shock and their role in multiple organ dysfunction. Clin Immunol. 2005;116:158–65.
30. Venet F, Chung CS, Monneret G, Huang X, Horner B, Garber M, et al. Regulatory T cell populations in sepsis and trauma. J Leukoc Biol. 2007;83:523–35.

31. Hotchkiss RS, Tinsley KW, Swanson PE, Schmieg Jr RE, Hui JJ, Chang KC, et al. Sepsis-induced apoptosis causes progressive profound depletion of B and CD4+ T lymphocytes in humans. J Immunol. 2001;166:6952–63.
32. Ledere JA, Rodrick ML, Mannick JA. The effects of injury on the adaptive immune response. Shock. 1999;11:153–9.
33. Ayala A, Deol ZK, Lehman DL, Herdon CD, Herdon CD, Chaudry IH. Polymicrobial sepsis but not low dose endotoxin infusion causes decreased splenocyte IL-2/IFN-gamma release while increasing IL-4/IL-10 production. J Surg Res. 1994;56:579–85.
34. Aziz M, Jacob A, Yang WL, Matsuda A, Wang P. Current trends in inflammatory and immuno-modulatory mediators in sepsis. J Leukoc Biol. 2013;93:329–42.
35. Castellheim A, Brekke OL, Espevik T, Harboe M, Mollnes TE. Innate immune responses to danger signals in systemic inflammatory response syndrome and sepsis. Scand J Immunol. 2009;69:479–91.
36. Adib-Conquy M, Cavaillon JM. Stress molecules in sepsis and systemic inflammatory response syndrome. FEBS. 2007;581:3723–33.
37. Spittler A, Razenberger M, Kupper H, et al. Relationship between interleukin-6 plasma concentration in patients with sepsis, monocyte phenotype, monocyte phagocytic properties, and cytokine production. Clin Infect Dis. 2000;31:1338–42.
38. Osuchowski MF, Welch K, Siddiqui J, Kaul M, Hackl W, Boltz-Nitulescu G, et al. Circulating cytokine/inhibitor profiles reshape the understanding of the SIRS/CARS continuum in sepsis and predict mortality. J Immunol. 2006;177:1967–74.
39. Cummings CJ, Martin TR, Frevert CW, Quan JM, Wong VA, Mongovin SM, et al. Expression and function of the chemokine receptors CXCR1 and CXCR2 in sepsis. J Immunol. 1999;162:2341.
40. Cooke JA, Wise WC, Butler RR, Reines HD, Rambo W, Halushka PV. The potential role of thromboxane and prostacyclin in endotoxic and septic shock. Am J Emerg Med. 1982;2:28–37.
41. Ayala A, Chung C, Grutkoski P, Song GY. Mechanisms of immune resolution. Crit Care Med. 2003;31(8):S558–71.

Chapter 5
Sepsis-Induced Immune Suppression

Nicholas Csikesz and Nicholas S. Ward

Introduction

Newton's third law is commonly quoted as "for every action, there is an equal and opposite reaction." This concept was largely ignored in the initial theories regarding the body's response to overwhelming infection, which was characterized as a surge of inflammation that arises to eliminate invading pathogens, and may injure the host organism along with it. This leads to the concept that it may be possible to ameliorate the organ damage in sepsis by reining in this unmitigated inflammatory response. Indeed, many early preclinical studies showed some initial promise in mitigating sepsis mortality in animals by limiting the pro-inflammatory response. However, a large number of clinical trials in humans of a variety of anti-inflammatory therapies failed to demonstrate any improvement in the high mortality associated with sepsis [1].

In 1996, Roger Bone invoked Isaac Newton in a landmark editorial discussing possible explanations for the failure of anti-inflammatory therapies in sepsis [2]. Bone and others recognized that there was a growing body of evidence demonstrating immunosuppression following other forms of inflammation such as surgery or trauma. He reviewed the existing evidence showing that the immune response to sepsis is not nearly as straightforward as was originally held. In addition to the pro-inflammatory response to sepsis, there is a concomitant anti-inflammatory response. He postulated that the balance between these two intertwined responses largely

N. Csikesz (✉)
Alpert Medical School of Brown University, Rhode Island Hospital,
593 Eddy Street, Providence, RI 02903, USA
e-mail: ncsikesz@lifespan.org

N.S. Ward
Division of Pulmonary, Critical Care, and Sleep Medicine, Alpert/Brown Medical School,
Providence, RI, USA
e-mail: nward@lifespan.org

© Springer International Publishing AG 2017
N.S. Ward, M.M. Levy (eds.), *Sepsis*, Respiratory Medicine,
DOI 10.1007/978-3-319-48470-9_5

determines the outcome in sepsis and coined the term "Compensatory Anti-inflammatory Response Syndrome" (CARS) to describe the anti-inflammatory response.

Thus was created a more nuanced view of sepsis as a pathologic dysregulation of the immune system with both pro- and anti-inflammatory effects. Bone hypothesized that overwhelming infection disrupts the body's normal homeostasis such that at different points within the time course of infection pro-inflammatory or anti-inflammatory forces may predominate, either of which can be pathologic and contribute to mortality. The most straightforward theory resulting from these ideas holds that the early course of sepsis is characterized by the traditional pro-inflammatory response, with capillary leak, organ dysfunction, and (if left unchecked) death. This is then followed by a period of immune suppression during which the body is susceptible to secondary infections (and subsequent death) before returning to homeostasis. The relative strength of the pro- and anti-inflammatory responses likely depends on the host and the pathogen, as well as on external interventions (i.e., medical care), resulting in multiple potential immunologic responses.

Two terms critical to the discussion of this topic are immunosuppression and immunoparalysis. For the purposes of this chapter, immunosuppression should be considered to be the active anti-inflammatory responses (such as increased secretion of anti-inflammatory cytokines, and increases in immune suppressor cell populations). Immunoparalysis should be considered the loss of any discernible function that occurs in some cell populations in this process, i.e., anergy. There is now overwhelming evidence demonstrating the clinical importance of sepsis-induced immune suppression along with the general idea of an initial pro-inflammatory state giving way to a later anti-inflammatory state. Almost 2/3 of deaths due to sepsis occur after hospital day 5, during a phase marked by an increase in the percentage of positive cultures due to normally nonpathogenic organisms [3]. Critically ill patients have also been shown to have high rates of reactivation of dormant viruses such as cytomegalovirus (CMV) and herpes simplex virus (HSV) [4, 5]. This chapter will review the current understanding of sepsis-induced immune suppression.

Cytokines in Sepsis-Induced Immune Suppression

Cytokines play a significant role in mediating the immune response of the body. While specific pathways of activation of individual cytokines are nuanced, many can be generally labeled as either pro-inflammatory or anti-inflammatory. Some well characterized pro-inflammatory cytokines include interleukin 1 (IL-1), IL-6, IL-12, tumor necrosis factor α (TNFα), and interferon γ (IFNγ). Anti-inflammatory cytokines include IL-4, IL-10, and transforming growth factor β (TGFβ) although these cytokines can have proinflammatory effects in other conditions [6, 7]. Both pro- and anti-inflammatory cytokine production is stimulated early on in response to infection.

An illustrative study demonstrating this was done by Novotny et al. [8]. Measurements of IL-6 and IL-10 were taken from human patients with postoperative sepsis as well as in a murine model of septic peritonitis. The initial immune response in both study populations was characterized by concomitant increases in IL-6 and IL-10. Further, the relationship was exponential such that a linear increase in the pro-inflammatory cytokine IL-6 correlated with an exponential increase in the anti-inflammatory cytokine IL-10. This suggests that the body engages in an immediate attempt to rein in the pro-inflammatory response that is unleashed in response to infection.

IL-10 is currently thought to be the most important of the anti-inflammatory cytokines [6]. It was first characterized around 1990 when it was shown to regulate T-cell populations [9, 10]. It has now been established that IL-10 has multiple immunosuppressive roles, with most important being the downregulation of TNF [11]. In animal models of sepsis, the administration of IL-10 has been shown to have both positive [12–14] and negative [15, 16] effects on outcome, which likely depend on the time of administration and the severity of the infection. In one carefully done animal model, Ashare and colleagues [17] followed levels of pro-inflammatory and anti-inflammatory cytokines throughout the whole course of sepsis in mice. They found that bacterial levels in tissue correlated with IL-10 levels and that if the pro-inflammatory response was blocked by pretreatment with IL-1 receptor antagonist, bacterial levels were higher, as was mortality. Similarly, Song and colleagues [18] showed that blocking IL-10 activity early had no effect on mortality, whereas blocking it late (12 h) after sepsis improved mortality. This suggests that in the pro-inflammatory milieu of early sepsis, IL-10 does not have a major role, whereas in the later phase of disease when immunosuppression predominates, its effect is more pronounced.

The Role of Immune Cells in Sepsis-Induced Immunosuppression

Impaired Immune Cell Function and Programmed Cell Death in Sepsis

Activated by triggers such as antigens or inflammatory cytokines, immune cells speed the death and clearance of infectious organisms in sepsis. This immune protection comes at a cost however, as immune cell activity can lead to tissue and organ injury through the release of anti-infective products such as oxidants. As the sepsis inflammatory cascade develops, the body begins the process of inhibiting these immune cells through two processes, deactivation of immune cell function and apoptosis.

Some of the earliest studies in impaired immunity in states of inflammation noted impaired immune cell function manifest as anergy [19]. Later studies were able to characterize an array of immune cell dysfunction that accompanies severe inflammation (reviewed below). Cell death is a common process and can occur via two pathways, apoptosis or necrosis. Apoptosis, or programmed cell death, is a carefully regulated process by which the body can allow for cell turnover without inducing inflammation (as occurs with necrosis) [20]. Apoptosis of immune effector cells is an important mechanism by which the body regulates the intensity and duration of a pro-inflammatory state. Many animal and human studies in sepsis have shown extensive apoptosis of immune effector cells including B and CD4+ T lymphocytes, dendritic cells, and epithelial cells [21–24]. Additionally, the subsequent burden that clearing these apoptic cells plays on the remaining immune cells is thought to be a major contributor to immunoparalysis.

Neutrophils

Neutrophils play a critical role in the body's response to infection, so it is not surprising that they are intricately involved in the balance between pro- and anti-inflammatory pathways in sepsis [25]. In contrast to many other immune cells, the apoptosis of neutrophils is down-regulated in sepsis [26, 27]. This was shown by Tamayo et al. in a prospective observational study of 80 septic patients and 25 healthy controls [27]. The rates of neutrophil apoptosis were decreased at 24 h, 5 days, and 12 days after diagnosis of sepsis in comparison to controls. There was no difference seen between survivors and non-survivors of sepsis.

Additionally, immature neutrophils are released in a large number from the bone marrow, resulting in the neutrophilia with bandemia seen in many patients presenting with sepsis [28]. These immature neutrophils are immunologically active. This was shown in a prospective observational study by Drifte et al. [28]. Whole blood from 33 ICU patients with sepsis, 12 ICU patients with SIRS, and 32 healthy volunteers was taken and immune function was assessed in vitro. Immature neutrophils were able to engage in phagocytosis and bacterial killing via production of reactive oxygen species, although less efficiently than mature neutrophils. Interestingly, immature neutrophils exhibited a more pro-inflammatory state, as evidenced by an elevated TNF-alpha/IL-10 ratio. This is important as mature neutrophils have been shown to be involved in the anti-inflammatory response of sepsis via the production of IL-10 [29]. This balance between a pro-inflammatory and anti-inflammatory state in neutrophils has been shown to predict the development of secondary infections that are so often the actual cause of mortality in sepsis. Stephan et al. studied in vitro neutrophil function in patients with sepsis 4 days after they had been admitted [30]. They found that those patients who subsequently developed a nosocomial infection exhibited impaired phagocytosis and bacteriocidal killing at day 4.

Antigen Presenting Cells

Dendritic Cells

Antigen presenting phagocytes, including dendritic cells and macrophages, play a critical role in the immune response to infection [20, 31, 32]. Tinsley et al. investigated dendritic cell populations in a murine model of sepsis [24]. They found a rapid proliferation in follicular dendritic cells in the first 36 h after infection that was followed by extensive apoptosis, resulting in a net decrease in dendritic cell numbers by 48 h. Fujita et al. identified a subset of regulatory dendritic cells that activate anti-inflammatory pathways via the secretion of IL-10 [32]. Additional studies have also identified a shift in phenotype of dendritic cells toward an anti-inflammatory pathway in patients with sepsis-induced immunosuppression [33, 34]. These findings are in keeping with the model of sepsis as a balance between pro- and anti-inflammatory immune responses.

Multiple studies have examined the importance of dendritic cells to the immune response to sepsis. In a straightforward study, Guisset et al. measured peripheral blood dendritic cell counts in patients with sepsis [35]. They found that an early decrease in dendritic cell numbers correlated strongly with subsequent mortality and hypothesized that this may be a useful prognostic biomarker in septic patients. Toliver-Kinsky et al. have extensively studied the ability of a dendritic cell growth factor, FLT3 ligand, to impact murine resistance to pseudomonal infection in burns. They have shown that FLT3 ligand improves murine resistance to infection via improved neutrophil function in a dendritic-cell-dependent manner [36, 37].

Monocytes/Macrophages

In contrast to dendritic cells, macrophage populations are not reduced in response to sepsis [31]. However, numerous studies have demonstrated that monocytes/macrophages effectively undergo "cellular reprogramming" with a transition from a pro-inflammatory, immune activating response to an immunosuppressing anti-inflammatory response [38, 39]. Indeed, the impaired monocyte response to lipopolysaccharide (LPS), the immunogenic cell membrane component of gram-negative bacteria, seen in sepsis, labeled "endotoxin tolerance," is considered to be a hallmark of the disorder. These alterations in monocyte function were shown in a study by Munoz et al. using plasma from patients in the ICU with sepsis or non-septic shock [40]. Monocytes isolated from patients with sepsis exhibited impaired release of IL-1, IL-6, and TNF-alpha in response to LPS exposure. Further, sepsis survivors recovered their capacity to respond to LPS exposure whereas non-survivors did not. Monneret et al., while investigating the anti-inflammatory response in sepsis, showed a down-regulation of HLA-receptor expression on monocytes which correlated strongly with levels of the anti-inflammatory cytokine IL-10 [41].

Lymphocytes

Natural Killer Cells

Lymphopenia is a frequent finding in sepsis with reductions in all lymphocyte sub-types [42]. In addition to a reduction in cell number, there is also evidence for cellular reprogramming similar to that seen in antigen presenting cells. Natural Killer (NK) cells are part of the innate immune response and were originally described based on their ability to kill leukemic cells [43]. They play an important role in the early response to infection, largely through production of IFNγ. Similarly to other lymphocyte populations, a reduction in NK cell numbers has been demonstrated in septic patients [42, 44]. A higher percentage of NK cells correlates with improved survival in septic patients [45]. Sepsis may result in NK cell tolerance to antigen stimulation, resulting in impaired production of IFNγ [44, 46, 47].

Chiche et al. demonstrated the clinical importance of this in a study of CMV reactivation in septic patients in the ICU [48]. Patients with sepsis admitted to the ICU were followed prospectively with serial monitoring of NK cell function while assessing for CMV reactivation. At baseline there was no difference in NK cell effector function between cases and controls. However, prior to CMV reactivation, there was a decrease in the ability of NK cells to secrete IFN-gamma (and elevations in serum IL-10 and IL-15 levels).

CD4+ T_H Cells

CD4+ helper T cells are typically divided into two distinct subtypes, Th1 and Th2, based on their pattern of cytokine secretion in response to stimulation. Th1 cells release pro-inflammatory cytokines including TNF-a, IFN-g, and IL-2, whereas Th2 cells release anti-inflammatory cytokines including IL-4 and IL-10 [6]. Sepsis has been shown in some studies to result in a shift toward a pro-Th2 response with the release of more anti-inflammatory cytokines, whereas other studies have shown an overall suppression of both Th1 and Th2 cells [6, 39]. These findings are consistent with the development of both immune suppression and immunoparalysis.

A third population of helper T cells, Th17 cells, has also been identified as playing an important role in sepsis-induced immune suppression. These cells are important in protecting against extracellular bacterial and fungal infections via secretion of IL-17 and IL-22. Th17 cells are also decreased in septic patients and loss of effective Th17 function is thought to contribute to the occurrence of secondary fungal infections in sepsis-induced immune suppression [39, 42, 49].

γδ T Cells

γδ T cells are present in high numbers in the intestinal mucosa and can be considered first line defenders against particular pathogens. In 2005, Venet et al. showed that γδ T cells decrease in patients with sepsis [50]. In the largest study to date, Andreu-Ballester et al. studied 135 patients with sepsis from an emergency department and intensive care unit. All the γδ T cell populations decreased significantly as the septic picture worsened. Almost 20% of patients died and the γδ T cells were significantly reduced in those septic patients who died. In this study, γδ T cells showed the largest decrease of any T cell population and the reduction correlated with sepsis severity [51].

Regulatory T Cells

Regulatory T cells (T_{Reg}), formerly known as suppressor T cells, are a subpopulation of CD4+ T cells that play an important role in modulating the immune response [39]. T_{Reg} levels are elevated in patients with sepsis compared to controls, and higher levels (along with more immunoparalysis) are seen in non-survivors compared to survivors [52, 53]. Several studies have attempted to elucidate the mechanisms by which T_{Reg} cells may directly contribute to immunoparalysis. T_{Reg} cells have been shown to redirect monocytes and macrophages into an anti-inflammatory alternative activating macrophages (AAM) pathway. This was partly through T_{Reg} production of IL-10, but also through a cytokine-independent pathway [54]. T_{Reg} cells also inhibit the memory γδ T cell production of IFN-γ in response to antigen challenge [55].

Predicting Clinical Outcomes with Biomarkers of Sepsis-Induced Immunosuppression

There have been many efforts to study the timing and magnitude of the immunosuppressive response in relation to patient outcomes which would create effective biomarkers for prognosis and therapies [56]. In 1983, Keane et al. studied lymphocytes cultured from 31 patients with severe trauma. They found that, overall, lymphocyte response to stimulation with mitogens was markedly reduced from controls. Furthermore, responses were lower and the duration of suppression longer in those patients who became infected, and the suppression of response preceded the onset of infection. Extremely low responses were found in three patients who later died [19].

More commonly, studies of patient's monocytes and their own HLA receptor down regulation have shown promise as a biomarker [57–66]. Asadulla et al. studied 57 neurosurgical patients and found that HLA-DR expression was lower in 14 patients who developed infection, compared with patients with an uncomplicated postoperative course [57]. Out of ten patients with less than 30% HLA-DR positive monocytes, nine developed infection. They hypothesized that the mechanism of this down regulation was high levels of endogenous cortisol as the effect coincided with high ACTH and cortisol concentrations and similar down regulation was seen in other patients who received high doses of exogenous corticosteroids. Subsequent studies supported the theory that the magnitude of HLA-DR receptor down regulation predicted a variety of other poor outcomes such as sepsis in liver transplant patients [58], however that study was confounded by exogenous steroids in some patients [60]. Allen et al. found HLA levels predicted sepsis in pediatric cardiac surgery patients [67]. In a small study of septic adults, Su et al. found that levels of HLA-DR positive monocytes <30% were more predictive of mortality than APACHE II scores [65].

The predictive power of monocyte deactivation has not been shown consistently, however and more recent studies have yielded different results. In 2003, three papers were published that seemed to contradict earlier findings. Hynninen et al. evaluated the HLA-DR expression of 61 patients with sepsis at admission and showed no predictive power of HLA expression for survival [61]. Another study of 70 septic patients also found no correlation between HLA expression and infectious or mortality outcomes [63]. Interestingly, this study showed that if patients' monocytes were stimulated with G-CSF ex-vivo, their HLA expression increased. The third study looked at 85 cardiac surgery patients. HLA expression was measured at presurgery, immediately after and 1 day later. Their data showed that while all patients' HLA levels declined after surgery, the magnitude of the response did not correlate with sepsis/SIRS, or other infectious complications [62]. Reasons for the different results are unclear but may be the result of small sample sizes, timing, or well-described variation caused by the different laboratory techniques used. In one study, the same samples were analyzed in two different labs and differed by as much as 20% [62].

Other studies have looked at anti-inflammatory cytokine levels as predictors of poor outcomes; most of these studies have been on human patients and bore mixed results. These data likely reflect the varied magnitudes and time courses of both pro and anti-inflammatory cytokine expression in real patients. In 1998, Doughty et al. sampled 53 pediatric ICU patients and found that high IL-10 levels correlated with three or more organ dysfunction and mortality [68]. Ahlstrom found no predictive value in IL-10 levels in patients with SIRS [64] but Simmons et al. found that IL-10 levels did correlate with mortality in a sample of 93 critically ill patients with acute renal failure [69]. Perhaps the most interesting data comes from two studies that looked at the ratio of IL-10 to TNF. In a large study of over 400 patients admitted to the hospital for fever, van Dissel et al. showed that a higher IL-10 to TNF ratio was predictive of mortality [70]. A similar study by Gogos et al. in a population of patients with mixed sepsis showed the same results [56].

A postmortem study by Boomer et al. compared patients who died in the intensive care unit (ICU) from severe sepsis with control patients who died of other causes. They found evidence of both immunosuppression and immunoparalysis in patients who died of sepsis. There was a marked change in the balance between suppressor cell populations and immunogenic cell lines including splenic CD4, CD8, and HLA-DR cells. Additionally, they found that patients who died of sepsis had <10% of the levels of both pro-inflammatory cytokines (TNF-α, IFN-γ, IL-6) and anti-inflammatory (IL-10) cytokines compared to patients dying of other causes [71].

Potential Therapeutic Interventions in Sepsis-Induced Immune Suppression

Decades of research in sepsis-induced immunosuppression has fostered the concept that both the pro and anti-inflammatory responses are necessary for recovery from an overwhelming infection and that it is the imbalance of these forces that can lead to organ injury and death. This has led some investigators to explore manipulation of these systems to improve outcomes. While some animal studies in this field have shown positive results, many have not and it is clear that in a system as complicated as sepsis the timing and dose of any agent used to affect the degree of pro or anti-inflammatory response are crucial factors.

Some of the first agents used to manipulate the balance of immunosuppression were androgens and estrogens. The idea for hormonal therapy came from earlier studies showing that testosterone seemed to have a negative impact on sepsis and trauma outcomes and is believed to act through augmenting postinjury immunosuppression [72]. Two subsequent studies by the same investigators showed that administration of the estrogen-like drug DHEA reduced the immunosuppression and improved mortality in septic mice [73, 74]. By far, most of the studies that have tried to manipulate the balance of inflammation have involved using anti-inflammatory cytokines that are here reviewed.

Interleukin-10

In animal models of sepsis, the administration of IL10 has been shown to have both positive [12–14] and negative [15, 16] effects on outcome which likely are dependent on the time of administration and the severity of the infection. In one carefully done animal model, Ashare et al. followed levels of pro-inflammatory cytokines and anti-inflammatory cytokines throughout the whole course of sepsis in mice. They found that bacterial levels in tissue correlated with IL-10 levels and that if the complementary pro-inflammatory response was blocked by pretreatment with IL-1 receptor antagonist, bacterial levels were higher as was mortality [17]. Similarly, Song et al. showed that blocking IL-10 activity early had no effect on mortality, blocking it late (12 h) after sepsis improved mortality [18]. These studies help illustrate how IL10 helps maintain a careful balance of the immune system in inflammation; thus, manipulation of it is so dangerous.

Interleukin 7 (IL-7)

Interleukin 7 may be the immunomodulatory agent that is closest to clinical utility in sepsis as it has shown positive results in animal trials of sepsis as well as has been shown to be safe in clinical trials in humans for other disease processes. IL-7 plays a critical role in T cell function. Mutations in IL-7 are one of the causes of severe combined immunodeficiency (SCID) [75–77]. In a murine model of sepsis, IL-7 has been shown to prevent loss of T-cells by both decreasing T-cell apoptosis and increasing T-cell proliferation. This prevented the loss of delayed type hypersensitivity (DTH) response and improved overall survival [78, 79]. A phase I/IIA study in humans with HIV and persistent lymphopenia despite combination anti-retroviral therapy demonstrated sustained increases in CD4 and CD8 T cells without signs of a hyper-inflammatory response or other adverse effects [80].

Interleukin 15 (IL-15)

IL-15 is closely related to IL-7 [78]. It is an anti-apoptotic cytokine that is regarded as a promising immunomodulatory therapy in cancer [81]. In murine models of sepsis, it has been shown to block apoptosis through the BCL-2 pathway, resulting in improved IFNγ production and reversal of sepsis-induced immunosuppression, which leads to improved survival [82]. Technical challenges related to rapid renal clearance of its recombinant form have limited its efficacy in human studies to date, but further trials are ongoing [81].

Programmed Cell Death Receptor-1 (PD-1) and Programmed Cell Death Ligand-1 (PD-L1)

PD-1 and PD-L1 are part of a family of co-inhibitory cell surface molecules that have been studied as another promising immunomodulatory therapy. PD-1 is expressed by activated T-cells and PD-L1 by epithelial, endothelial, and antigen presenting cells. PD-1/PD-L1 binding is thought to be part of the negative feedback loop that is triggered by an activation of the immune system. In the presence of prolonged antigen presence, this may lead to T cell exhaustion. Blocking the PD-1/PD-L1 pathway has shown extreme promise in cancer immunotherapy in human trials [83, 84]. In studies of human septic patients, PD-1 and PD-L1 expression has been shown to be upregulated in T cells and monocytes respectively [85, 86]. Further, levels of expression of PD-1 and PD-L1 correlated with increased secondary infections and mortality [86]. In murine models of bacterial sepsis as well as in both primary and secondary fungal sepsis, blockade of this pathway has resulted in improved survival [87, 88]. Human studies of anti-PD-1 and anti-PD-L1 have not yet been performed.

Granulocyte Macrophage Colony-Stimulating Factor (GM-CSF)

Loss of immune cells is an important factor in sepsis-induced immune suppression. Stimulating immune cell production has been looked at as a therapeutic target. Initial studies focused on granulocyte stimulating factor (G-CSF), which resulted in a marked increase in neutrophil number, but no change in clinical outcomes [89, 90]. Given the loss of cell types other than neutrophil as well as the importance of non-neutrophil immune cells in fighting the secondary viral and fungal infections that are common in sepsis-induced immune suppression, subsequent studies have focused on inducing a broader immune response with GM-CSF. Two such studies in humans have shown promising results, and are also notable for their use of a biomarker-based approach for identifying patients in the immunosuppressed phase of sepsis [91, 92]. While neither study was powered to show a difference in mortality, both showed improvement in markers of immune function (specifically TNF-α production) in patients treated with GM-CSF.

Interferon-Gamma

IFNγ is a key downstream mediator activating the innate immune response. IFNγ levels are decreased in patients with sepsis-induced immune suppression. Administration of IFNγ in uncontrolled studies has been shown to restore immune function [93, 94]. At least five studies have examined the use of gamma interferon which has been shown in-vivo to reverse monocyte deactivation [95, 96]. Two very similar small trials were done on human subjects with sepsis [93, 97]. In both studies, subjects with sepsis and monocyte HLA-DR expression of 30% or less were given interferon gamma. Both groups reported increases in HLA-DR expression, usually after just one dose. One of the studies also examined the monocytes ex-vivo and showed that interferon improved monocyte cytokine production as well [93]. A third human trial was different in that it sought to study the effects of Interferon gamma regionally [98]. In this study, the authors selected 21 patients with severe trauma and alveolar macrophage dysfunction as determined by a bronchoalveolar lavage sample showing macrophage HLA-DR expression of 30% or less. Interferon gamma was administered via inhalation. They found about 50% of the subjects had an increase in their alveolar macrophage HLA-DR expression. These patients had a lower incidence of pneumonia but no other differences in outcomes. The small numbers and lack of a control population in all three of these studies limit the conclusions that can be drawn, especially since HLA-DR expression is known to increase as patients recover. A small randomized controlled trial of IFNγ in sepsis is ongoing (ClinicalTrials.gov number: NCT01649921).

Conclusion

Sepsis-induced immune suppression is likely a major contributor to the morbidity and mortality associated with sepsis. It is characterized by a decrease in immune effector cell number as well as loss of function, which results in increased susceptibility to secondary infections. Potential therapies to augment the immune response show promise as a means to decrease sepsis-related mortality but large randomized controlled trials have not yet been done.

References

1. Freeman BD, Natanson C. Anti-inflammatory therapies in sepsis and septic shock. Expert Opin Investig Drugs. 2000;9(7):1651–63.
2. Bone RC. Sir Isaac Newton, sepsis, SIRS, and CARS. Crit Care Med. 1996;24(7):1125–8.
3. Otto GP, Sossdorf M, Claus RA, Rödel J, Menge K, Reinhart K, et al. The late phase of sepsis is characterized by an increased microbiological burden and death rate. Crit Care. 2011;15(4):R183.
4. Luyt CE, Combes A, Deback C, Aubriot-Lorton MH, Nieszkowska A, Trouillet JL, et al. Herpes simplex virus lung infection in patients undergoing prolonged mechanical ventilation. Am J Respir Crit Care Med. 2007;175(9):935–42.
5. Limaye AP, Kirby KA, Rubenfeld GD, Leisenring WM, Bulger EM, Neff MJ, et al. Cytomegalovirus reactivation in critically ill immunocompetent patients. JAMA. 2008;300(4):413–22.
6. Ward NS, Casserly B, Ayala A. The compensatory anti-inflammatory response syndrome (CARS) in critically ill patients. Clin Chest Med. 2008;29(4):617–25. viii
7. Schulte W, Bernhagen J, Bucala R. Cytokines in sepsis: potent immunoregulators and potential therapeutic targets—an updated view. Mediators Inflamm. 2013;2013:165974.
8. Novotny AR, Reim D, Assfalg V, Altmayr F, Friess HM, Emmanuel K, et al. Mixed antagonist response and sepsis severity-dependent dysbalance of pro- and anti-inflammatory responses at the onset of postoperative sepsis. Immunobiology. 2012;217(6):616–21.
9. MacNeil IA, Suda T, Moore KW, Mosmann TR, Zlotnik A. IL-10, a novel growth cofactor for mature and immature T cells. J Immunol. 1990;145(12):4167–73.
10. O'Garra A, Stapleton G, Dhar V, Pearce M, Schumacher J, Rugo H, et al. Production of cytokines by mouse B cells: B lymphomas and normal B cells produce interleukin 10. Int Immunol. 1990;2(9):821–32.
11. Oberholzer A, Oberholzer C, Moldawer LL. Interleukin-10: a complex role in the pathogenesis of sepsis syndromes and its potential as an anti-inflammatory drug. Crit Care Med. 2002;30(1 Supp):S58–63.
12. Berg DJ, Kuhn R, Rajewsky K, Müller W, Menon S, Davidson N, et al. Interleukin-10 is a central regulator of the response to LPS in murine models of endotoxic shock and the Shwartzman reaction but not endotoxin tolerance. J Clin Invest. 1995;96(5):2339–47.
13. Howard M, Muchamuel T, Andrade S, Menon S. Interleukin 10 protects mice from lethal endotoxemia. J Exp Med. 1993;177(4):1205–8.
14. van der Poll T, Jansen PM, Montegut WJ, Braxton CC, Calvano SE, Stackpole SA, et al. Effects of IL-10 on systemic inflammatory responses during sublethal primate endotoxemia. J Immunol. 1997;158(4):1971–5.
15. Remick DG, Garg SJ, Newcomb DE, Wollenberg G, Huie TK, Bolgos GL. Exogenous interleukin-10 fails to decrease the mortality or morbidity of sepsis. Crit Care Med. 1998;26(5):895–904.

16. Steinhauser ML, Hogaboam CM, Kunkel SL, Lukacs NW, Strieter RM, Standiford TJ. IL-10 is a major mediator of sepsis-induced impairment in lung antibacterial host defense. J Immunol. 1999;162(1):392–9.
17. Ashare A, Powers LS, Butler NS, Doerschug KC, Monick MM, Hunninghake GW. Anti-inflammatory response is associated with mortality and severity of infection in sepsis. Am J Physiol Lung Cell Mol Physiol. 2005;288(4):L633–40.
18. Song GY, Chung CS, Chaudry IH, Ayala A. What is the role of interleukin 10 in polymicrobial sepsis: anti-inflammatory agent or immunosuppressant? Surgery. 1999;126(2):378–83.
19. Keane RM, Birmingham W, Shatney CM, Winchurch RA, Munster AM. Prediction of sepsis in the multitraumatic patient by assays of lymphocyte responsiveness. Surg Gynecol Obstet. 1983;156(2):163–7.
20. Green DR, Beere HM. Apoptosis. Gone but not forgotten. Nature. 2000;405(6782):28–9.
21. Hotchkiss RS, Swanson PE, Freeman BD, Tinsley KW, Cobb JP, Matuschak GM, et al. Apoptotic cell death in patients with sepsis, shock, and multiple organ dysfunction. Crit Care Med. 1999;27(7):1230–51.
22. Hotchkiss RS, Schmieg Jr RE, Swanson PE, Freeman BD, Tinsley KW, Cobb JP, et al. Rapid onset of intestinal epithelial and lymphocyte apoptotic cell death in patients with trauma and shock. Crit Care Med. 2000;28(9):3207–17.
23. Hotchkiss RS, Tinsley KW, Swanson PE, Schmieg Jr RE, Hui JJ, Chang KC, et al. Sepsis-induced apoptosis causes progressive profound depletion of B and CD4+ T lymphocytes in humans. J Immunol. 2001;166(11):6952–63.
24. Tinsley KW, Grayson MH, Swanson PE, Drewry AM, Chang KC, Karl IE, et al. Sepsis induces apoptosis and profound depletion of splenic interdigitating and follicular dendritic cells. J Immunol. 2003;171(2):909–14.
25. Kovach MA, Standiford TJ. The function of neutrophils in sepsis. Curr Opin Infect Dis. 2012;25(3):321–7.
26. Fialkow L, Fochesatto Filho L, Bozzetti MC, Milani AR, Rodrigues Filho EM, Ladniuk RM, et al. Neutrophil apoptosis: a marker of disease severity in sepsis and sepsis-induced acute respiratory distress syndrome. Crit Care. 2006;10(6):R155.
27. Tamayo E, Gomez E, Bustamante J, Gómez-Herreras JI, Fonteriz R, Bobillo F, et al. Evolution of neutrophil apoptosis in septic shock survivors and nonsurvivors. J Crit Care. 2012;27(4):415. e1–11.
28. Drifte G, Dunn-Siegrist I, Tissieres P, Pugin J. Innate immune functions of immature neutrophils in patients with sepsis and severe systemic inflammatory response syndrome. Crit Care Med. 2013;41(3):820–32.
29. Kasten KR, Muenzer JT, Caldwell CC. Neutrophils are significant producers of IL-10 during sepsis. Biochem Biophys Res Commun. 2010;393(1):28–31.
30. Stephan F, Yang K, Tankovic J, Soussy CJ, Dhonneur G, Duvaldestin P, et al. Impairment of polymorphonuclear neutrophil functions precedes nosocomial infections in critically ill patients. Crit Care Med. 2002;30(2):315–22.
31. Hotchkiss RS, Tinsley KW, Swanson PE, Grayson MH, Osborne DF, Wagner TH, et al. Depletion of dendritic cells, but not macrophages, in patients with sepsis. J Immunol. 2002;168(5):2493–500.
32. Fujita S, Seino K, Sato K, Sato Y, Eizumi K, Yamashita N, et al. Regulatory dendritic cells act as regulators of acute lethal systemic inflammatory response. Blood. 2006;107(9):3656–64.
33. Poehlmann H, Schefold JC, Zuckermann-Becker H, Volk HD, Meisel C. Phenotype changes and impaired function of dendritic cell subsets in patients with sepsis: a prospective observational analysis. Crit Care. 2009;13(4):R119.
34. Pastille E, Didovic S, Brauckmann D, Rani M, Agrawal H, Schade FU, et al. Modulation of dendritic cell differentiation in the bone marrow mediates sustained immunosuppression after polymicrobial sepsis. J Immunol. 2011;186(2):977–86.
35. Guisset O, Dilhuydy MS, Thiebaut R, Lefèvre J, Camou F, Sarrat A, et al. Decrease in circulating dendritic cells predicts fatal outcome in septic shock. Intensive Care Med. 2007;33(1):148–52.

36. Toliver-Kinsky TE, Cui W, Murphey ED, Lin C, Sherwood ER. Enhancement of dendritic cell production by fms-like tyrosine kinase-3 ligand increases the resistance of mice to a burn wound infection. J Immunol. 2005;174(1):404–10.

37. Bohannon J, Fang G, Cui W, Sherwood E, Toliver-Kinsky T. Fms-like tyrosine kinase-3 ligand alters antigen-specific responses to infections after severe burn injury. Shock. 2009;32(4):435–41.

38. Cavaillon JM, Adib-Conquy M. Bench-to-bedside review: endotoxin tolerance as a model of leukocyte reprogramming in sepsis. Crit Care. 2006;10(5):233.

39. Hotchkiss RS, Monneret G, Payen D. Sepsis-induced immunosuppression: from cellular dysfunctions to immunotherapy. Nat Rev Immunol. 2013;13(12):862–74.

40. Munoz C, Carlet J, Fitting C, Misset B, Bleriot JP, Cavaillon JM. Dysregulation of in vitro cytokine production by monocytes during sepsis. J Clin Invest. 1991;88(5):1747–54.

41. Monneret G, Finck ME, Venet F, Debard AL, Bohé J, Bienvenu J, et al. The anti-inflammatory response dominates after septic shock: association of low monocyte HLA-DR expression and high interleukin-10 concentration. Immunol Lett. 2004;95(2):193–8.

42. Venet F, Davin F, Guignant C, Larue A, Cazalis MA, Darbon R, et al. Early assessment of leukocyte alterations at diagnosis of septic shock. Shock. 2010;34(4):358–63.

43. Chiche L, Forel JM, Thomas G, Farnarier C, Vely F, Bléry M, et al. The role of natural killer cells in sepsis. J Biomed Biotechnol. 2011;2011:986491.

44. Forel JM, Chiche L, Thomas G, Mancini J, Farnarier C, Cognet C, et al. Phenotype and functions of natural killer cells in critically-ill septic patients. PLoS One. 2012;7(12):e50446.

45. Giamarellos-Bourboulis EJ, Tsaganos T, Spyridaki E, Mouktaroudi M, Plachouras D, Vaki I, et al. Early changes of CD4-positive lymphocytes and NK cells in patients with severe Gram-negative sepsis. Crit Care. 2006;10(6):R166.

46. Souza-Fonseca-Guimaraes F, Parlato M, Fitting C, Cavaillon JM, Adib-Conquy M. NK cell tolerance to TLR agonists mediated by regulatory T cells after polymicrobial sepsis. J Immunol. 2012;188(12):5850–8.

47. Souza-Fonseca-Guimaraes F, Parlato M, Philippart F, Misset B, Cavaillon JM, Adib-Conquy M, et al. Toll-like receptors expression and interferon-gamma production by NK cells in human sepsis. Crit Care. 2012;16(5):R206.

48. Chiche L, Forel JM, Thomas G, Farnarier C, Cognet C, Guervilly C, et al. Interferon-gamma production by natural killer cells and cytomegalovirus in critically ill patients. Crit Care Med. 2012;40(12):3162–9.

49. Monneret G, Venet F, Kullberg BJ, Netea MG. ICU-acquired immunosuppression and the risk for secondary fungal infections. Med Mycol. 2011;49(Suppl 1):S17–23.

50. Venet F, Bohe J, Debard AL, Bienvenu J, Lepape A, Monneret G. Both percentage of gammadelta T lymphocytes and CD3 expression are reduced during septic shock. Crit Care Med. 2005;33(12):2836–40.

51. Andreu-Ballester JC, Tormo-Calandin C, Garcia-Ballesteros C, Pérez-Griera J, Amigó V, Almela-Quilis A, et al. Association of gammadelta T cells with disease severity and mortality in septic patients. Clin Vaccine Immunol. 2013;20(5):738–46.

52. Monneret G, Debard AL, Venet F, Bohe J, Hequet O, Bienvenu J, et al. Marked elevation of human circulating CD4+CD25+ regulatory T cells in sepsis-induced immunoparalysis. Crit Care Med. 2003;31(7):2068–71.

53. Venet F, Chung CS, Kherouf H, Geeraert A, Malcus C, Poitevin F, et al. Increased circulating regulatory T cells (CD4(+)CD25(+)CD127(−)) contribute to lymphocyte anergy in septic shock patients. Intensive Care Med. 2009;35(4):678–86.

54. Tiemessen MM, Jagger AL, Evans HG, van Herwijnen MJ, John S, Taams LS. CD4+CD25+Foxp3+ regulatory T cells induce alternative activation of human monocytes/macrophages. Proc Natl Acad Sci U S A. 2007;104(49):19446–51.

55. Li L, Wu CY. CD4+ CD25+ Treg cells inhibit human memory gammadelta T cells to produce IFN-gamma in response to M tuberculosis antigen ESAT-6. Blood. 2008;111(12):5629–36.

56. Gogos CA, Drosou E, Bassaris HP, Skoutelis A. Pro-versus anti-inflammatory cytokine profile in patients with severe sepsis: a marker for prognosis and future therapeutic options. J Infect Dis. 2000;181(1):176–80.

57. Asadullah K, Woiciechowsky C, Docke WD, Egerer K, Kox WJ, Vogel S, et al. Very low monocytic HLA-DR expression indicates high risk of infection—immunomonitoring for patients after neurosurgery and patients during high dose steroid therapy. Eur J Emerg Med. 1995;2(4):184–90.
58. van den Berk JM, Oldenburger RH, van den Berg AP, Klompmaker IJ, Mesander G, van Son WJ, et al. Low HLA-DR expression on monocytes as a prognostic marker for bacterial sepsis after liver transplantation. Transplantation. 1997;63(12):1846–8.
59. Denzel C, Riese J, Hohenberger W, Born G, Köckerling F, Tschaikowsky K, et al. Monitoring of immunotherapy by measuring monocyte HLA-DR expression and stimulated TNFalpha production during sepsis after liver transplantation. Intensive Care Med. 1998;24(12):1343–4.
60. Haveman JW, van den Berg AP, van den Berk JM, Mesander G, Slooff MJ, de Leij LH, et al. Low HLA-DR expression on peripheral blood monocytes predicts bacterial sepsis after liver transplantation: relation with prednisolone intake. Transpl Infect Dis. 1999;1(3):146–52.
61. Hynninen M, Pettila V, Takkunen O, Orko R, Jansson SE, Kuusela P, et al. Predictive value of monocyte histocompatibility leukocyte antigen-DR expression and plasma interleukin-4 and -10 levels in critically ill patients with sepsis. Shock. 2003;20(1):1–4.
62. Oczenski W, Krenn H, Jilch R, Watzka H, Waldenberger F, Köller U, et al. HLA-DR as a marker for increased risk for systemic inflammation and septic complications after cardiac surgery. Intensive Care Med. 2003;29(8):1253–7.
63. Perry SE, Mostafa SM, Wenstone R, Shenkin A, McLaughlin PJ. Is low monocyte HLA-DR expression helpful to predict outcome in severe sepsis? Intensive Care Med. 2003;29(8):1245–52.
64. Ahlstrom A, Hynninen M, Tallgren M, Kuusela P, Valtonen M, Orko R, et al. Predictive value of interleukins 6, 8 and 10, and low HLA-DR expression in acute renal failure. Clin Nephrol. 2004;61(2):103–10.
65. Su L, Zhou DY, Tang YQ, Wen Q, Bai T, Meng FS, et al. Clinical value of monitoring CD14+ monocyte human leukocyte antigen (locus) DR levels in the early stage of sepsis. Zhongguo Wei Zhong Bing Ji Jiu Yi Xue. 2006;18(11):677–9.
66. Zhang YT, Fang Q. Study on monocyte HLA-DR expression in critically ill patients after surgery. Zhonghua Wai Ke Za Zhi. 2006;44(21):1480–2.
67. Allen ML, Peters MJ, Goldman A, Elliott M, James I, Callard R, et al. Early postoperative monocyte deactivation predicts systemic inflammation and prolonged stay in pediatric cardiac intensive care. Crit Care Med. 2002;30(5):1140–5.
68. Doughty L, Carcillo JA, Kaplan S, Janosky J. The compensatory anti-inflammatory cytokine interleukin 10 response in pediatric sepsis-induced multiple organ failure. Chest. 1998;113(6):1625–31.
69. Simmons EM, Himmelfarb J, Sezer MT, Chertow GM, Mehta RL, Paganini EP, et al. Plasma cytokine levels predict mortality in patients with acute renal failure. Kidney Int. 2004;65(4):1357–65.
70. van Dissel JT, van Langevelde P, Westendorp RG, Kwappenberg K, Frolich M. Anti-inflammatory cytokine profile and mortality in febrile patients. Lancet. 1998;351(9107):950–3.
71. Boomer JS, To K, Chang KC, Takasu O, Osborne DF, Walton AH, et al. Immunosuppression in patients who die of sepsis and multiple organ failure. JAMA. 2011;306(23):2594–605.
72. Angele MK, Wichmann MW, Ayala A, Cioffi WG, Chaudry IH. Testosterone receptor blockade after hemorrhage in males. Restoration of the depressed immune functions and improved survival following subsequent sepsis. Arch Surg. 1997;132(11):1207–14.
73. Angele MK, Catania RA, Ayala A, Cioffi WG, Bland KI, Chaudry IH. Dehydroepiandrosterone: an inexpensive steroid hormone that decreases the mortality due to sepsis following trauma-induced hemorrhage. Arch Surg. 1998;133(12):1281–8.
74. Catania RA, Angele MK, Ayala A, Cioffi WG, Bland KI, Chaudry IH. Dehydroepiandrosterone restores immune function following trauma-haemorrhage by a direct effect on T lymphocytes. Cytokine. 1999;11(6):443–50.
75. Roifman CM, Zhang J, Chitayat D, Sharfe N. A partial deficiency of interleukin-7R alpha is sufficient to abrogate T-cell development and cause severe combined immunodeficiency. Blood. 2000;96(8):2803–7.

76. Puel A, Leonard WJ. Mutations in the gene for the IL-7 receptor result in T(−)B(+)NK(+) severe combined immunodeficiency disease. Curr Opin Immunol. 2000;12(4):468–73.
77. Puel A, Ziegler SF, Buckley RH, Leonard WJ. Defective IL7R expression in T(−)B(+)NK(+) severe combined immunodeficiency. Nat Genet. 1998;20(4):394–7.
78. Hutchins NA, Unsinger J, Hotchkiss RS, Ayala A. The new normal: immunomodulatory agents against sepsis immune suppression. Trends Mol Med. 2014;20(4):224–33.
79. Unsinger J, McGlynn M, Kasten KR, Hoekzema AS, Watanabe E, Muenzer JT, et al. IL-7 promotes T cell viability, trafficking, and functionality and improves survival in sepsis. J Immunol. 2010;184(7):3768–79.
80. Levy Y, Lacabaratz C, Weiss L, Viard JP, Goujard C, Lelièvre JD, et al. Enhanced T cell recovery in HIV-1-infected adults through IL-7 treatment. J Clin Invest. 2009;119(4):997–1007.
81. Ochoa MC, Mazzolini G, Hervas-Stubbs S, de Sanmamed MF, Berraondo P, Melero I. Interleukin-15 in gene therapy of cancer. Curr Gene Ther. 2013;13(1):15–30.
82. Inoue S, Unsinger J, Davis CG, Muenzer JT, Ferguson TA, Chang K, et al. IL-15 prevents apoptosis, reverses innate and adaptive immune dysfunction, and improves survival in sepsis. J Immunol. 2010;184(3):1401–9.
83. Topalian SL, Hodi FS, Brahmer JR, Gettinger SN, Smith DC, DF MD, et al. Safety, activity, and immune correlates of anti-PD-1 antibody in cancer. N Engl J Med. 2012;366(26):2443–54.
84. Brahmer JR, Tykodi SS, Chow LQ, Hwu WJ, Topalian SL, Hwu P, et al. Safety and activity of anti-PD-L1 antibody in patients with advanced cancer. N Engl J Med. 2012;366(26):2455–65.
85. Zhang Y, Li J, Lou J, Zhou Y, Bo L, Zhu J, et al. Upregulation of programmed death-1 on T cells and programmed death ligand-1 on monocytes in septic shock patients. Crit Care. 2011;15(1):R70.
86. Guignant C, Lepape A, Huang X, Kherouf H, Denis L, Poitevin F, et al. Programmed death-1 levels correlate with increased mortality, nosocomial infection and immune dysfunctions in septic shock patients. Crit Care. 2011;15(2):R99.
87. Chang KC, Burnham CA, Compton SM, Rasche DP, Mazuski RJ, JS MD, et al. Blockade of the negative co-stimulatory molecules PD-1 and CTLA-4 improves survival in primary and secondary fungal sepsis. Crit Care. 2013;17(3):R85.
88. Zhang Y, Zhou Y, Lou J, Li J, Bo L, Zhu K, et al. PD-L1 blockade improves survival in experimental sepsis by inhibiting lymphocyte apoptosis and reversing monocyte dysfunction. Crit Care. 2010;14(6):R220.
89. Root RK, Lodato RF, Patrick W, Cade JF, Fotheringham N, Milwee S, et al. Multicenter, double-blind, placebo-controlled study of the use of filgrastim in patients hospitalized with pneumonia and severe sepsis. Crit Care Med. 2003;31(2):367–73.
90. Nelson S, Belknap SM, Carlson RW, Dale D, De Boisblanc B, Farkas S, et al. A randomized controlled trial of filgrastim as an adjunct to antibiotics for treatment of hospitalized patients with community-acquired pneumonia. CAP Study Group. J Infect Dis. 1998;178(4):1075–80.
91. Meisel C, Schefold JC, Pschowski R, Baumann T, Hetzger K, Gregor J, et al. Granulocyte-macrophage colony-stimulating factor to reverse sepsis-associated immunosuppression: a double-blind, randomized, placebo-controlled multicenter trial. Am J Respir Crit Care Med. 2009;180(7):640–8.
92. Hall MW, Knatz NL, Vetterly C, Tomarello S, Wewers MD, Volk HD, et al. Immunoparalysis and nosocomial infection in children with multiple organ dysfunction syndrome. Intensive Care Med. 2011;37(3):525–32.
93. Docke WD, Randow F, Syrbe U, Krausch D, Asadullah K, Reinke P, et al. Monocyte deactivation in septic patients: restoration by IFN-gamma treatment. Nat Med. 1997;3(6):678–81.
94. Nalos M, Santner-Nanan B, Parnell G, Tang B, McLean AS, Nanan R. Immune effects of interferon gamma in persistent staphylococcal sepsis. Am J Respir Crit Care Med. 2012;185(1):110–2.
95. Hershman MJ, Appel SH, Wellhausen SR, Sonnenfeld G, Polk Jr HC. Interferon-gamma treatment increases HLA-DR expression on monocytes in severely injured patients. Clin Exp Immunol. 1989;77(1):67–70.

96. Bundschuh DS, Barsig J, Hartung T, Randow F, Döcke WD, Volk HD, et al. Granulocyte-macrophage colony-stimulating factor and IFN-gamma restore the systemic TNF-alpha response to endotoxin in lipopolysaccharide-desensitized mice. J Immunol. 1997;158(6):2862–71.
97. Kox WJ, Bone RC, Krausch D, Döcke WD, Kox SN, Wauer H, et al. Interferon gamma-1b in the treatment of compensatory anti-inflammatory response syndrome. A new approach: proof of principle. Arch Intern Med. 1997;157(4):389–93.
98. Nakos G, Malamou-Mitsi VD, Lachana A, Karassavoglou A, Kitsiouli E, Agnandi N, et al. Immunoparalysis in patients with severe trauma and the effect of inhaled interferon-gamma. Crit Care Med. 2002;30(7):1488–94.

Chapter 6
Molecular Targets for Therapy

Andre C. Kalil and Steven M. Opal

Introduction

Defining potential molecular targets for sepsis therapeutics has proven to be a real challenge in translating laboratory findings into effective clinical treatments. A myriad of possible targets have been proposed from preclinical studies but they often have overlapping pathologic functions, can differ depending upon the causative microbial pathogen, site of infection, and status of the immune response of the host at the time of treatment is initiated. When attempting to modulate the host response in critically ill patients during an ongoing systemic infection, the capacity to do harm is substantial and the net effects of such interventions on host defenses and antimicrobial clearance mechanisms in individual patients are highly variable. Finding a final common pathway that drives sepsis pathophysiology has been elusive and has limited progress in developing new sepsis therapeutics. Current aims to improve outcomes in sepsis are now focused upon regulation of the coagulation system; maintenance and repair of endothelial surfaces and the blood compartment; epithelial membrane integrity; regulating the dysfunctional systemic immune response in sepsis; and bolstering host defenses against microbial toxins and virulence.

A.C. Kalil, MD, MPH (✉)
Infectious Disease Division, Department of Internal Medicine,
University of Nebraska Medical Center, Omaha, NE, USA
e-mail: AKalil@unmc.edu

S.M. Opal, MD
Infectious Disease Division, Memorial Hospital of RI, Alpert Medical School
of Brown University, 111 Brewster Street, Pawtucket, RI 02860, USA
e-mail: Steven_Opal@brown.edu

© Springer International Publishing AG 2017   89
N.S. Ward, M.M. Levy (eds.), *Sepsis*, Respiratory Medicine,
DOI 10.1007/978-3-319-48470-9_6

Molecular Targets for Sepsis Therapies Within the Endothelium and Coagulation System

The hemostatic system is among the oldest human evolutionary tools for humans to defend themselves against invasions from microorganisms such as bacteria and fungi by isolating them through the formation of micro clots, triggering an inflammatory response, and then allowing the immune system to act more effectively within these locations [1]. However, the derangement of this hemostatic system may lead to serious coagulation disturbances, including disseminated intravascular coagulation, microvascular thrombosis, hypoperfusion, organ failure, and death; accordingly, correct modulation of this clotting system could reduce the development of organ failure and death in patients with severe sepsis [2]. Thrombin and other serine proteases of the clotting system are highly injurious when generated in the intravascular space and are pro-thrombotic and pro-inflammatory mediators. There are three main regulators of the coagulation system during sepsis: tissue factor pathway inhibitor, protein C, and antithrombin. These three coagulation inhibitors work simultaneously on limiting the excessive thrombin generation. When any of these molecules becomes qualitatively or quantitatively dysfunctional, a hypercoagulable state evolves during sepsis. Therefore, concentrates and recombinant forms of these molecules have been administered to humans with the intent to improve outcomes of patients with sepsis-induced hypercoagulable states. We discuss the evidence in favor of and against the use of these molecular targets as potential therapies system during sepsis and severe sepsis.

Antithrombin

Antithrombin is a direct inhibitor of thrombin and serine proteases factors Xa and IXa, and leads to the formation of thrombin–anti-thrombin (TAT) complexes. Antithrombin becomes depleted in patients with sepsis and its function is further compromised by the reduction of glycosaminoglycans on the endothelial surface during sepsis. High doses of antithrombin concentrates (plasma-derived) have been used in clinical trials with the goal to achieve supra-physiologic plasma levels in patients with sepsis and/or DIC. A large phase III clinical trial (KyberSept) [3] in patients with severe sepsis showed no survival benefits with antithrombin; however, the concomitant use of heparin and the heterogeneous population with and without DIC may have precluded the detection of potential benefits.

A Cochrane systematic review [4] concluded that anti-thrombin was not associated with significant mortality reduction (RR = 0.96, 95% CI 0.89–1.03), and a similar study done by the same authors [5] with the use of trial sequential analysis, reached similar conclusions; in addition, they concluded that the sample size of their meta-analysis was large enough to conclude that antithrombin was not associated with a 10% relative death reduction, but the available evidence could not rule out a potential 5% relative death reduction. Another meta-analysis performed by

Wiederman and Kaneider [6] evaluated only studies and patient subgroups that received antithrombin, had both severe sepsis and DIC, and did not receive heparin. They concluded that there was a significant (35%) reduction in the relative odds of death (OR = 0.65, 95% CI 422–0.998; p = 0.049). However, their analysis was based on the pooling of post-hoc subgroup data, which may have introduced both multiplicity (higher probability of false-positive) and selection bias since the randomization process for the subgroups was not followed as in the original studies. Bleeding adverse events were more common in the large clinical trials as well as in the Cochrane meta-analysis: RR = 1.52 (95% CI 1.30–1.78), and the concomitant use of heparin further increased the rate of bleeding: RR = 1.77 (95% CI 1.43–2.18).

Many factors may have confounded the antithrombin trial results: baseline disease severity, baseline level of sepsis-induced coagulopathy, heparin interaction, and rate of antithrombin alpha-form in the concentrate formulations; thus, more evidence is needed to better define the role of antithrombin in patients with severe sepsis and coagulopathy. A new recombinant form of antithrombin (KW-3357) is currently being evaluated in a clinical trial in Japan.

Recombinant Tissue Factor Pathway Inhibitor (TFPI)

Tissue Factor (TF) is the major initiator of coagulation in vivo and plays an integral role in blood coagulation and thrombin generation. TF signaling proceeds with the sequential generation of coagulation mediators (FVIIa, FXa, and FIIa: active serine proteases) and fibrin production, all of which further enhance the pro-inflammatory state via interactions with protease activated receptors (PAR1–4) [7]. TFPI is an endogenous serine protease inhibitor that inactivates factor Xa and VIIa/tissue factor complex in a Xa-dependent way. Two clinical trials on the use of a recombinant form of TFPI (Tifacogin) have been performed in humans with severe sepsis [8, 9]. The phase II trial [8] showed a nonsignificant trend to lower 28-day mortality by 13% (28% vs. 41%; p = 0.14), but the small sample size of the study precluded further interpretation. Subsequently, a larger phase III trial was executed, and the overall 28-day mortality was not different between TFPI (32.4% [N = 880]) and placebo (33.9% [N = 874]); p = 0.88. Because heparin displaces TFPI from biding glycosaminoglycans on the surface of endothelial cells, a subgroup analysis was done for the presence versus the absence of heparin; the results suggested a potential survival benefit for patients who received TFPI without concomitant heparin: 34.6% vs. 42.7% (p = 0.05). Different baseline INR levels (lower or higher than 1.5) were not associated with changes in survival benefits. However, bleeding as adverse events were more frequent in patients who received TFPI (24%) compared to placebo (19%), p = 0.008. Questions about the optimal dose of TFPI, best population target (sepsis-induced coagulopathy), ideal ratio between TFPI-alpha and TFPI-beta, and its overall efficacy and safety remain ill defined.

Recombinant Human Activated Protein C

Protein C is a vitamin K-dependent protein, which is activated by proteolysis on the thrombin-thrombomodulin complex and by the endothelial protein C receptor. The activated form of protein C decreases thrombin generation by an irreversible inhibition of the acceleration factors of the coagulation system Factor Va and VIIIa. A recombinant human form of activated protein C (drotrecogin alfa activated) has anticoagulant, anti-inflammatory, profibrinolytic, and cytoprotective effects. Several experimental studies in mice, rats, and baboons have shown the in vivo effect of activated protein C and suggest that the cytoprotective effects of activated Protein C are more important than its anticoagulant effects [10–12]. Two large meta-analyses have recently been performed; the study by Marti-Carvajal et al. [13] included only randomized trials and reached the conclusion that recombinant activated protein C was not associated with mortality reduction (RR = 0.97, 95% CI 0.78–1.22), while the study by Kalil and LaRosa [14] concluded this therapy was significantly associated with mortality reduction (RR = 0.82, 95% CI 0.78–0.87) in patients with severe sepsis. The major difference between these two meta-analyses was related to the evaluation of all available evidence, including analytical and controlled studies that were included only in Kalil and LaRosa's study. Both meta-analyses showed significant increase in bleeding adverse events with activated protein C compared to controls. The discordant results between two of the largest phase III trials—PROWESS [15] and PROWESS-SHOCK [16], were likely due to highly significant clinical and statistical heterogeneity between these studies [17]. Thus, the final verdict on the efficacy of recombinant activated protein C in patients with severe sepsis is yet to be handed down.

Thrombomodulin

Thrombomodulin promotes the thrombin-mediated activation of protein C and during severe sepsis and septic shock this molecule is downregulated, which corroborates to a pro-coagulant and pro-inflammatory state. A recombinant form of soluble thrombomodulin has been approved for clinical use in Japan since 2008 based on a RCT which enrolled 234 patients with hematologic malignancy or infection [18]; their results showed a higher rate of DIC resolution: 66.1% in experimental therapy vs. 49.9% in the control group ($p < 0.05$), and no differences were noted in bleeding rates. Subsequently, a phase II placebo-controlled RCT was performed in patients with severe sepsis [19], and the results showed no significant differences in mortality (21.6% vs. 17.8%) or bleeding rates (5.1% vs. 4.6%). However, a subgroup of patients with evidence of coagulation activation (thrombocytopenia and elevated international normalized ratio [INR]) appeared to benefit from soluble thrombomodulin. A large phase III trial is currently enrolling patients with severe sepsis and coagulopathy to further evaluate the efficacy and safety of recombinant thrombomodulin.

Heparin

Heparins bind to antithrombin and lead to conformational changes that augment its anticoagulant activity by several hundred times. A clinical trial on the effect of heparin on the survival of patients with sepsis was completed in 2009 and no significant 28-day survival benefit was observed [20] (14% vs. 16%; $p = 0.652$). Another study, the XPRESS trial [21] showed a trend for survival benefit with prophylactic doses of heparin (28.3% vs. 31.9%; $p = 0.08$). Several other studies have been performed and a just published systematic review and meta-analysis by Zarychanski et al. [22] showed significant mortality reduction with the use of heparin (unfractionated—8 trials, and low molecular weight—1 trial) compared to placebo or usual care: RR = 0.88 (95% CI, 0.77–1.00; $p = 0.05$). The authors noticed poor reporting of bleeding side effects in most studies, but suggested up to twofold increase in bleeding events. The Canadian Critical Care Trials Group is planning to perform a phase III RCT on the efficacy of heparin in patients with severe sepsis.

Heparin has a number of other anti-inflammatory effects that might be of therapeutic value n sepsis independent of its anticoagulant properties by activating antithrombin. During blood stream infection, neutrophils aggregate and discharge their DNA into an intricate network of fibers called neutrophil extracellular traps (NETs) [23]. These NETs function as intravascular nets that physically capture bacteria in the circulation. In the process of forming NETs, extracellular histones are released from the nucleus, which are strongly positively charged and induce generalized inflammation via activation of the pattern recognition receptor Toll-like receptor 4 [24, 25]. Heparin is among the strongest negatively charged molecules known in human biology and can avidly bind and inactivate histone signaling [26, 27]. Even non-anticoagulant forms of heparin bind to circulating histones and are highly protective in animal models of sepsis [23]. The degree to which this and other anti-inflammatory effects of heparin account for its potential protective effects in septic patients is unknown at present.

The Vascular Endothelium as a Target for Sepsis Therapeutics

The endothelial surface regulates intravascular inflammation and to a lesser extent extravascular inflammatory responses during sepsis [28, 29]. The innate immune system and coagulation pathways coevolved to collaborate in protecting the host from the simultaneous risk of exsanguination and invasive microbial infection following any break in the integument. The interface between clotting and inflammation is particularly critical in sepsis [2]. Dysfunction or disruption of the endothelial barrier by injury or apoptosis exposed the fluid phase of the blood compartment to subendothelial sources of tissue factor (TF), the main initiator of coagulation activation in sepsis. Activated monocytes and macrophages are major sources of TF in severe sepsis. Even activated endothelial cells themselves can express TF along their cell surface when exposed to high levels TNF or interleukin-1β. TF binds circulating factor VII and this TF:FVIIa complex and activate factor X with generation of thrombin and fibrin. TF can also reside on microparticles (MPs) shed from hematopoietic and endothelial cells. MPs can activate both coagulation and inflammation in sepsis [30].

Platelet adhesion to activated endothelial cells is increased in sepsis by alterations in von Willebrand factor. Final assembly of von Willebrand factor multimers occurs on endothelial surfaces. Large multimers of von Willebrand factor, occur in sepsis which avidly bind to platelet glycoprotein Ibα under conditions of shear force [31]. These large von Willebrand factor multimers are normally cleaved by a protease known as ADAMTS 13 (a disintegrin and metalloproteinase with a thrombospondin type 1 motif, member 13). Sepsis induces an acquired deficiency of ADAMTS13, resulting in ultra-large von Willebrand factor multimers and platelet adhesion to injured endothelium [30, 31]. Expression of P-selectin on adherent platelet surfaces link platelets to leukocytes and endothelial cells, further amplifying TF expression on monocytes [32].

Thrombin and other activated clotting factors cleave a set of unusual seven-transmembrane receptors known as protease-activated receptors (PARs) [33]. Four PARs exist in humans and can either promote or disrupt endothelial barrier function, depending on which G-protein-linked intracellular signaling pathway is activated. Thrombin bound to PAR1 in early sepsis contributes to endothelial dysfunction by GTPase RhoA-dependent cytoskeletal derangements in endothelial cells and induces endothelial cell contraction and rounding [30, 33]. Endothelial cell contraction disables extracellular membrane barrier function thereby increasing vascular permeability. Macromolecules such as large proteins and white cells can now exit the circulation into the extravascular space. Over time thrombin-PAR1 complexes transactivate PAR2 and form PAR1–PAR2 heterodimers on endothelium. This reverses the net effect of thrombin generation to an endothelial barrier protection effect. This is mediated by PAR1–PAR2 switching of intracellular GTPase signaling from the RhoA-mediated barrier disruptive pathway to a PAR2-mediated Rac1 endothelial barrier protective function. This two way competing pathway can be manipulated to a therapeutic advantage with agents that target specific PARs [34–36].

Endothelial barrier function prevents vascular leak, maintains an anticoagulant surface and prevents macromolecules from exiting the microcirculation. Endothelial barriers are maintained by adherens junctions, consisting of vascular endothelial (VE)-cadherin, and tight junctions (the zona occludens), formed by occludins and claudins [33]. Intracellular actin filament networks maintain endothelial cell apposition and this is further supported by transmembrane Robo4-slit proteins [37, 38]. Several treatment options designed to retain endothelial barrier function are now under preclinical and clinical investigation (see Table 6.1).

Table 6.1 New treatment options targeting coagulation and the endothelium in sepsis

Molecule	Mechanism(s) of action	Current status
Heparin and non-anticoagulant heparin	Activate antithrombin, binds histones, blocks endothelial cell adhesion	Nonanticoagulant heparin preclinical; heparin-P III
Recombinant antithrombin	Limits coagulation; anti-inflammatory limits WBC migration and adherence	P II study in Japan
Non-anticoagulant Activated Protein C	Cytoprotective activities, limits Endothelial cell apoptosis	Preclinical studies
Anti-HMGB1 mAb	Blocks HMGB1-mediated loss of endothelial barrier function	Preclinical studies
Fibrinopeptide Bβ_{15-42} (FXO6)	Fibrin split product binds VE-cadherin and stabilizes Endothelial junctions	P II clinical trials
Pepducins	Lipidated peptides promote PAR2-Rac-mediated endothelial barrier function	Preclinical studies and early clinical studies
VEGF receptor mAb	Prevents loss of VE-cadherin from endothelial junctions	Early clinical trials
Recombinant human thrombomodulin	Prevents endothelial apoptosis; degrades C5a, limits neutrophil binding	Available in Japan, in Phase III clinical trials

P phase of clinical trial, *HMGB1* high-mobility group box 1, *PAR2* protease-activated receptor 2, *Rac* an intracellular signaling molecule from a subfamily of guanosine triphosphatases (GTPase), *VEGF* vascular endothelial growth factor, *VE* vascular endothelium, *mAb* monoclonal antibody. See Refs. 29, 33, 37, 39 for review

Epithelial Barrier Protection as a Therapeutic Target in Sepsis

Loss of epithelial mucosal barrier protection contributes to initiation and amplification of systemic immune dysfunction in sepsis [39–41]. Mucosal ischemia and inflammatory changes are commonplace is septic shock patients and these events can perturb endothelial function and the resident microflora that inhabit these mucous membranes. Epithelial membranes play an essential role in normal physiology. Epithelial cells separate the parenchymal tissues from the external milieu and are polarized with an apical surface and a basolateral surface. The feature selective semipermeable membranes that determine the rate of water, solute, and macromolecule flow, and segregate the endogenous microbiota, now referred to as the resident microbiome, from host tissues [42].

The microbiome of the gut is best known by less complex microbiomes are now recognized in the lower airways, oropharynx, skin, and genitourinary tract [42–44]. The gut microbiome contains 100-fold more expressed genes that the entire complement of expressed human genes. The microbiome consists of over 10^{14} bacterial cells with is home to thousands of different species of bacteria, viruses, Archea, fungi, and commensal protozoan parasites. Changes in the microbiome certainly occur in critical illness and the relevance of these alterations on the human host is only beginning to be understood. Attempts to regulate and reestablish a healthy microbiome might represent a novel strategy to promote the resolution of sepsis in patients with persistent critical illness (PCI) [41, 45].

This might be feasible by probiotics (the placement of favorable bacterial strains or fungi along the epithelium to reestablish a healthy microbiome) or prebiotics (the process of placing a nonabsorbable complex polysaccharides or other macromolecules to alter the substrates for metabolism on the microbiome population and alter its makeup of microorganisms). These efforts have already produced some limited success, particularly in preventing necrotizing enterocolitis in critically ill neonates and preventing recurrent respiratory infections in children [46]. Many other possible benefits could accrue by regulating the microbiome. Some preliminary studies suggest that probiotics or prebiotics could be useful to prevent colonization and infections from multidrug-resistant, nosocomial gram-negative bacterial pathogens [47–51] and recurrent *Clostridium difficile*-associated colitis [52].

Another therapeutic option is to repair damaged epithelial cells or reestablish the structure and functional junctions between adjacent epithelial cells. In the gut epithelium cells are held together by intercellular adhesion molecules including occludin, ZO-1, and claudin [39, 53]. Growth factors such as granulocyte-macrophage colony stimulating factor [53] and hepatocyte growth factor [54], along with specific cytokines including interleukin-11 [55], IL-22 [56], and other epithelial growth factors [57, 58] can reduce epithelial apoptosis, strengthen tight junctions, and stimulate growth promote growth and repair and strengthen epithelial tight junctions. New epithelial barrier defensive strategies to prevent or to treat sepsis are presented in Table 6.2.

Table 6.2 New sepsis agents targeting the epithelium

Therapeutic agent	Mechanism(s) of action	Developmental status
GM-CSF	Epithelial and myeloid cell growth factor, limits colonic inflammation and facilitates injury repair	Preclinical and pilot studies in humans [53]
Hepatocyte growth factor (HGF)	Epithelial growth factors, cytoprotective for intestinal epithelium	Preclinical studies [54]
Interleukin-11 and Interleukin-22	Epithelial growth factor promotes tight junctions and prevents epithelial permeability and apoptosis	Preclinical studies and pilot clinical studies [55, 56]
Regulate the microbiome	Tightens epithelial junctions, stimulates intestinal immunity, limits MDR pathogens and *C. difficile*	Preclinical studies [51, 52]
Insulin-like growth factor-1	Prevents sepsis-induced excess gut epithelial permeability and apoptosis	Preclinical studies [57]
TNFAIP3	Maintains tight junction occludins and epithelial barrier during sepsis	Preclinical investigations [58]
Anti-HMGB1 mAb	Limits gut permeability and lowers cytokine response following I/R	Preclinical investigations [59]

GM-CSF granulocyte-macrophage colony stimulating factor, *MDR* multidrug resistant, *TNFAIP3* tumor necrosis factor alpha-induced protein 3, *HMGB1* high mobility group box, *I/R* ischemia reperfusion injury

Other Promising New Therapeutic Targets to Treat Sepsis

High Mobility Group Box 1

HMGB1 is a nuclear 30 kDa DNA binding protein that is secreted from activated immune effector cells and cells undergoing necrosis [59–61]. The disulfide form of HMGB1 signals through the LPS receptor MD2-TLR4 (myeloid differentiation 2 toll-like receptor 4) [61]. HMGB1 disrupts endothelial barriers, and promotes the release of large quantities of IL-1 alpha and beta from endothelial cells [62–64]. HMGB1 induces major defects in gut epithelial barrier function and induces mucosal hyper-permeability in shock states [59]. HMGB1 also contributes to mitochondrial injury and cellular apoptosis [61]. Compelling evidence now supports the important role of HMGB1 in the perpetuation of septic shock in its later phases. Remarkably, HMGB1 also appears to play a role in the rather common occurrence of cognitive decline as a late complication of severe sepsis, at last in mouse models [65]. Antibodies to HMGB1 and other inhibitory strategies to block HMGB1 actions are protective in experimental sepsis. Hopefully therapies that specifically target HMGB1 will be tested in human clinical trials in sepsis in the near future.

Another anti-HMGB1 approach is blocking its activity at the tissue receptor level. The receptor of advanced glycated end products (RAGE) is another HMGB1 binding and signaling protein expressed on the surface of hematopoietic cells and other tissues. Administration of a soluble inhibitor of RAGE known as sRAGE is effective in preventing organ damage and lethality in animal models of sepsis [66].

Plasma levels of a ubiquitous human protein called gelsolin fall rapidly in severe sepsis and the loss of this protein impairs actin clearance, reduces phagocytosis, and promotes inflammatory cytokine generation [67]. Recombinant gelsolin is available and could be a potential novel therapy for severe sepsis. There are a number of innovative hemoperfusion devices that function as blood purification strategies. One column is in phase III testing uses fixed polymyxin which binds endotoxin and other inflammatory molecules [68]. Another column adsorbs cytokines from the circulation and is available clinically in some European and Asian countries [69, 70]. Another uses the complement related pattern recognition receptor mannose binding lectin to bind endotoxin and bacterial, viral, and fungal pathogens [71]. Another promising blood purification strategy is heparin bound columns that avidly bind to many bacterial pathogens to clear bacteremic infections [72]. These devices might be particularly useful in clearance of blood stream infections with multidrug-resistant bacteria no longer susceptible to standard antimicrobial agents.

Oral administration of protease inhibitors to prevent increased gut permeability from pancreatic enzymes are in clinical trials at present [73]. Non-absorbed agents like transexamic acid and related protease inhibitors remain in the gut lumen and protect the intestinal epithelium from protease-mediated excess permeability during septic shock. Other novel sepsis therapies are designed as mitochondrial sparing agents to prevent intrinsic pathway activation of cellular apoptosis [74, 75]. Considerable interest has recently developed in readily available methods of regulating the host inflammatory status by immunometabolism approaches [76, 77].

Table 6.3 Other molecular targets and treatments to prevent or manage sepsis

Therapeutic agent	Mechanism(s) of action	Developmental status
Recombinant gelsolin	Clears extracellular actin, immunomodulatory activity	Early clinical trials in pneumonia and sepsis [67]
Polymyxin B perfusion columns, other blood purification strategies	Clears bacterial LPS, inflammatory cytokines, HMGB1, MDR pathogens, inflammatory mediators	In early trials to phase 3 clinical trials [68–72]
Orally administered protease inhibitors	Block pancreatic enzyme-mediated gut injury and increased permeability	In phase 2 trials [73]
Mitochondrial sparing agents	Improves cellular energetics and limits intrinsic pathway apoptosis	Preclinical investigations [74, 75]
Immuno-nutrition strategies	Can induce inhibitory phenotype of macrophages and lymphocytes	Preclinical investigations [76, 77]
mAb to PCSK9	Promote clearance of LPS and other pathologic lipids by the LDL receptor	Preclinical and early human studies [78, 79]
Pro-resolving agents	Promote resolution of inflammation, tissue repair, clear inflammatory cells	Preclinical investigations [80]

LPS lipopolysaccharide, *mAb* monoclonal antibody, *HMGB1* high mobility group box 1, *MDR* multidrug resistant, *PCSK9* pro-protein convertase subtilisin kexin type 9, *LDL* low density lipoprotein

Targeting specific proteases including PCSK9 (proprotein convertase subtilisin kexin type 9) appear promising as methods to improve hepatic clearance of bacterial endotoxin and removal of other injurious host-derived and pathogen-derived lipid mediators from the circulation in sepsis [78, 79]. Moreover, evidence now exists that recovery from sepsis and initiation of tissue repair is not a passive process of simply the lack of active inflammation. Resolution from sepsis is not a passive event but an active, organized process mediated by specific, lipooxygenase-derived, lipid signaling molecules such as resolvins or protectins [80]. Synthetic proresolving agonists might prove useful to prime the resolution phase of sepsis. The current status of these and other promising agents are listed on Table 6.3.

Immune Regulation and Immune Reconstitution as a Molecular Target

A myriad of immunologic findings clear demonstrate that sepsis-induced immune dysfunction occurs in many patients with prolonged sepsis and PCI [39, 41]. Reduced T cell and B cell functions, reduced lymphocyte proliferative capacity excess apoptosis, T cell exhaustion and dysregulated innate immune responses are readily demonstrable and likely have important adverse clinical consequences [81]. Reduced expression of major histocompatibility complex (MHC) class II antigens on antigen presenting cells frequently occur in severe sepsis [82]. Opportunistic viral infections are reactivated in the majority of patients with severe sepsis after prolonged ICU care [83, 84] and closely replicate the occurrence of systemic opportunistic viral infections observed in organ transplant recipients [85]. Disseminated cytomegalovirus infection and herpes simplex infection occur regularly in severe sepsis patient. Opportunistic bacterial and fungal infections also occur at high frequency in septic patients [82].

A number of therapeutic strategies to limit immune dysfunction or reconstitute immune function following sepsis are now in early clinical development. These include the T cell growth factor and thymic conditioning factor known as thymosin alpha 1 [86], inhibitors of inhibitory control mechanisms such as anti-programmed cell death ligand (PDL1) antibody [81], or anti-B and T lymphocyte attenuator (BTLA) [82], or other immune support and T cell growth factors such as interleukin-7 and IL-15 [87, 88]. Mesenchymal stem cells have remarkable immune regulation activities and might prove useful to manage selected patients with septic shock [89]. Immunostimulatory oligodeoxynucleotides appear capable of restoring immune competence in experimental models of sepsis and might find their way into clinical trials in the future [90, 91].

What is not clear at present is whether sepsis-induced immune suppression is primarily a physiologic, compensatory defense mechanism to control an overly exuberant systemic immune response in sepsis, or a pathological state of immune suppression increasing the risk of secondary infections [92]. When, if ever, does this compensatory anti-inflammatory state move from a necessary immune control mechanism of net benefit to patients to a state of immunosuppression that puts the patient at excess risk from opportunistic infection? It seems likely that status of the dysregulated immune function in sepsis will vary between individual patients and over time in the same septic patient. Interventions designed to regulate the systemic immune response will need to be carefully conducted in controlled clinical studies with regular monitoring of immune function to safely use these immune response modifiers [93].

Finally, short peptide inhibitors of the CD28 homodimer interface during cell activation between the costimulatory signals on antigen presenting cells and T lymphocytes look promising in experimental studies in toxic shock syndromes and necrotizing soft tissue infections [94, 95]. A recent phase II trial with a CD28 inhibitory peptide known as AB103 was successful in a phase II trial in patients with necrotizing fasciitis and is scheduled to enter phase III trials by the end of 2015 [96].

Conclusions

With the ever-increasing knowledge of the molecular and cellular mediators of sepsis have come remarkable new targets for interventions. Recovery and maintenance of epithelial and endothelial barriers are just some of the promising new targets for new therapies for sepsis. Other experimental agents currently in development promote cell survival by targeting mitochondria and cellular energetics. New strategies that bolster immune defenses should be tested at this time when progressive antimicrobial resistance among bacterial and fungal pathogens threatens to efficacy of our most effective weapon against sepsis antibiotics. We anticipate that novel agents targeting new molecular mediators, combined with appropriate biomarker-driven trials using innovations in genomic medicine, will bring a new generation of adjuvant therapies to benefit patients in septic shock.

References

1. Cinel I, Opal SM. Molecular biology of inflammation and sepsis: a primer. Crit Care Med. 2009;37(1):291–304. PubMed PMID: 19050640
2. van der Poll T, Opal SM. Host-pathogen interactions in sepsis. Lancet Infect Dis. 2008;8(1):32–43. PubMed PMID: 18063412
3. Warren BL, Eid A, Singer P, Pillay SS, Carl P, Novak I, et al. Caring for the critically ill patient. High-dose antithrombin III in severe sepsis: a randomized controlled trial. JAMA. 2001;286(15):1869–78. PubMed PMID: 11597289
4. Afshari A, Wetterslev J, Brok J, Moller AM. Antithrombin III for critically ill patients. Cochrane Database Syst Rev. 2008;3:CD005370.PubMed PMID: 18646125
5. Afshari A, Wetterslev J, Brok J, Moller A. Antithrombin III in critically ill patients: systematic review with meta-analysis and trial sequential analysis. BMJ. 2007;335(7632):1248–51. PubMed Central PMCID: 2137061
6. Wiedermann CJ, Kaneider NC. A systematic review of antithrombin concentrate use in patients with disseminated intravascular coagulation of severe sepsis. Blood Coagul Fibrinolysis. 2006;17(7):521–6. PubMed PMID: 16988545
7. Chu AJ. Tissue factor, blood coagulation, and beyond: an overview. Int J Inflamm. 2011;2011:367284. PubMed Central PMCID: 3176495
8. Abraham E, Reinhart K, Svoboda P, Seibert A, Olthoff D, Dal Nogare A, et al. Assessment of the safety of recombinant tissue factor pathway inhibitor in patients with severe sepsis: a multicenter, randomized, placebo-controlled, single-blind, dose escalation study. Crit Care Med. 2001;29(11):2081–9. PubMed PMID: 11700399
9. Abraham E, Reinhart K, Opal S, Demeyer I, Doig C, Rodriguez AL, et al. Efficacy and safety of tifacogin (recombinant tissue factor pathway inhibitor) in severe sepsis: a randomized controlled trial. JAMA. 2003;290(2):238–47. PubMed PMID: 12851279
10. Taylor Jr FB, Chang A, Esmon CT, D'Angelo A, Vigano-D'Angelo S, Blick KE. Protein C prevents the coagulopathic and lethal effects of *Escherichia coli* infusion in the baboon. J Clin Invest. 1987;79(3):918–25. PubMed Central PMCID: 424237
11. Li W, Zheng X, Gu J, Hunter J, Ferrell GL, Lupu F, et al. Overexpressing endothelial cell protein C receptor alters the hemostatic balance and protects mice from endotoxin. J Thromb Haemost. 2005;3(7):1351–9. PubMed PMID: 15978090
12. Murakami K, Okajima K, Uchiba M, Johno M, Nakagaki T, Okabe H, et al. Activated protein C attenuates endotoxin-induced pulmonary vascular injury by inhibiting activated leukocytes in rats. Blood. 1996;87(2):642–7. PubMed PMID: 8555486
13. Marti-Carvajal AJ, Sola I, Lathyris D, Cardona AF. Human recombinant activated protein C for severe sepsis. Cochrane Database Syst Rev. 2012;3:CD004388.PubMed PMID: 22419295
14. Kalil AC, LaRosa SP. Effectiveness and safety of drotrecogin alfa (activated) for severe sepsis: a meta-analysis and metaregression. Lancet Infect Dis. 2012;12(9):678–86. PubMed PMID: 22809883
15. Bernard GR, Vincent JL, Laterre PF, LaRosa SP, Dhainaut JF, Lopez-Rodriguez A, et al. Efficacy and safety of recombinant human activated protein C for severe sepsis. N Engl J Med. 2001;344(10):699–709. PubMed PMID: 11236773
16. Ranieri VM, Thompson BT, Barie PS, Dhainaut JF, Douglas IS, Finfer S, et al. Drotrecogin alfa (activated) in adults with septic shock. N Engl J Med. 2012;366(22):2055–64. PubMed PMID: 22616830

17. Kalil AC, Florescu DF. Severe sepsis: are PROWESS and PROWESS-SHOCK trials comparable? A clinical and statistical heterogeneity analysis. Crit Care. 2013;17(4):167. PubMed Central PMCID: 3706817
18. Saito H, Maruyama I, Shimazaki S, Yamamoto Y, Aikawa N, Ohno R, et al. Efficacy and safety of recombinant human soluble thrombomodulin (ART-123) in disseminated intravascular coagulation: results of a phase III, randomized, double-blind clinical trial. J Thromb Haemost. 2007;5(1):31–41. PubMed PMID: 17059423
19. Vincent JL, Ramesh MK, Ernest D, LaRosa SP, Pachl J, Aikawa N, et al. A randomized, double-blind, placebo-controlled, Phase 2b study to evaluate the safety and efficacy of recombinant human soluble thrombomodulin, ART-123, in patients with sepsis and suspected disseminated intravascular coagulation. Crit Care Med. 2013;41(9):2069–79. PubMed PMID: 23979365
20. Jaimes F, De La Rosa G, Morales C, Fortich F, Arango C, Aguirre D, et al. Unfractionated heparin for treatment of sepsis: a randomized clinical trial (The HETRASE Study). Crit Care Med. 2009;37(4):1185–96. PubMed PMID: 19242322
21. Levi M, Levy M, Williams MD, Douglas I, Artigas A, Antonelli M, et al. Prophylactic heparin in patients with severe sepsis treated with drotrecogin alfa (activated). Am J Respir Crit Care Med. 2007;176(5):483–90. PubMed PMID: 17556722
22. Zarychanski R, Abou-Setta AM, Kanji S, Turgeon AF, Kumar A, Houston DS, et al. The efficacy and safety of heparin in patients with sepsis: a systematic review and metaanalysis. Crit Care Med. 2014; Dec 9. PubMed PMID: 25493972
23. Wildhagen K, García de Frutos P, Reutelingsperger C, Schrijver R, Areste C. Ortega-Gomez et al. Nonanticoagulant heparin prevents histone-mediated cytotoxicity in vitro and improves survival in sepsis. Blood. 2014;123(7):1098–101. PubMed PMID: 24264231.
24. Brinkman V, Reichard U, Goosmann C, Fauler B, Uhlemann Y, Weiss DS, et al. Neutrophil extracellular traps kill bacteria. Science. 2004;303(5663):1532–5. Pub Med PMID: 15001782.
25. Clark SR, Ma AC, Tavener SA, McDonald B, Goodarzi Z, Kelly MM, et al. Platelet TLR4 activates neutrophil extracellular traps to ensnare bacteria in septic blood. Nat Med. 2007;13(4):463–9. Pub Med PMID: 17384648.
26. Xu J, Zhang X, Pelayo R, Monestier M, Ammollo CT, Semeraro F, et al. Extracellular histones are major mediators of death in sepsis. Nat Med. 2009;15(11):1318–21. Pub Med PMID: 19855397.
27. Saffarzadeh M, Juenemann C, Queisser MA, Lochnit G, Barreto G, Galuska SP, et al. Neutrophil extracellular traps directly induce epithelial and endothelial cell death: a predominant role of histones. PLoS One. 2012;7(2):e32366. PubMed PMID: 22389696.
28. Aird WC. The role of the endothelium in severe sepsis and multiple organ dysfunction syndrome. Blood. 2003;101(10):3765–77. PubMed PMID: 12543869
29. Schouten M, Wiersinga WJ, Levi M, van der Poll T. Inflammation, endothelium, and coagulation in sepsis. J Leukoc Biol. 2008;83(3):536–45. PubMed PMID: 19751574
30. Levi M, van der Poll T. Endothelial injury in sepsis. Intensive Care Med. 2013;39(10):1839–42. PubMed PMID: 23925547
31. Bockmeyer CL, Claus RA, Budde U, Kentouche K, Schneppenheim R, Losche W, et al. Inflammation-associated ADAMTS13 deficiency promotes formation of ultra-large von Willebrand factor. Haematologica. 2008;93(1):137–40. PubMed PMID: 18166799
32. de Stoppelaar SF, van 't Veer C, van der Poll T. The role of platelets in sepsis. Thromb Haemost. 2014;112(4):666–77. PubMed PMID: 24966015
33. Opal SM, van der Poll T. Endothelial barrier dysfunction in septic shock. J Intern Med. 2015;277(3):277–93. doi:10.1111/joim.12331. PubMed PMID: 25418337
34. Sevigny LM, Zhang P, Bohm A, Lazarides K, Perides G, Covic L, et al. Interdicting protease-activated receptor-2-driven inflammation with cell-penetrating pepducins. Proc Natl Acad Sci U S A. 2011;108(20):8491–6. PubMed PMID: 21536878
35. Covic L, Gresser AL, Talavera J, Swift S, Kuliopulos A. Activation and inhibition of G protein-coupled receptors by cell-penetrating membrane-tethered peptides. Proc Natl Acad Sci U S A. 2002;99(2):643–8. PubMed PMID: 11805322

36. Kaneider NC, Leger AJ, Agarwal A, Nguyen N, Perides G, Derian C, et al. 'Role reversal' for the receptor PAR1 in sepsis-induced vascular damage. Nat Immunol. 2007;8(12):1303–12. PubMed PMID: 179657:1303–12.

37. Lee WL, Slutsky AS. Sepsis and endothelial permeability. N Engl J Med. 2010;363(7):689–91. PubMed PMID: 20818861

38. London NR, Zhu W, Bozza FA, Smith MC, Greif DM, Sorensen LK, et al. Targeting Robo4-dependent Slit signaling to survive the cytokine storm in sepsis and influenza. Sci Transl Med. 2010;2:23ra19. PubMed PMID: 20375003

39. Cohen J, Vincent J-L, Adhikari FR, Machado F, Angus D, Calandra T, et al. Sepsis: a roadmap for future research. Lancet Infect Dis. 2015;15:581–614.

40. Dominguez J, Samocha A, Liang Z, Burd EM, Farris AB, Coopersmith CM. Inhibition of IKKB in enterocytes exacerbates sepsis-induced intestinal injury and worsens mortality. Crit Care Med. 2013;41:e275–85. PubMed PMID: 23939348.

41. Deutchman CS, Tracey KJ. Sepsis: current dogma and new perspectives. Immunity. 2014;40:463–75. PubMed PMID: 24745331

42. Human Microbiome Project C. Structure, function and diversity of the healthy human microbiome. Nature. 2012;486(7402):207–14. PubMed PMID: 22699609

43. Pearce MM, Hilt EE, Rosenfeld AB, Zilliox JM, Thomas-White K, Fok C, et al. The female urinary microbiome: a comparison of women with and without urgency urinary incontinence. mBio. 2014;5:1–12. PubMed PMID: 25006228.

44. Blaser MJ. The microbiome revolution. J Clin Invest. 2014;124(10):4162–5. PubMed PMID: 25271724

45. Fink M, Warren H. Strategies to improve drug development for sepsis. Nat Rev Drug Discov. 2014;10:1–18. PubMed PMID: 25190187

46. Nair V, Soraisham A. Probiotics and prebiotics: role in prevention of nosocomial sepsis in preterm infants. Int J Pediatr. 2013;2013:1–8. Article 874726, PubMed PMID: 23401695

47. Weichert S, Schroten H, Adam R. The role of prebiotics and probiotics in prevention and treatment of childhood infectious diseases. Pediatr Infect Dis J. 2012;31(8):859–62. PubMed PMID: 22801095

48. Novak J, Katz J. Probiotics and prebiotics for gastrointestinal infections. Curr Infect Dis Rep. 2006;8(2):103–9. PubMed PMID: 16524546

49. Strunk T, Koilmann T, Patola S. Probiotics to prevent early-life infection. Lancet Infect Dis. 2015;15:378–9. PubMed PMID: 25942569

50. Besselink MG, van Santvoort HC, Renooij W, de Smet MB, Fischer K, Timmerman HM, et al. Intestinal barrier dysfunction in a randomized trial of a specific probiotic composition in acute pancreatitis. Ann Surg. 2009;250:712–9. PubMed PMID: 19801929.

51. Zaborin A, Defazio J, Kade M, Deatherage Kaiser BL, Belogortseva N, Camp II DG, et al. Phosphatecontaining Polyethylene glycol polymers prevent lethal sepsis by multidrug-resistant pathogens. Antimicrob Agents Chemother. 2014;58:966–77. PubMed PMID: 24277029.

52. Buffie C, Bucci V, Stein R, McKenney P, Ling L, Gobourne A, et al. Precision microbiome reconstitution restores tile acid mediated resistance to Clostridium difficile. Nature. 2014. doi:10.1038/nature13828. PubMed PMID: 25337874.

53. Egea L, McAllister C, Lakhdari O, Minev I, Shenouda S, Kagnoff MF, et al. GM-CSF produced by non-hematopoietic cells in required for early epithelial cell proliferation and repair of injured colonic mucosa. J Immunol. 2013;190(4):1702–13. PubMed PMID: 233258.

54. Liu Y. Hepatocyte growth factor promotes renal epithelial cell survival by dual mechanisms. Am J Physiol. 1999;277(4 Pt 2):F624–33. PubMed PMID: 10516287

55. Opal SM, Keith JC, Jhung J, Parejo N, Marchese E, Maganti V, et al. Orally administered recombinant human interleukin-11 is protective in experimental neutropenic sepsis. J Infect Dis. 2003;187:70–6. PubMed PMID: 12508148.

56. Xu MJ, Feng D, Wang H, Guan Y, Yan X, Gao B, et al. IL-22 ameliorates renal ischemia-reperfusion injury by targeting proximal tubule epithelium. J Am Soc Nephrol. 2014;25:967–77. PubMed: 24459233.

57. Hunninghake GW, Doerschug KC, Nymon AB, Schmidt GA, Meyerholz DK, Ashare A, et al. Insulin-like growth factor-1 levels contribute to the development of bacterial translocation in sepsis. Am J Respir Crit Care Med. 2010;182:517–25. PubMed PMID: 20413631.

58. Kolodziej L, Lodolce J, Chang J, Schneider J, Grimm W, Bartulis S, et al. TNFAIP3 maintains intestinal barrier function and supports epithelial cell tight junctions. PLoS One. 2011;6:1–11. PubMed PMID: 22031828.

59. Yang R, Harada T, Mollen KP, Prince JM, Levy RM, Englert JA, et al. Anti-HMGB1 neutralizing antibody ameliorates gut barrier dysfunction and improves survival after hemorrhagic shock. Mol Med. 2006;12:105–14. PubMed PMID: 16953558.

60. Qin S, Wang H, Yuan R, Li H, Ochani M, Ochani K, et al. Role of HMGV1 in apoptosis-mediated sepsis lethality. J Exp Med. 2006;203:1637–42. PubMed PMID: 16818669.

61. Li J, Kokkola R, Tabibzadeh S, Yang R, Ochani M, Qiang X, et al. Structural basis for the proinflammatory cytokine activity of high mobility group box 1. Mol Med. 2003;9:37–45. PubMed PMID: 12765338.

62. Fiuza C, Bustin M, Talwar S, Tropea M, Gertenberger E, Shelhamer JH, et al. Inflammation-promoting activity of HMGB1 on human microvascular endothelial cells. Blood. 2003;101:2652–60. PubMed PMID: 14684474

63. Wolfson RK, Chiang ET, Garcia JGN. HMGB1 induces human lung endothelial cell cytoskeletal rearrangement and barrier disruption. Microvasc Res. 2011;81(2):189–97. PubMed PMID: 21146549

64. Huang W, Liu Y, Li L, Zhang R, Liu W, Wu J, et al. HMGB1 increases permeability of the endothelial cell monolayer via RAGE and Src family tyrosine kinases. Inflammation. 2012;35(1):350–62. PubMed PMID: 21494799

65. Chavan SS, Huerta PT, Robbiati S, Valdes-Ferrer SI, Ochani M, Dancho M, et al. HMGB1 Mediates cognitive impairment in sepsis survivors. Mol Med. 2012;18:930–7. PubMed PMID: 22634723.

66. Jeong SJ, Lim BJ, Park S, Choi D, Kim HW, Ku NS, et al. The effect of sRAGE-Fc fusion protein attenuates inflammation and decreases mortality in a murine cecal ligation and puncture model. Inflamm Res. 2012;61:1211–8. PubMed PMID: 22777145.

67. DiNubile M. Adjunctive treatment of severe sepsis. Lancet Infect Dis. 2013;13:917–8. PubMed PMID: 24156894

68. Cruz DN, Perazella MA, Bellomo R, de Cal M, Polanco N, Corradi V, et al. Effectiveness of polymyxin B-immobilized fiber column in sepsis: a systematic review. Crit Care. 2007;11(2):R47. PubMed PMID: 17448226.

69. Basu R, Pathak S, Goyal J, Chaudhry R, Goel R, et al. Use of a novel hemoadsorption device for cytokine removal as adjuvant therapy in a patient with septic shock with multi-organ dysfunction: a case study. Indian J Crit Care Med. 2014;18(12):822–4. PubMed PMID: 25538418

70. Honore P, Jacobs R, Joannes-Boyau O, De Regt J, De Waele E. Newly designed CRRT membranes for sepsis and SIRS—a pragmatic approach for bedside intensivists summarizing the more recent advances: a systematic structured review. ASAIO J. 2013;59(2):99–106. PubMed PMID: 23438770

71. Kang JH, Super M, Yung DW, Cooper RM, Domansky K. An extracorporeal blood-cleansing device for sepsis therapy. Nat Med. 2014;20(10):1211–6. PubMed PMID: 25216635

72. McCrea K, Wart R, LaRosa S. Removal of Carbapenem-Resistant Enterobacteriaceae (CRE) from blood by heparin-functional hemoperfusion media. PLoS One. 2014;9(12):e114242.

73. Delano FA, Hoyt DB, Schmid-Schonbein GW. Pancreatic digestive enzyme blockade in the intestine increases survival after experimental shock. Sci Transl Med. 2013;5:169ra11. PubMed PMID: 23345609

74. Brealey D, Brand M, Hargreaves I, Heales S, Land J, Smolenski R, et al. Association between mitochondrial dysfunction and severity and outcome of septic shock. Lancet. 2002;360:219–23. PubMed PMID: 1133657

75. Singer M. The role of mitochondrial dysfunction in sepsis-induced multi-organ failure. Virulence. 2014;5:66–72. PubMed PMID: 24185508

76. Maldonado A, Gerriets V, Rathmell J. Matched and mismatched metabolic fuels in lymphocyte function. Semin Immunol. 2012;24:405–13. PubMed PMID: 23290889

77. McGettrick A, O'Neill A. How metabolism generates signals during innate immunity and inflammation. J Biol Chem. 2013;288:22893–8. PubMed PMID: 23798679

78. Artenstein A, Opal SM. Proprotein convertases in health and disease. N Engl J Med. 2011;365:2507–18. PubMed PMID: 22204726

79. Walley KR, Thain KR, Russell JA, Reilly MP, Meyer NJ, Ferguson JF, et al. PCSK9 is a critical regulator of the innate immune response and septic shock outcome. Sci Transl Med. 2014;6:1–10. PubMed PMID: 25320235.

80. Spite M, Norling LV, Summers L, Yang R, Cooper D, Petasis NA, et al. Resolvin D2 is a potent regulator of leukocytes and controls microbial sepsis. Nature. 2009;461:1287–91. PubMed PMID: 19865173.

81. Hotchkiss R, Monneret G, Payen D. Sepsis-induced immunosuppression: from cellular dysfunctions to immunotherapy. Nat Rev Immunol. 2013;13:862–74. PubMed PMID: 24232462

82. Hotchkiss RS, Opal SM. Immunotherapy for sepsis: a new approach against an ancient foe. N Engl J Med. 2010;363(1):87–9. PubMed PMID: 20592301

83. Kalil AC, Florescu DR. Prevalence and mortality associated with cytomegalovirus infection in nonimmunosuppressed patients in the intensive care unit. Crit Care Med. 2009;37(8):2350–8. PubMed PMID: 18531944

84. Walton AH, Muenzer JT, Rasche D, Boomer JS, Sato B, Brownstein BH, et al. Reactivation of multiple viruses in patients with sepsis. PLoS One. 2014;9(6):e98819.PubMed PMID: 24919177

85. DeVlaminck I, Khush K, Strehl C, Kohli B, Luikart H, Neff NF, et al. Temporal response of the human virome to immunosuppression and antiviral therapy. Cell. 2013;155:1178–87. PubMed PMID: 24267896.

86. Wu J, Zhou L, Liu J, Ma G, Kou Q, He Z, et al. The efficacy of thymosin alpha 1 for severe sepsis (ETASS): a multicenter, single-blind, randomized and controlled trial. Crit Care. 2013;17(1):R8. PubMed PMID: 23327199.

87. Unsinger J, Burnham CA, McDonough J, Morre M, Prakash PS, Caldwell CC, et al. Interleukin 7 ameliorates immune dysfunction and improves survival in a two hit model of fungal sepsis. J Infect Dis. 2012;206(4):606–16. PubMed PMID: 22693226.

88. Inoue S, Unsinger J, Davis CG, Muenzer JT, Ferguson TA, Chang K, et al. IL-15 prevents apoptosis, reverses innate and adaptive immune dysfunction, and improves survival in sepsis. J Immunol. 2010;184:1401–9. PubMed PMID: 20026737.

89. Walter J, Ware L, Matthay M. Mesenchymal stem cells: mechanisms of potential therapeutic benefit in ARDS and sepsis. Lancet. 2014;2:1016–26. PubMed PMID: 25465643

90. Chahin A, Opal S, Zorzopulos J, Jobes D, Migdady Y, et al. The noval immunotherapeutic oligodeoxynucleotide IMT504 protects neutropenic animals from fatal Pseudomonas aeruginosa bacteremia and sepsis. Antimicrob Agents Chemother. 2015;59(2):1225–9. PubMed PMID: 25512413.

91. Elias F, Flo J, Lopez RA, Zorzopulos J, Montaner A, Rodriguez JM, et al. Strong cytosine quanosine-independent immunostimulation in humans and other primates by synthetic oligodeoxynucleotides with PyNTTTTGT motifs. J Immunol. 2003;171(7):3697–704. PubMed PMID: 14500668.

92. Cavaillon J-M, Eisen D, Annane D. Is boosting the immune system in sepsis appropriate? Crit Care Med. 2014;18:216. PubMed PMID: 24886820

93. Osuuchowski M, Connett J, Welch K, Granger J, Remick D, et al. Stratification is the key: inflammatory biomarkers accurately direct immunomodulatory therapy in experimental sepsis. Crit Care Med. 2009;37:1576–72. PubMed PMID: 24238100.

94. Ramachandran G, Kaempfer R, Chung CS, Shirvan A, Chahin AB, Palardy J, et al. CD 28 homodimer interface mimetic peptide as a novel inhibitor in experimental models of gram negative sepsis. J Infect Dis. 2014. PubMed PMID: 25305323.

95. Ramachandran G, Tulapurkar ME, Harris KM, Arad G, Shivran A, Shemesh R, et al. A peptide antagonist of CD 28 signaling attenuates toxic shock and necrotizing soft tissue infection induced by *Streptococcus pyogenes*. J Infect Dis. 2013;206(12):1869–77. PubMed PMID: 23493729

96. Bulger EM, Maier RV, Sperry J, Joshi M, Henry S, Moore FA, et al. A novel drug for treatment of necrotizing soft tissue infections: results of a phase 2a randomized controlled trial of AB103, a CD28 co-stimulatory receptor modulator. JAMA Surg. 2014. doi:10.1001/jamasurg.2013.4841. PubMed PMID:24740134.

Part III

Chapter 7
Mechanisms of Organ Dysfunction and Altered Metabolism in Sepsis

Douglas R. Closser, Mathew C. Exline, and Elliott D. Crouser

Sepsis Overview

The term "sepsis" was first described by Hippocrates (c.a. 460–370 BC) in reference to blood putrefaction (septicemia) and fever, and the connection between sepsis and bacteria was made by French chemist Louis Pasteur (1822–1895). No treatment has been shown to prevent the onset or hasten recovery of failed organ systems during sepsis, which often persists long after the infection has been eliminated and ultimately leads to the death of the patient. Mechanisms linking host-pathogen interactions to organ dysfunction remain poorly understood and related insights may provide the key to more effectively treating sepsis-induced organ failures. This chapter will discuss the current theories of sepsis-induced organ failure and potential future therapies that might be derived from new understanding of the pathophysiology of sepsis.

Severe Sepsis and Organ Dysfunction

As discussed in preceding chapters, sepsis is historically defined as the presence of two of the four systemic inflammatory response syndrome (SIRS) criteria and a known or suspected infection. The definition of sepsis is limited by the nonspecific nature of the SIRS criteria which can be manifested in many diseases and even in healthy subjects undergoing physical or emotional stress. It is also limited by the difficulty in detecting or confirming infections.

D.R. Closser, MD • M.C. Exline, MD • E.D. Crouser, MD (✉)
Division of Pulmonary, Critical Care, and Sleep Medicine, The Ohio State
University Wexner Medical Center, Columbus, OH 43210, USA
e-mail: closser15@gmail.com; matthew.exline@osumc.edu; elliott.crouser@osumc.edu

© Springer International Publishing AG 2017
N.S. Ward, M.M. Levy (eds.), *Sepsis*, Respiratory Medicine,
DOI 10.1007/978-3-319-48470-9_7

As displayed in Table 7.1, any vital organ can be adversely affected by sepsis. The extreme diversity of presentations both in terms of severity of organ dysfunction and heterogeneity of organ involvement has historically prompted investigators to look for systemic and unifying mechanisms of organ dysfunction, rather than considering organ-specific mechanisms. In this regard, circulating toxins released from infectious organisms and activated immune cells and/or alterations in the distribution of vital metabolic substrates are most commonly incriminated in the pathogenesis of sepsis-induced organ failures. However, these simplistic models of disease have not held up to scientific scrutiny, and new paradigms are emerging to explain the vital organ dysfunction in the context of sepsis.

The Spectrum of Organ Damage during Human Sepsis and Septic Shock

Before considering the likely mechanisms contributing to organ failures during human sepsis, which is most often gleaned from animal models, it is important to first establish what is observed to exist in humans. Beyond the physiological (e.g., fever, tachycardia, tachypnea, hypotension, lactic acidosis) and peripheral immune (e.g., leukocytosis or leukopenia) manifestations of sepsis, relatively little is known about the mechanisms contributing directly to organ failures in humans. Unfortunately, meaningful real-time analyses of the altered cells and tissues of failing organs are not feasible in living humans in the hospital setting, and mechanisms must be inferred from tissue specimens derived from nonvital organs (e.g., blood, skeletal muscle), imaging studies, or from post-mortem examinations.

Post-mortem examination of failed organs in the context of sepsis is logistically complicated and rarely feasible within a timeframe that would provide useful information. This is mainly due to the rapid degradation of the tissues and the need for immediate tissue harvesting. Several studies have overcome these obstacles and have provided critical insights into the likely mechanisms of sepsis-induced organ failures. An interesting series of investigations performed in the late 1970s sought to determine the ultrastructural changes in vital organs in the context of acute, overwhelming, and ultimately fatal septic shock [1, 2]. For example, one of the septic patients selected for these studies developed refractory shock with multiple organ failures and death within 24 h of acute bowel perforation. This scenario is uncommon in modern ICUs due to rapid resuscitation protocols. Nonetheless, ultrastructural analysis of the vital organs in those who died acutely of septic shock revealed widespread endoplasmic reticulum (ER) and mitochondrial swelling and disruption of mitochondrial structures with evidence of extensive cell necrosis. By contrast, those who survived the early phase of shock only to die of sustained multiple organ failures had evidence of extensive autophagocytosis, which is in keeping with attempts to remove damaged cellular components to avoid cell death. It was further noted that delayed deaths in septic shock were associated with a discrepancy between profound organ failure and the paucity of ultrastructural abnormalities.

Table 7.1 Features of organ failure in sepsis

Organ	Clinical findings	Histopathology	Reversible mechanisms	Irreversible mechanisms
Lungs	• Pulmonary edema • Hypoxemia • Hypercarbia or hypocarbia	• Edema (alveolar + interstitial) • Lamellar bodies • Type I pneumonocyte necrosis/apoptosis • Inflammation (early) • Fibrosis (late)	• Endothelial damage • Surfactant deficiency • Epithelial damage/dysfunction • Vasoregulatory defects	• Pulmonary fibrosis • Pulmonary hypertension • Ventilation-perfusion mismatch
Heart	• Normal or ↓ LVEF • Dilated right ventricle • Mild troponin elevation • Arrhythmias (atrial > ventricular) • Abnormal T2 signal by MRI	• Minimal myocyte damage • Minimal edema • Minimal inflammatory cell infiltration	• Changes in calcium regulation • Oxidative stress • "Hibernation" through HIF-1α pathway • Mitochondrial dysfunction	• Myocardial remodeling

Kidneys	• Elevated BUN and creatinine
	• Decreased GFR
	• Abnormal casts by urinalysis
		• Moderate to severe acute tubular necrosis
		• Minimal glomerulosclerosis
		• Minimal edema
		• Minimal apoptosis
		• Intact vasculature
			• Hypoperfusion
			  – Regional vasoregulation
			  – Systemic hypotension
			• Oxidative stress
			• Mitochondrial defects
			• Endothelial dysfunction
				• Glomerulosclerosis (rare)

Liver	• Reduced albumin • Elevated transaminases • Mild cholestasis • Coagulopathy • Hypoglycemia (less common)	• Edema • Minimal periportal inflammation • Necrosis (uncommon except in septic shock) • Minimal inflammatory cell infiltration	• Reprogramming of metabolic pathways • Mitochondrial autophagy • Oxidative stress • Endothelial injury • Activation of Kupffer cells by gut microbial leakage • Suppression of complement • Impaired microbial clearance	• Irreversible injury is unusual
Brain	• Altered mental status (delirium) • Nonspecific EEG alterations • Status epilepticus • Cerebral infarction • Leukoencephal-opathy	• Usually normal • Localized cell death observed in fatal septic shock	• Oxidative stress • Mitochondrial dysfunction • Endothelial damage (e.g., blood-brain barrier defects) • Inflammation	• Localized cell death (rarely) • White matter changes • Cause of long-term cognitive dysfunction

These early observations were substantiated in a more recent study by Takasu et al. wherein immediate autopsy was performed on patients who survived the early phases of severe sepsis or septic shock and had died thereafter during "chronic sepsis" (on average ~6 days after sepsis onset). Despite ongoing hemodynamic instability and renal dysfunction at the time of death, these patients were noted to have moderate degrees of mitochondrial swelling and autophagocytosis in the heart and kidneys with minimal cell death or signs of irreversible damage (e.g., fibrosis) [3]. In a comparable study, cardiac magnetic resonance imaging performed on severe sepsis survivors in a late stage of the disease (on average 6 days after sepsis onset) demonstrated a dramatic increase in mid-myocardial T2 signal intensity, in a non-ischemic pattern (i.e., sparing the endomyocardium), which implies altered metabolism or inflammation [4]. These findings are consistent with other observations in septic humans and animals, discussed in the following sections, challenging the notion that impaired tissue perfusion is primarily responsible for altered organ function in the setting of sepsis.

Host-Pathogen Interactions and Induction of Organ Failures

The observed nearly simultaneous or rapidly sequential failing of organs during sepsis implies a common and widespread process. Though systemic oxygen and other energy substrate deliveries (e.g., glucose, ketones) may be impaired under extreme circumstances with refractory septic shock, systemic blood flow is typically high and indices of tissue hypoxia are lacking during most cases of established sepsis-induced organ failures. It follows that circulating factors other than oxygen, glucose, or other metabolic substrates are contributing to organ damage and dysfunction during sepsis.

The concept of "blood poisoning" originally applied to microbial factors that are either directly or indirectly (through activation of immune cells) toxic to systemic organs. Among the first bacterial toxins to be carefully described in septic humans is a component of streptococcal bacteria that directly inhibits the action of coenzyme diphosphopyridine nucleotide (DPN). This compound inhibits numerous metabolic pathways, including constituents of the citric acid cycle, which is vital for mitochondrial oxidative metabolism [5]. There have been many other bacterial toxins described, exhibiting an array of cytopathic effects and pathological manifestations. These include virulence factors introduced into eukaryotic cells by gram-negative organisms via a direct intercellular type III secretion mechanism. Exoenzymes-S and -T are potentially cytotoxic through inhibition of vital signaling pathways (e.g., RAS) and disruption of the cytoskeleton [6]. PA-I lectin/adhesin potently disrupts vital barrier functions to allow the translocation of bacteria across epithelial barriers (e.g., the gut) [7]. A comprehensive review of this topic is beyond the scope of this chapter; however, a summary of the putative mechanisms linking host-pathogen interactions to organ failures is provided in Fig. 7.1.

Bacteria, viruses, and other pathogens commonly promote cell and organ damage indirectly through the activation of an intense immune response. This leads to the destruction of the pathogen and simultaneously causes "collateral damage" to the host.

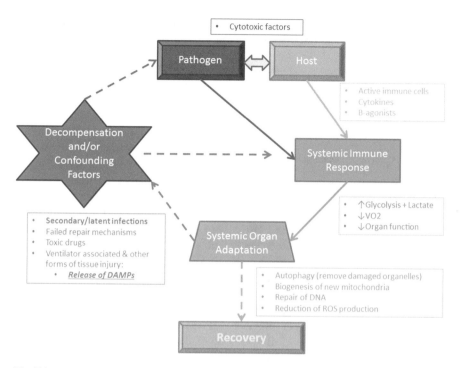

Fig. 7.1 Mechanisms of host-pathogen interaction in sepsis-related organ failure

Eukaryotic organisms have evolved a system by which common pathogen-associated molecular patterns (PAMPs) are identified to elicit a brisk counter-response by components of the immune system. The pattern recognizing receptors of the immune system, including Toll-like receptors (TLRs), nucleotide-binding oligomerization domain (NOD)-like receptors (NLRs), are somewhat specific in terms of the PAMPs to which they respond. The pattern of receptor activations leads to specialized immune responses designed to overcome the invasive features of each pathogen.

In the context of organ damage induced indirectly by the immune response to PAMPs, an important breakthrough in understanding these mechanisms was provided by Kevin Tracey and colleagues in the late 1980s. This study was the first to provide convincing evidence that tumor necrosis factor-alpha (TNFα) was produced by the host in response to bacterial infection and that release of this immune mediator was sufficient to produce a systemic inflammatory response and related organ injury equivalent to that induced by the infection itself [8]. This observation spawned a generation of research aimed to suppress the immune response during the early phases of sepsis. Despite numerous encouraging preclinical studies in animals wherein early inhibition of TNFα or other inflammatory mediators was shown to be protective, no single immune-modulating agent has proven effective in human sepsis clinical trials. The explanations for these failures are unclear, but presumably relates to the timing of therapy relative to the onset of sepsis in humans, which is often delayed by hours or days, and the complex nature of the host-immune response.

In addition to PAMPs and the robust immune response, tissue damage is capable of perpetuating the immune response through the release of host factors, referred to as "danger associated molecular patterns (DAMPs)." DAMPs are mimics of bacterial PAMPs. For instance, mitochondria are derived from bacterial ancestors and retain many bacterial features, including N-formylated proteins, hypomethylated CpG DNA, cardiolipin, ATP, and mitochondrial transcription factor A (TFAM). All of these components are immunogenic in humans. Endogenous DAMPs are normally sequestered within intact host cells only to be released during cell damage or apoptosis. There are a number of DAMPs that have been reported in the context of trauma or tissue inflammation (e.g., arthritis), but only a few are implicated in the context of sepsis. Among these, mitochondrial factors have been detected systemically during severe sepsis in animals and mitochondrial DNA is shown to serve as a biomarker of mortality in septic humans [9, 10]. However, the contribution of mitochondrial and non-mitochondrial DAMPs to the pathogenesis of sepsis-induced organ failures remains to be more clearly defined.

While it appears evident from this discussion that early intervention to prevent excessive activation of the immune response in the setting of sepsis would help reduce organ damage, there is little evidence supporting this approach in the clinical setting. Despite numerous animal studies showing that pretreatment or early treatment with anti-TNFα agents or inhibitors of PAMPS or their receptors is protective against sepsis-induced organ failures, none of the subsequent human trials (>30 randomized controlled trials) have shown a benefit to these anti-inflammatory approaches. Indeed, most patients have passed through the "hyperimmune" phase of sepsis by the time they present to the healthcare providers, which explains why these strategies are ineffective. Thus, the focus has turned to the mechanisms responsible for organ failures in the later stages of sepsis during which most mortality is observed.

Theories of Sepsis-Induced Organ Dysfunction

Oxygen Debt Versus Altered Oxygen Utilization

Early models of ICU care were based upon the premise that organ failures were primarily caused by inadequate energy substrate delivery. An influential clinical observation published in the journal *Science* in 1964 and coauthored by Max H. Weil, one of the founding members of the Society of Critical Care Medicine, demonstrated a dramatic correlation between lactic acidosis severity and mortality in critically ill patients [11]. Since lactic acidosis often is associated with systemic hypotension and with the development of organ failures, it was logical to assume that the latter was a consequence of tissue hypoperfusion or "oxygen debt." This paradigm strongly influenced patient management in the ICU setting for the past 50 years, such as the standardized use of monitoring parameters relating to tissue oxygen delivery (pulse oximetry, central venous oxygen probes), evolution of invasive (e.g., pulmonary artery catheters) and noninvasive measures of cardiac output, and efforts to monitor blood lactate levels. These parameters were used to guide therapies designed to optimize systemic oxygen delivery, based upon Eq. (7.1), wherein oxygen delivery (DO_2) is directly related to cardiac output (CO; Eq. 7.1a) and the amount of oxygen present in the blood (VO_2; Eq. 7.1b). However, it is becoming evident with time and further study that septic shock is distinct from other forms of shock and new research calls into the question the role of tissue hypoxia as a primary mechanism of organ failures in those with severe sepsis.

$$DO_2 = CO \times VO_2 \tag{7.1}$$

$$CO = stroke\ volume \times heart\ rate \tag{7.1a}$$

$$VO_2 = \left[\begin{array}{c} \left(Hgb\ g/100ml \times 1.34ml\ O_2/gm\ Hgb \times SpO_2 \times 0.01 \right) \\ +\left(0.003\ ml/mmHg \times PaO_2 \right) \end{array} \right] \tag{7.1b}$$

Based upon the common finding of lactic acidosis in the context of severe sepsis and septic shock, it has long been assumed and is presently taught in medical schools worldwide that lactic acidosis equates with inadequate tissue perfusion and portends ischemic organ injury and related organ failures. Many of the components of the Surviving Sepsis Management Bundle endorsed by the Society of Critical Care Medicine and many other institutions are focused on timely monitoring of blood lactate and correction of hemodynamic variables during the early phases of sepsis. Collectively, these measures to optimize hemodynamic parameters and to reverse lactic acidosis during sepsis are referred to as "Early Goal-Directed Therapy" (EGDT). However, a number of studies conducted in patients with established severe sepsis (with organ failures) failed to show a benefit to enhancing or "optimizing" systemic oxygen delivery either through the use of ionotropic therapies or by increasing the oxygen carrying capacity of the blood [12, 13]. In fact, the use of ionotropic agents showed a trend toward increased sepsis mortality. Likewise, efforts to optimize systemic oxygen delivery using pulmonary artery catheters to guide therapy have not been shown to improve mortality [14]. Most recently, the efficacy of EGDT has been questioned by a large study published in the *New England Journal of Medicine* showing no clinical benefit relative to standard care [15, 16]. Finally, efforts to augment tissue perfusion by addressing potential mismatching of perfusion with energy substrate utilization at the microvascular level (i.e., microcirculatory dysfunction) with a potent vasodilator (nitric oxide) have shown no benefit in the setting of sepsis-induced organ failures and did not reduce lactate levels [17, 18]. These studies imply that impaired tissue perfusion at either macro- or micro-circulatory levels is not the primary cause of organ failures during sepsis.

The apparent disconnect between lactic acidosis and tissue perfusion is obviated when one considers the challenges of interpreting lactic acidosis in critically ill patients. In this regard, pyruvate is a critical metabolite of glucose metabolism that serves as a substrate for the efficient formation of high energy phosphates through aerobic respiration. The conversion of pyruvate to lactate is favored in the setting of impaired mitochondrial respiration, disruption of the citric acid cycle, or inhibition of pyruvate dehydrogenase (PDH). In the context of tissue hypoxia, the ratio of lactate to pyruvate is relatively high, whereas there is a relative increase in pyruvate in the setting of cytopathic alterations, such as PDH inhibition or mitochondrial dysfunction. Research studies conducted in septic humans confirm that the lactate/pyruvate profile is not in keeping with the tissue hypoxia paradigm, and is more consistent with inhibition of PDH, and/or altered mitochondrial respiration [19]. Indeed, animal models indicate that both PDH inhibition and altered mitochondrial respiration, as well as inhibited lactate clearance by the liver and kidneys, may all contribute to elevated lactate levels during severe sepsis.

Given that the profile of lactic acidosis during sepsis is not adequately explained by tissue hypoxia and assuming that tissue hypoxia is deleterious to organ function, how do we interpret measures of tissue oxygen delivery in the clinical setting? Systemic oxygen during sepsis is commonly elevated and is characterized by increased cardiac output, low systemic vascular resistance, and enhanced tissue blood flow (e.g., warm, hyperemic skin). Adequate tissue oxygen delivery during septic shock is supported by measures of effluent venous blood (SvO_2) and by indirect measures of tissue oxygenation in animal sepsis models [20]. Moreover, serum derived from patients with sepsis is capable of altering mitochondrial and cellular respiration in normal human cells, indicating the presence of circulating factors capable of altering oxygen metabolism at the cell and tissue level, and independent of blood flow or tissue energy substrate availability [21].

Additional clinical evidence favoring a cytopathic cause of organ failures during sepsis is provided by recent well-publicized clinical trials. As noted previously, a large study (1600 septic patients) performed in Australia demonstrated that early, aggressive resuscitation measures designed to optimize systemic oxygen delivery using EGDT in the early phase of sepsis had no effect on any patient outcome (e.g., mortality, duration of organ support) [15]. Other studies have indicated that the only interventions that significantly alter the clinical course of sepsis are early antibiotics and strategies to reduce ventilator-associated lung injury [22, 23].

Furthermore, human studies show that altered mitochondrial function, particularly Complex I-activity, and related changes in high energy phosphate levels are highly predictive of sepsis mortality [24, 25]. Based upon the existing evidence, it can be said that current sepsis protocols, which include intravascular volume resuscitation to optimize systemic blood flow and related oxygen delivery, provide adequate hemodynamic support during sepsis. Moreover, progress toward preventing and reversing organ failures in the context of sepsis should consider other disease mechanisms.

Systemic Inflammation, Organ Injury, and the "Cytokine Storm"

Another compelling explanation for the pathogenesis of sepsis-induced organ dysfunction is the concept of an "inflammatory storm," often attributed to Dr. Lewis Thomas in his 1972 article [26]. The concept is that it is not the pathogen that results in organ-failure, but rather it is the host's immune response to infection and resulting "collateral damage" that is responsible. This theory was strongly supported by investigations carried out by Kevin Tracey's group in the 1980s showing for the first time that cytokines, such as TNFα, are capable of recapitulating the systemic inflammatory response as occurs in the setting or experimental sepsis or endotoxemia [8]. The theory was further supported by preclinical studies showing that suppression of TNFα prior to onset of sepsis, conferred potent protection in terms of mortality [27]. However, subsequent clinical trials have shown no benefit of anti-TNFα antibodies or other proinflammatory molecule inhibitors (e.g., activated protein C) in septic humans [28]. This is presumably because the recognition and treatment of sepsis in humans is often delayed such that the therapeutic window is missed.

With advances in the supportive care of critically ill patients within the past 20 years, many more septic patients survive the acute hyper-inflammatory phase of sepsis only to die days or weeks later. The cause of delayed deaths in septic patients is currently unknown. It is noted that as many as 50% of these patients develop secondary infections with organisms that are not typically pathogenic in immune competent hosts (e.g., candida species) [29, 30]. Additionally, reactivation of latent infections, such as CMV, has been shown to significantly increase mortality risk [31]. The cause of immune suppression is complex and discussed in another chapter. It is unclear if immune suppression and related secondary infections further delay or exacerbate organ failures. However, it is apparent that suppression of the immune response is not a viable treatment for patients during the late phases of sepsis, which represents a growing majority of hospitalized and institutionalized sepsis patients. Thus, other mechanisms to reverse organ failures need to be considered. If such therapies could be identified there is hope that septic patients will be liberated from life support devices and discharged from ICUs and hospitals, such that the associated risks of secondary infections would be minimized.

Mechanisms of Altered Metabolism during Sepsis

The Early "Cytopathic" Phase of Sepsis

The early phase of sepsis is often associated with dramatic changes in the patient as they progress from localized infection to severe sepsis or septic shock (Table 7.2). In cases of acutely fatal septic shock, there is widespread tissue damage evident during histological and ultrastructural analyses in vital organs [1]. However, the

Table 7.2 Common clinical manifestations of sepsis, severe sepsis, and septic shock

Clinical findings	Localized infection	Sepsis	Severe sepsis	Septic shock
Symptoms	• Fever • Localized symptoms at the site of infection	• Fever • Chills • Rigors • Malaise • Diaphoresis • Hypokinetic • Dyspnea • Loss of appetite • +/− Localizing symptoms	• Altered mental status • Oliguria	• Moribund
Vital signs	• Fever • Otherwise stable	• Fever or hypothermia • Tachycardia • Tachypnea	• Meet multiple SIRS criteria with normal blood pressure	• Meet multiple SIRS criteria • Hypotension
Exam findings	• Localizing signs of infection	• Acutely ill appearing • Anxious, alert and responsive • +/− accessory respiratory muscle use, crackles on lung exam • Warm extremities • Normal pulses	• Somnolent or disoriented	• Unresponsive or delirious • Warm extremities (occasionally cool extremities) • Thready pulses

severity and extent of vital organ injury is probably much less in most septic patients. As will be discussed in the following sections, those who survive the early phase of sepsis and go on to die days or weeks later have little evidence of cell death or irreversible cell or tissue damage. Despite the relatively favorable histology findings, none of the treatments currently available have demonstrable benefits in terms of reversing organ damage. Thus, a better understanding of the mechanisms contributing to organ failures during the late phase of sepsis will likely be required to identify novel treatments.

Metabolic Compensation During Established Sepsis

Mitochondria are vital for the function of cells and organs, and are vulnerable to injury during sepsis. In addition to their well-known functions relating to aerobic energy metabolism, mitochondria are the major source of potentially toxic reactive oxygen species (ROS) and are critical regulators of cell death. Mitochondria are dynamic in that new ones are produced to match the metabolic needs of the cell. Similarly, senescent or damaged mitochondria or unneeded mitochondria (e.g., during fasting) are efficiently removed during the lifespan of most cells.

This mitochondrial turnover allows for the adaptation of cells to the environment. Changes in mitochondrial mass and increases in mitochondrial turnover are common during acute illnesses, such as the acute phase of sepsis. Autophagy selectively targets de-energized mitochondria and leads to reduced mitochondrial mass and net improvement in cellular efficiency [9].

Whereas many inflammatory mediators likely contribute to altered metabolism, TNFα is a prototypical mediator of the sepsis syndrome [27] and is capable of causing profound mitochondrial dysfunction. TNFα is released from activated mononuclear cells in response to various pathogen-associated mediators, such as lipopolysaccharide, and the release of TNFα is further regulated by the sympathetic and parasympathetic nervous systems [32]. TNFα binds to a number of TNF receptors, which promotes the intracellular release of ceramide and also the production of reactive oxygen species (ROS) formation, which are known to favor mitochondria dysfunction. TNF receptor activation promotes NF-kB pro-inflammatory pathways in various immune cells including PMNs and monocytes, which strongly induces ROS formation leading to mitochondrial DNA damage and inhibition of mitochondrial complex activities in exposed cells. Inhibition of mitochondrial complexes favors diversion of electrons through the Q-cycle to produce even more ROS. Ultimately, the formation of ROS exceeds the robust mitochondrial antioxidant mechanisms (manganese superoxide dismutase, glutathione reductase) which can trigger a catastrophic mitochondrial deenergization relating to the opening of mitochondrial "permeability transition pores" (PTP) [33]. The resulting mitochondrial permeability transition leads to dissolution of the electrochemical gradient required to form ATP and these deenergized mitochondria are targeted for removal via "self-ingestion" (i.e., autophagy) by lysosomes. Widespread induction of the mitochondrial PTP involving many mitochondria simultaneously can promote necrotic or programmed cell death (apoptosis). Finally, TNFα also inhibits mitochondrial biogenesis, in part through induction of HIF1a by inflammatory mechanisms [34, 35]. Thus, systemic TNFα release in the early phase of sepsis leads to a net reduction in mitochondrial mass and impaired mitochondrial function. It is also apparent that inflammatory mediators, such as TNFα, can alter the status of mitochondria during sepsis thereby influencing the viability and function of cells and vital organs through the induction of cell death, as noted above. In keeping with the notion that mitochondrial depletion contributes to organ failures, animal models of sepsis indicate that restoration of mitochondrial populations through biogenesis pathways is essential for recovery from sepsis [36].

Altered Function of Other Metabolic Pathways During Sepsis

In addition to changes in mitochondrial mass, qualitative changes in mitochondrial function and a shift toward glycolytic pathways are regulated by various hormones, enzymes, and regulatory pathways within the cells. Oxidant stress, particularly reactive derivatives of nitric oxide and superoxide anion (peroxynitrite), promote glycolysis by activating the rate-limiting step of the pentose pathway, glucose-6-phosphate dehydrogenase. The pentose pathway, in turn, leads to the formation of NADPH in favor of NADH. Whereas NADH is the substrate for high-energy phosphate formation mitochondrial oxidative phosphorylation, NADPH is vital for the formation and repair of proteins, DNA, and lipids. Consequently, by diverting glycolytic intermediates from the Kreb's cycle to suppress aerobic mitochondrial respiration, the cells and tissues transition to a state of reduced oxygen consumption and lower ATP production. This is commonly referred to (e.g., in the context of cancer) as the "Warburg effect." Under these circumstances, the cells and tissues are less reliant upon oxidative metabolism, thereby reducing oxidative stress and promoting the formation of reducing equivalents (e.g., Lactic acid, NADPH) that favor cell repair [37]. The Warburg effect and related mediators, such as HIF1α, are shown to be induced under conditions modeling sepsis [38] and confer cytoprotection in vital organs and inhibit inflammation under conditions of acute cell stress [39, 40]. However, HIF-1α activation in immune cells is shown to perpetuate pro-inflammatory pathway activation as well [41]. This serves as to remind us of the complex mechanisms at play during sepsis and why attempts to block any specific molecular target have failed to improve outcomes.

In addition to altered glucose metabolism, sepsis promotes the mobilization of free fatty acids (FFA) from fat stores and amino acids from skeletal muscle. FFA may be converted to ketones by the liver or directly metabolized by tissues to promote mitochondrial ATP formation. Amino acids released from muscle, particularly glutamine, are variably converted to acute phase proteins or deaminated to form urea by the liver [42]. Alternatively, amino acids can also serve as a mitochondrial energy substrate or can be recycled for the purpose of replacing damaged proteins in other vital organs. Thus, nonvital fat and skeletal muscle is scavenged to preserve vital organs (Fig. 7.2).

The notion of "multiple organ failure" versus "multiple organ success" refers to the benefits of adopting a lower resting metabolic state (impaired organ function) and associated alterations of the metabolic profile to promote tissue repair following the early phases of sepsis [43]. In this regard, and in contrast to current practice patterns wherein adrenergic agonists are commonly used to provide hemodynamic support in the setting of severe sepsis and septic shock, a recent clinical trial provides evidence that beta-adrenergic inhibition reduces metabolic demand (VO_2), reduces fluid resuscitation requirements, protects against organ damage, and appears to reduce mortality in these patients [44, 45]. Moreover, measures to aggressively correct hyperglycemia resulting in transient hypoglycemia or efforts to fully correct protein catabolism by providing enteral protein-rich diets appear to be associated with increased mortality [46].

Organ-Specific Mechanisms

In addition to the global changes in cellular metabolism incriminated in the pathogenesis of organ failure, the mechanisms specifically contributing to altered organ function may vary from one organ to the next. Moreover, host factors, including age

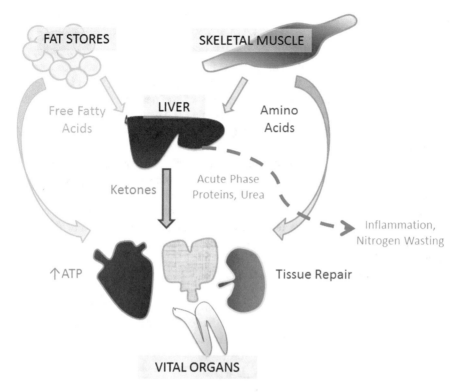

Fig. 7.2 Altered lipid and protein metabolism in sepsis

and comorbid disease, contribute significantly to organ failures during sepsis. In this regard, it is interesting to note that genetic variations associated with enhanced mitochondrial function are the only known genetic predictors of sepsis mortality [47]. Hence, it is likely that global metabolic alterations combined with organ-specific mechanisms conspire to promote organ failures. Other chapters address the organ-specific mechanisms that lead to impaired function, but the lung is special in that damage to the vascular endothelium is sufficient to cause impaired lung function due to altered vascular permeability and increased lung fluid (non-cardiogenic pulmonary edema). Support for the role of vascular injury (e.g., tissue edema or impaired blood flow) in other vital organs is not as convincing. Recent studies of the heart provide convincing evidence in support of the concept that altered energy substrate delivery, the accepted paradigm, does not primarily promote organ failure or damage in the context of sepsis.

Cardiac Dysfunction

Severe sepsis is commonly associated with reduced LVEF and troponin release. Troponin elevation predicts mortality even in the absence of atherosclerotic coronary disease and irrespective of hemodynamic status (e.g., shock) [48, 49]. This indicates that myocardial damage may be a manifestation of a more global process affecting multiple organs. In this regard, the concept of "demand ischemia" has been applied to the condition of myocardial injury in the setting of severe sepsis. "Demand ischemia" is based on the premise that increased oxygen demands relating to the septic response (i.e., tachycardia, increased cardiac output) lead to ischemic injury. However, recent post-mortem analyses of the heart in the setting of fatal sepsis show no evidence of myocardial ischemia [3]. Histologic analysis of cardiac tissues shows no significant myocardial cell death by necrosis or apoptosis compared to matching ICU controls. Ultrastructural evaluation (electron microscopy) of the heart demonstrates moderate mitochondrial swelling and damage but the appearance of the contractile units and all other cardiomyocyte structures largely appeared normal [3]. In keeping with the post-mortem findings, in vitro cardiac magnetic resonance imaging performed within days after the onset of sepsis revealed a non-ischemic injury pattern characterized by epicardial and mid-myocardial T2 elevation. This pattern of T2 elevation is in contrast to ischemic heart disease which is associated with an endomyocardial T2 pattern [4]. Thus, the mechanism of cardiac injury in the context of severe sepsis is unlikely to relate to irreversible ischemic damage (e.g., necrosis), and other explanations need to be considered.

The experimental evidence provided from animal models of sepsis points to multiple potential mechanisms contributing to non-ischemic myocardial injury and dysfunction (Fig. 7.3). A recent review by Antonucci et al. nicely summarizes many

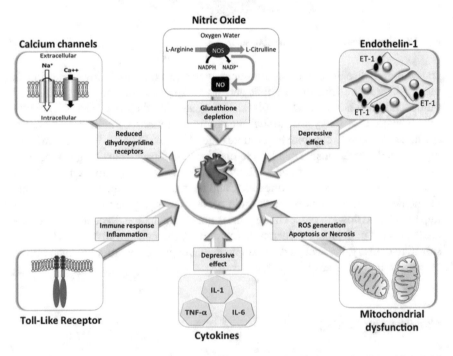

Fig. 7.3 Mechanisms of cardiac dysfunction in severe sepsis. Figure previously published by Antonucci et al. [50]

of these mechanisms, and further suggests that a single therapeutic treatment is unlikely to normalize myocardial function or prevent myocardial injury [50]. Given the extensive research relating to cardiac dysfunction during sepsis, a full review of all proposed mechanisms of myocardial injury and dysfunction is beyond the scope of this chapter. Suffice it to say that more research is needed to explain the early damage and adaptations of the heart to the stress of sepsis, a condition that is associated with a nearly twofold higher risk of all-cause mortality [51, 52].

Evidence that Metabolic Alterations Contribute to Dysfunction of Other Vital Organs

Other chapters will address organ-specific mechanisms of injury and altered function during sepsis. However, this chapter focuses on critical metabolic pathways that are common to all vital organs and are likely to contribute independently to altered organ function.

The kidneys are particularly sensitive to injury during sepsis, and some degree of renal dysfunction is detected in a majority of patients with sepsis. Multiple mechanisms including inflammation, oxidative stress, mitochondrial injury, and hypoperfusion all likely contribute to AKI during sepsis [53]. AKI in setting of experimental sepsis is characterized by acute alterations of parenchymal mitochondrial function and inactivation of endogenous mitochondrial antioxidant functions (e.g., manganese superoxide dismutase) [54]. Protection is conferred through induction of mitochondrial biogenesis or by targeting antioxidants to mitochondria [54, 55]. Given that delivery of mitochondrial targeted antioxidants and treatments designed to promote mitochondrial biogenesis are feasible, it is reasonable to expect that such therapies could prove to be protective against AKI during sepsis.

Altered mentation is the most common central nervous system clinical manifestation of sepsis. However, little data exists regarding the mechanisms causing encephalopathy during sepsis. There is evidence of neuronal apoptosis in specific regions of the brain in fatal cases of septic shock [56]. Other studies incriminate alterations of the blood-brain barrier relating to endothelial damage as a mechanism contributing to inflammatory cytokine release into the brain [57]. Additionally, regional disruption of vasoregulation and induction of coagulation pathways may occasionally lead to the formation of hemorrhagic lesions [57]. Animal models also support the notion that oxidative stress leads to metabolic reprogramming of neurons to favor cellular repair (e.g., of DNA damage) while suppressing ATP formation via mitochondrial oxidative phosphorylation [58]. This altered metabolic profile is equivalent to the "Warburg effect" that occurs in the context of other pathological conditions.

The mechanisms of gastrointestinal damage during sepsis are complex, and include oxidative damage to the contractile units and epithelium [59]. The source of reactive oxidant species includes activated immune cells, damaged mitochondria, and the intracellular release of highly reactive free iron. The ensuing damage to the gut epithelium, with attendant release of "danger signals," can promote the conversion of non-pathogenic colonizing bacteria into invasive and pathogenic organisms [59]. As such, preservation of intestinal barrier function may be of primary importance during the progression and recovery from multiple organ failure during sepsis.

Clinical Implications of Sepsis-Related Metabolism Alterations

Accepting that sepsis induces alterations of metabolism favoring cell and tissue repair at the cost of impaired organ function, it follows that certain patient populations would be predisposed to organ failures during sepsis based upon the concept of a metabolic "threshold" below which vital organs begin to fail. Direct support for this concept is provided by compelling population-based genetic data, showing that mitochondrial DNA (mtDNA) genetic variants promoting altered mitochondrial function are highly predictive of death due to sepsis. In this regard, mtDNA haplotype associated with enhanced mitochondrial respiration, including haplotype H in Europeans and haplotype R in Chinese populations, are highly protective (OR ~ 0.5) [60, 61]. In contrast, the mtDNA allele 4216C is associated with sepsis of greater severity in the setting of burn injury [62]. In addition to these genetic mtDNA variants, it is well recognized that the humans acquire mtDNA damage and associated loss of mitochondrial function with age, and the elderly are at greatly increased risk of severe sepsis compared to younger adults and children [63]. Together with data showing that altered mitochondrial function is predictive of sepsis mortality, these data strongly suggest that conditions associated with altered metabolic reserve predispose to organ failure and death in the context of sepsis.

Altered glucose metabolism also has important implications for the management of sepsis. Glycolysis is promoted in the setting of sepsis and even mild hypoglycemia in septic patients portends higher mortality and increased risk for ICU complications [64, 65]. Indeed, the severity of hypoglycemia correlates strongly with mortality risk and with adverse neurological outcome [66]. Since mitochondrial function is reduced during sepsis, inferring increased reliance on glycolysis to maintain adequate ATP production, it follows that the combination of sepsis-induced inhibition of mitochondrial ATP formation together with the lack of glucose as a substrate for glycolytic ATP production would result in critically reduced tissue ATP levels. Tissue ATP depletion, in turn, is shown to be associated with increased sepsis mortality [24].

There are many other clinical implications of altered metabolism during sepsis as relates to patient management. These include the potentially important effects of commonly used medications that influence metabolic pathways (e.g., antimicrobial agents, hypoglycemic medications, lipid altering drugs), the implications relating to changes in dietary requirements, and controversies relating to early mobilization of critically patients, all of which have unclear implications in terms of metabolic adaptation during sepsis. Finally, it is further unclear how the early management of septic patients influences organ recovery and quality-of-life in sepsis survivors. Extensive research is needed to resolve these controversies and to better understand the mechanisms of organ failure, repair, and recovery in the context of severe sepsis.

References

1. Cowley RA, Mergner WJ, Fisher RS, Jones RT, Trump BF. The subcellular pathology of shock in trauma patients: studies using the immediate autopsy. Am Surg. 1979;45(4):255–69.
2. Sato T, Kamiyama Y, Jones RT, Cowley RA, Trump BF. Ultrastructural study on kidney cell injury following various types of shock in 26 immediate autopsy patients. Adv Shock Res. 1978;1:55–69.
3. Takasu O, Gaut JP, Watanabe E, To K, Fagley RE, Sato B, et al. Mechanisms of cardiac and renal dysfunction in patients dying of sepsis. Am J Respir Crit Care Med. 2013;187(5):509–17.
4. Siddiqui Y, Crouser ED, Raman SV. Nonischemic myocardial changes detected by cardiac magnetic resonance in critical care patients with sepsis. Am J Respir Crit Care Med. 2013;188(8):1037–9.
5. Carlson AS, Kellner A, Bernheimer AW, Freeman EB. A streptococcal enzyme that acts specifically upon diphosphopyridine nucleotide: characterization of the enzyme and its separation from streptolysin O. J Exp Med. 1957;106(1):15–26.
6. Sundin C, Henriksson ML, Hallberg B, Forsberg A, Frithz-Lindsten E. Exoenzyme T of Pseudomonas aeruginosa elicits cytotoxicity without interfering with Ras signal transduction. Cell Microbiol. 2001;3(4):237–46.
7. Patel NJ, Zaborina O, Wu L, Wang Y, Wolfgeher DJ, Valuckaite V, et al. Recognition of intestinal epithelial HIF-1alpha activation by Pseudomonas aeruginosa. Am J Physiol Gastrointest Liver Physiol. 2007;292(1):G134–42.
8. Tracey KJ, Beutler B, Lowry SF, Merryweather J, Wolpe S, Milsark IW, et al. Shock and tissue injury induced by recombinant human cachectin. Science. 1986;234(4775):470–4.
9. Crouser ED, Julian MW, Huff JE, Struck J, Cook CH. Carbamoyl phosphate synthase-1: a marker of mitochondrial damage and depletion in the liver during sepsis. Crit Care Med. 2006;34(9):2439–46.
10. Nakahira K, Kyung SY, Rogers AJ, Gazourian L, Youn S, Massaro AF, et al.. Circulating mitochondrial DNA in patients in the ICU as a marker of mortality: derivation and validation. PLoS Med. 2013;10(12):e1001577; discussion e1001577.
11. Broder G, Weil MH. Excess lactate: an index of reversibility of shock in human patients. Science. 1964;143(3613):1457–9.
12. Gattinoni L, Brazzi L, Pelosi P, Latini R, Tognoni G, Pesenti A, et al. A trial of goal-oriented hemodynamic therapy in critically ill patients. SvO2 Collaborative Group. N Engl J Med. 1995;333(16):1025–32.
13. Hayes MA, Timmins AC, Yau EH, Palazzo M, Hinds CJ, Watson D. Elevation of systemic oxygen delivery in the treatment of critically ill patients. N Engl J Med. 1994;330(24):1717–22.
14. Shah MR, Hasselblad V, Stevenson LW, Binanay C, O'Connor CM, Sopko G, et al. Impact of the pulmonary artery catheter in critically ill patients: meta-analysis of randomized clinical trials. JAMA. 2005;294(13):1664–70.
15. Peake SL, Delaney A, Bailey M, Bellomo R, Cameron PA, Cooper DJ, et al. Goal-directed resuscitation for patients with early septic shock. N Engl J Med. 2014;371(16):1496–506.
16. Yealy DM, Kellum JA, Huang DT, Barnato AE, Weissfeld LA, Pike F, et al. A randomized trial of protocol-based care for early septic shock. N Engl J Med. 2014;370(18):1683–93.

17. Boerma EC, Koopmans M, Konijn A, Kaiferova K, Bakker AJ, van Roon EN, et al. Effects of nitroglycerin on sublingual microcirculatory blood flow in patients with severe sepsis/septic shock after a strict resuscitation protocol: a double-blind randomized placebo controlled trial. Crit Care Med. 2010;38(1):93–100.

18. Trzeciak S, Glaspey LJ, Dellinger RP, Durflinger P, Anderson K, Dezfulian C, et al. Randomized controlled trial of inhaled nitric oxide for the treatment of microcirculatory dysfunction in patients with sepsis. Crit Care Med. 2014;42(12):2482–92.

19. Gore DC, Jahoor F, Hibbert JM, DeMaria EJ. Lactic acidosis during sepsis is related to increased pyruvate production, not deficits in tissue oxygen availability. Ann Surg. 1996;224(1):97–102.

20. Hotchkiss RS, Karl IE. Reevaluation of the role of cellular hypoxia and bioenergetic failure in sepsis. JAMA. 1992;267(11):1503–10.

21. Trentadue R, Fiore F, Massaro F, Papa F, Iuso A, Scacco S, et al. Induction of mitochondrial dysfunction and oxidative stress in human fibroblast cultures exposed to serum from septic patients. Life Sci. 2012;91(7–8):237–43.

22. Prabhu S. Ventilation with lower tidal volumes as compared with traditional tidal volumes for acute lung injury and the acute respiratory distress syndrome. The Acute Respiratory Distress Syndrome Network. N Engl J Med. 2000;342(18):1301–8.

23. Gaieski DF, Mikkelsen ME, Band RA, Pines JM, Massone R, Furia FF, et al. Impact of time to antibiotics on survival in patients with severe sepsis or septic shock in whom early goal-directed therapy was initiated in the emergency department. Crit Care Med. 2010;38(4):1045–53.

24. Brealey D, Brand M, Hargreaves I, Heales S, Land J, Smolenski R, et al. Association between mitochondrial dysfunction and severity and outcome of septic shock. Lancet. 2002;360(9328):219–23.

25. Svistunenko DA, Davies N, Brealey D, Singer M, Cooper CE. Mitochondrial dysfunction in patients with severe sepsis: an EPR interrogation of individual respiratory chain components. Biochim Biophys Acta. 2006;1757(4):262–72.

26. Thomas L. Germs. N Engl J Med. 1972;287(11):553–5.

27. Tracey KJ, Fong Y, Hesse DG, Manogue KR, Lee AT, Kuo GC, et al. Anti-cachectin/TNF monoclonal antibodies prevent septic shock during lethal bacteraemia. Nature. 1987;330(6149):662–4.

28. Ranieri VM, Thompson BT, Barie PS, Dhainaut JF, Douglas IS, Finfer S, et al. Drotrecogin alfa (activated) in adults with septic shock. N Engl J Med. 2012;366(22):2055–64.

29. Hotchkiss RS, Monneret G, Payen D. Sepsis-induced immunosuppression: from cellular dysfunctions to immunotherapy. Nat Rev Immunol. 2013;13(12):862–74.

30. Hotchkiss RS, Opal S. Immunotherapy for sepsis—a new approach against an ancient foe. N Engl J Med. 2010;363(1):87–9.

31. Heininger A, Haeberle H, Fischer I, Beck R, Riessen R, Rohde F, et al. Cytomegalovirus reactivation and associated outcome of critically ill patients with severe sepsis. Crit Care. 2011;15(2):R77.

32. Rosas-Ballina M, Ochani M, Parrish WR, Ochani K, Harris YT, Huston JM, et al. Slenic nerve is required for cholinergic intiinflammatory pathway control of TNF in endotoxemia. Proc Natl Acad Sci U S A. 2008;105(31):11008–13.

33. Exline MC, Crouser ED. Mitochondrial mechanisms of sepsis-induced organ failure. Front Biosci. 2008;13:5030–41.

34. Remels AH, Gosker HR, Schrauwen P, Hommelberg PP, Sliwinski P, Polkey M, et al. TNF-alpha impairs regulation of muscle oxidative phenotype: implications for cachexia? FASEB J. 2010;24(12):5052–62.

35. Scharte M, Han X, Uchiyama T, Tawadrous Z, Delude RL, Fink MP. LPS increases hepatic HIF-1alpha protein and expression of the HIF-1-dependent gene aldolase A in rats. J Surg Res. 2006;135(2):262–7.

36. MacGarvey NC, Suliman HB, Bartz RR, Fu P, Withers CM, Welty-Wolf KE, et al. Activation of mitochondrial biogenesis by heme oxygenase-1-mediated NF-E2-related factor-2 induction rescues mice from lethal *Staphylococcus aureus* sepsis. Am J Respir Crit Care Med. 2012;185(8):851–61.

37. Meloche J, Pflieger A, Vaillancourt M, Paulin R, Potus F, Zervopoulos S, et al. Role for DNA damage signaling in pulmonary arterial hypertension. Circulation. 2014;129(7): 786–97.
38. Cheng SC, Quintin J, Cramer RA, Shepardson KM, Saeed S, Kumar V, et al. mTOR- and HIF-1alpha-mediated aerobic glycolysis as metabolic basis for trained immunity. Science. 2014;345(6204):1250684.
39. Chin BY, Jiang G, Wegiel B, Wang HJ, Macdonald T, Zhang XC, et al. Hypoxia-inducible factor 1alpha stabilization by carbon monoxide results in cytoprotective preconditioning. Proc Natl Acad Sci U S A. 2007;104(12):5109–14.
40. Cicchillitti L, Di Stefano V, Isaia E, Crimaldi L, Fasanaro P, Ambrosino V, et al. Hypoxia-inducible factor 1-alpha induces miR-210 in normoxic differentiating myoblasts. J Biol Chem. 2012;287(53):44761–71.
41. Tannahill GM, Curtis AM, Adamik J, Palsson-McDermott EM, McGettrick AF, Goel G, et al. Succinate is an inflammatory signal that induces IL-1beta through HIF-1alpha. Nature. 2013;496(7444):238–42.
42. Druml W, Heinzel G, Kleinberger G. Amino acid kinetics in patients with sepsis. Am J Clin Nutr. 2001;73(5):908–13.
43. Singer M, De Santis V, Vitale D, Jeffcoate W. Multiorgan failure is an adaptive, endocrine-mediated, metabolic response to overwhelming systemic inflammation. Lancet. 2004;364 (9433):545–8.
44. Morelli A, Ertmer C, Westphal M, Rehberg S, Kampmeier T, Ligges S, et al. Effect of heart rate control with esmolol on hemodynamic and clinical outcomes in patients with septic shock: a randomized clinical trial. JAMA. 2013;310(16):1683–91.
45. Tang C, Yang J, Wu LL, Dong LW, Liu MS. Phosphorylation of beta-adrenergic receptor leads to its redistribution in rat heart during sepsis. Am J Physiol. 1998;274(4 Pt 2):R1078–86.
46. Investigators N-SS, Finfer S, Chittock DR, Su SY, Blair D, Foster D, et al. Intensive versus conventional glucose control in critically ill patients. N Engl J Med. 2009;360(13): 1283–97.
47. Lorente L, Iceta R, Martin MM, Lopez-Gallardo E, Sole-Violan J, Blanquer J, et al. Survival and mitochondrial function in septic patients according to mitochondrial DNA haplogroup. Crit Care. 2012;16(1):R10.
48. John J, Woodward DB, Wang Y, Yan SB, Fisher D, Kinasewitz GT, et al. Troponin-I as a prognosticator of mortality in severe sepsis patients. J Crit Care. 2010;25(2):270–5.
49. Kang EW, Na HJ, Hong SM, Shin SK, Kang SW, Choi KH, et al. Prognostic value of elevated cardiac troponin I in ESRD patients with sepsis. Nephrol Dial Transplant. 2009;24(5):1568–73.
50. Antonucci E, Fiaccadori E, Donadello K, Taccone FS, Franchi F, Scolletta S. Myocardial depression in sepsis: from pathogenesis to clinical manifestations and treatment. J Crit Care. 2014;29(4):500–11.
51. Bessiere F, Khenifer S, Dubourg J, Durieu I, Lega JC. Prognostic value of troponins in sepsis: a meta-analysis. Intensive Care Med. 2013;39(7):1181–9.
52. Sheyin O, Davies O, Duan W, Perez X. The prognostic significance of troponin elevation in patients with sepsis: a meta-analysis. Heart Lung. 2015;44(1):75–81.
53. Gomez H, Ince C, De Backer D, Pickkers P, Payen D, Hotchkiss J, et al. A unified theory of sepsis-induced acute kidney injury: inflammation, microcirculatory dysfunction, bioenergetics, and the tubular cell adaptation to injury. Shock. 2014;41(1):3–11.
54. Patil NK, Parajuli N, MacMillan-Crow LA, Mayeux PR. Inactivation of renal mitochondrial respiratory complexes and manganese superoxide dismutase during sepsis: mitochondria-targeted antioxidant mitigates injury. Am J Physiol Renal Physiol. 2014;306(7):F734–43.
55. Tran M, Tam D, Bardia A, Bhasin M, Rowe GC, Kher A, et al. PGC-1alpha promotes recovery after acute kidney injury during systemic inflammation in mice. J Clin Invest. 2011;121(10):4003–14.
56. Sharshar T, Gray F, Lorin de la Grandmaison G, Hopkinson NS, Ross E, Dorandeu A, et al. Apoptosis of neurons in cardiovascular autonomic centres triggered by inducible nitric oxide synthase after death from septic shock. Lancet. 2003;362(9398):1799–805.

57. Sharshar T, Annane D, de la Grandmaison GL, Brouland JP, Hopkinson NS, Francoise G. The neuropathology of septic shock. Brain Pathol. 2004;14(1):21–33.
58. Bozza FA, D'Avila JC, Ritter C, Sonneville R, Sharshar T, Dal-Pizzol F. Bioenergetics, mitochondrial dysfunction, and oxidative stress in the pathophysiology of septic encephalopathy. Shock. 2013;39(Suppl 1):10–6.
59. Mittal R, Coopersmith CM. Redefining the gut as the motor of critical illness. Trends Mol Med. 2014;20(4):214–23.
60. Baudouin SV, Saunders D, Tiangyou W, Elson JL, Poynter J, Pyle A, et al. Mitochondrial DNA and survival after sepsis: a prospective study. Lancet. 2005;366(9503):2118–21.
61. Yang Y, Shou Z, Zhang P, He Q, Xiao H, Xu Y, et al. Mitochondrial DNA haplogroup R predicts survival advantage in severe sepsis in the Han population. Genet Med. 2008;10(3):187–92.
62. Huebinger RM, Gomez R, McGee D, Chang LY, Bender JE, O'Keeffe T, et al. Association of mitochondrial allele 4216C with increased risk for sepsis-related organ dysfunction and shock after burn injury. Shock. 2010;33(1):19–23.
63. Martin GS, Mannino DM, Moss M. The effect of age on the development and outcome of adult sepsis. Crit Care Med. 2006;34(1):15–21.
64. Ebata T, Hirata K, Denno R, Gotoh Y, Azuma K, Ishida K, et al. Hepatic glycolytic intermediates and glucoregulatory enzymes in septic shock due to peritonitis: experimental study in rats. Nihon Geka Gakkai Zasshi. 1984;85(1):1–5.
65. Park S, Kim DG, Suh GY, Kang JG, Ju YS, Lee YJ, et al. Mild hypoglycemia is independently associated with increased risk of mortality in patients with sepsis: a 3-year retrospective observational study. Crit Care. 2012;16(5):R189.
66. Bagshaw SM, Bellomo R, Jacka MJ, Egi M, Hart GK, George C, et al. The impact of early hypoglycemia and blood glucose variability on outcome in critical illness. Crit Care. 2009;13(3):R91.

Chapter 8
Sepsis-Induced AKI

Hernando Gomez, Alex Zarbock, Raghavan Murugan, and John A. Kellum

Introduction

Sepsis is thought to be the primary etiology of acute kidney injury (AKI) in 40–50% of cases, making sepsis the most common cause of AKI in the critically ill [1]. Importantly, the development of AKI in the setting of sepsis increases the risk of death in hospital six to eightfold [1, 2], and among survivors, the risk of developing chronic kidney disease is also increased [3]. Despite this, the mechanisms by which sepsis causes AKI are not well understood, and hence current therapy remains reactive rather than preventive, and rather nonspecific. Given that the leading clinical conditions associated with AKI, namely, sepsis, major surgery, heart failure, and hypovolemia [1], are all associated with hypoperfusion, it is tempting to attribute all AKI to ischemia. However, an increasing body of evidence suggests that at least in a proportion of patients, AKI can occur in the absence of overt signs of hypoperfusion. Langenberg et al. showed, for example, that AKI developed in septic animals despite normal or increased renal blood flow [4]. In a human study, Prowle et al. were able to demonstrate that decreased renal blood flow (RBF) was not a universal finding even in patients with well-established sepsis-induced AKI [5]. Furthermore,

H. Gomez, MD • R. Murugan, MD • J.A. Kellum, MD (✉)
The Center for Critical Care Nephrology, University of Pittsburgh,
Pittsburgh, PA, USA

The CRISMA Center, Department of Critical Care Medicine,
University of Pittsburgh, Pittsburgh, PA, USA
e-mail: kellumja@upmc.edu

A. Zarbock, MD
Department of Anesthesiology, Intensive Care and Pain Medicine,
University of Münster, Münster, Germany

© Springer International Publishing AG 2017
N.S. Ward, M.M. Levy (eds.), *Sepsis*, Respiratory Medicine,
DOI 10.1007/978-3-319-48470-9_8

in a large-scale study, including more than 1800 patients with community-acquired pneumonia, Murugan et al. found that a fifth to a quarter of patients with non-severe pneumonia, who were never admitted to an ICU, and who never displayed overt signs of shock or hypoperfusion, still developed AKI [6]. Complementary to the insights from clinical and in vivo studies, in vitro experiments where hemodynamics are no longer relevant, have shown that incubation of human renal tubular epithelial cells with plasma from septic patients induces damage of tubular epithelial cells evidenced by the increased release of tubular enzymes, elevated permeability, and the decreased expression of key molecules for tubular functional integrity [7]. Taken together these data provide evidence that, at least in some patients, renal injury cannot be explained solely on the basis of the classic paradigm of hypoperfusion and that other mechanisms must come into play.

One of the limitations in advancing the understanding of sepsis-induced AKI is the lack of pathologic specimens available, given that the risk of performing biopsies in this patient population outweighs any potential benefit. Recent studies in septic animals and postmortem observations in septic humans have provided evidence of what sepsis-induced AKI actually looks like. Despite representing the latest stages of the disease, these kidneys were characterized by a strikingly bland histology with focal areas of tubular injury, which was also entirely discordant with the profound functional impairment seen pre-mortem. In addition, and contrary to prior understanding, necrosis and apoptosis were largely absent [8, 9], which not only argues in favor of the notion that sepsis-induced AKI is not equivalent to acute tubular necrosis (ATN), but supports the hypothesis that at least in the early stages, this phenotype may represent a concerted, organized, common underlying adaptive mechanism [9]. A consistent observation in these studies, regardless of species, disease stage, severity, or organ examined, appears to be the presence of three main alterations: inflammation [10, 11], diffuse microcirculatory flow abnormalities [12], and cellular bioenergetic adaptive responses to injury [9, 13]. The study and understanding of these three domains may provide a roadmap to unravel the mechanisms by which sepsis causes AKI and perhaps organ injury in general and may facilitate the development of more targeted therapies. In this chapter, we will first consider the current classification system for AKI and then briefly review the epidemiology; then we will review the roles various mechanisms may play in the genesis of sepsis-induced AKI and discuss potential therapeutic implications.

Definition of AKI in the Clinical Setting

The definition of AKI has undergone important transformations in recent years. The definition of AKI has been traditionally based on the assessment of renal function, and in particular, on the assessment of changes in glomerular filtration rate (GFR). Although practical at the bedside, this approach is limited by the fact that functional changes not necessarily reflect structural alterations [3]. This is particularly true in sepsis-induced AKI, where a dramatic alteration in renal function is associated with very bland histology [8, 9]. An additional limitation is the assessment of GFR through the quantification of creatinine. Although creatinine levels correlate well with GFR in steady-state conditions, AKI usually occurs in the setting of changing physiologic or pathologic conditions. Finally, the assessment of renal dysfunction based on glomerular function does not take into account the presence of tubular dysfunction, which has been increasingly recognized as an important pathophysiologic event, and to be at least as important as the alterations in GFR. Despite these limitations, the standardization of two measures of glomerular function has provided the scientific community with a tool, in a common language, to assess the occurrence of AKI. These measures are serum creatinine and urine output. Today, the evaluation of the presence and degree of severity of AKI can be standardized with tools like the KDIGO criteria [14].

The Epidemiology of Sepsis-Induced AKI

Sepsis is the leading cause of acute kidney injury (AKI) in acutely ill patients. Acute kidney injury occurs in as much as 40–50% of septic critically ill patients, which increases the risk of death six- to eightfold [1, 2, 15, 16], and also the risk of advancing to renal fibrosis and chronic kidney disease [3]. Importantly, a large proportion of patients who are usually considered to be less severely compromised and thus at lower risk, still develop AKI. Murugan et al. showed in a large cohort of patients admitted to the emergency department with non-severe community acquired pneumonia that 34% of these patients developed AKI many of whom never required admission to an ICU [6]. This suggests that AKI is not only related to shock states or critical illness, and that patients with non-life-threatening infections may also be at high risk of developing renal dysfunction and its short and long-term consequences.

Novel Concepts in the Pathophysiology of Sepsis-Induced AKI

Recent evidence suggests that the origin of most cases of AKI is multifaceted and that several, concurrent mechanisms may be at play. These mechanisms include inflammation, profound, heterogeneous distortion of microvascular flow at the peritubular and glomerular levels, and tubular epithelial cell injury and impairment. Given that these three major events occur early in the course of sepsis, and that cell death seldom occurs, we conceptualize early sepsis-induced AKI as the clinical and biochemical manifestation of tubular cell responses to injury. We further hypothesize that such response is, at least in part, adaptive in that it is driven by metabolic down-regulation and reprioritization of energy expenditure to avoid energy imbalance and favors individual cell survival processes (such as maintenance of membrane potential and cell cycle arrest), at the expense of organ function (i.e., tubular absorption and secretion of solutes).

The Renal Microcirculation during Sepsis-Induced AKI

Sepsis causes a profound alteration in microvascular blood flow distribution [12, 17]. Such alteration is characterized by an increase in the heterogeneity of regional blood flow distribution, a decrease in the proportion of capillaries with "nutritive" (or continuous) blood flow, and an increase in the proportion of capillaries with intermittent or no flow [12, 18]. The renal microcirculation is disturbed in a similar fashion, as has been recently described in different models of sepsis-induced AKI [11, 19, 20], even in the setting of normal or even increased RBF [21]. Multiple mechanisms seem to frame this characteristic microcirculatory derangement, including endothelial dysfunction, impaired red blood cell deformability, thinning and damage of the glycocalyx layer, increased leukocyte activation and recruitment, and activation of the coagulation cascade with fibrin deposition [18]. Importantly, these alterations in microcirculatory flow and endothelial function are thought to contribute directly to the development of organ dysfunction through multiple mechanisms.

Uncoupling of microcirculatory blood flow distribution from metabolic demand, with the creation of microvascular shunts, has been proposed to result in areas of hypoperfusion and hypoxia [22, 23]. In relation to this, the endothelium also provides an essential system of retrograde communication that allows the microcirculation to fine tune and couple blood flow distribution to metabolic demand, which is in essence the concept of regional autoregulation. Tyml et al. have shown that LPS-induced endothelial injury results in loss of such retrograde communication rate between microvessels 500 μm apart [23, 24], suggesting that sepsis may not only impair the response to vasoactive mediators but also, the capacity of peripheral microvascular beds to autoregulate.

Similarly, endothelial dysfunction results in increased vascular permeability and worsening interstitial edema [25, 26], with two important consequences. First, edema increases the diffusion distance oxygen has to travel to reach target cells [27] further creating areas at risk for hypoxia. Second, given that the kidney is an encapsulated organ, tissue edema contributes to increased venous output pressures, aggravating congestion and perpetuating microvascular perfusion alterations [28, 29].

Endothelial cells are also important determinants of vascular tone and play an important role in the responsiveness to vasoactive mediators [30]. Injury to the arterial and arteriolar endothelium has consistently shown to result in impaired responsiveness to vasoactive substances, which may explain the loss of vasomotor tone during sepsis.

Nitric oxide (NO) has also been shown to have a potential role in the genesis of microvascular dysfunction and in the pathophysiology of AKI. Although sepsis is characterized by global increased NO production [31], the expression of one of the most important catalyzers of its production, inducible NO synthase (iNOS), is rather heterogeneous [31]. Accordingly, it is possible that the heterogeneous expression of iNOS may result in heterogeneous regional concentrations of NO, which could result in the presence of vascular beds deprived of NO even in the setting of elevated systemic levels [32]. This is important as it is reminiscent of the characteristic heterogeneous pattern of microvascular dysfunction described in sepsis, and may relate pathophysiologically with areas of shunting and hypoxia [32]. Importantly, selective inhibition of iNOS not only can restore the renal microcirculatory derangements during sepsis, but is also associated with decreased functional manifestations of renal injury, suggesting that microcirculatory abnormalities may be in the mechanistic pathway of sepsis-induced AKI [19]. However, the interactions between NO, microvascular dysfunction, and AKI are not straightforward, as sepsis is also known to result in iNOS-dependent decrease in endothelial-derived NO synthase activity, which will also alter microvascular flow homeostasis [33, 34].

During sepsis, inflammation, oxidative stress, and the uncoupled eNOS [35] not only induce endothelial cell dysfunction but also damage the glycocalyx. The glycocalyx is a layer of organized glycosaminoglycan branches that protrudes from the surface of the endothelial cell membrane into the capillary lumen, and that has important biomechanical functions including maintenance of adequate capillary flow, oncotic and hydrostatic pressure gradient balance to limit filtration, and avoiding red and white cell adhesion [36]. Damage of the glycocalyx is thought to result in capillary leak, altered red blood cell flow, and increased adhesion and rolling of leukocytes after endothelial adhesion molecules are exposed, all of which contribute to the microvascular dysfunction phenotype characteristic of sepsis and to further inflammation.

Finally, sluggish peritubular flow may also result in amplification of the inflammatory signal. As demonstrated by Goddard et al. [37] in myocardial capillaries during a porcine model of endotoxemia, leukocytes decrease their velocities and increase their transit time in these areas of sluggish flow. In addition, there is evidence of upregulation of inflammatory molecules, such as intercellular adhesion molecule 1 and vascular cell adhesion molecule 1 [38, 39] in these peritubular capillaries that would contribute to leukocyte activation and prolonged leukocyte transit. This prolonged transit may directly translate into a greater time of exposure of the endothelium and neighboring tubular epithelial cells to activated, cytokine secreting leukocytes and to other pathogen and damage-associated molecular patterns (PAMPs and DAMPs, respectively) that ultimately amplify the inflammatory signal, and induce focal oxidative stress and tubular injury. The tubular epithelial cells exposed to this amplified signal then act as primary targets for this alarm, and trigger a response in the adjacent segments of the proximal tubule evidenced by the induction of oxidative stress and vacuolization. The lack of apoptosis and necrosis suggests this is an organized, adaptive response that ultimately signals other tubular cells to shut down in a paracrine fashion. Importantly, this provides an explanation for why only a few heterogeneous groups of tubular epithelial cells demonstrate the typical histopathologic changes.

Inflammation Propagates Renal Damage During Sepsis

A strong association between cytokine levels (interleukin (IL)-6, IL-10, and macrophage migration inhibitory factor) and the development of sepsis-induced AKI [6, 40] supports the hypothesis that systemic inflammation is an important mediator of this process. During sepsis, although the inflammatory response is fundamental to clear the infection and later promote tissue recovery, it can also result in tissue damage and organ dysfunction [41]. In addition to leukocytes, dendritic cells, and resident macrophages, tubular epithelial cells are capable of recognizing and responding to pathogens-associated molecular patterns (PAMPs) through pattern-recognition receptors including toll-like receptors (TLR), C-type lectin receptors, retinoic acid inducible gene 1-like receptors, and nucleotide-binding oligomerization domain-like receptors [42], which results in the up-regulation of inflammatory gene transcription and initiation of innate immunity. This response is also stimulated by endogenous substances released by injured cells and tissues known as damage-associated molecular patterns (DAMPs), which include DNA, RNA, histones, HMGB1, and S100 proteins, and which are recognized by these same receptors [43].

Pro-inflammatory mediators activate endothelial cells and induce up-regulation of adhesion molecules like E-selectin, which has been demonstrated to play a major role in leukocyte recruitment into the kidney during the late stages of sepsis-induced AKI [44]. Although not seen in all models of sepsis-induced AKI [45], elimination of neutrophils or blocking adhesion molecules that are required for neutrophil recruitment into the kidney completely abolished sepsis-induced AKI in a cecal ligation and puncture (CLP)-induced sepsis model [44]. This observation can be explained by the fact that leukocytes leaving peritubular capillaries have a close proximity to tubular epithelial cells and can directly activate tubular epithelial and dendritic cells by releasing pro-inflammatory mediators and DAMPs. The cycle is then perpetuated by the release of mediators like leukotriene B_4, and platelet-activating factor which increase vascular permeability and up-regulate the expression of adhesion molecules that promote further inflammation [46–48]. In addition, DAMPs, PAMPs, and pro-inflammatory cytokines that are readily filtered through the glomerulus can activate these tubular epithelial cells from within the tubule (Fig. 8.1) [46, 49]. It has been recently shown that mammalian tubular epithelial cells (including human) express TLR2 and TLR4, and that these cells are capable of recognizing inflammatory mediators such as lipopolysaccharide (LPS) in a TLR4-dependent manner [50–53]. Furthermore, Krüger et al. [50] demonstrated that damaged human tubules stain positively for the TLR4 ligand, HMGB1, and that in vitro stimulation of human tubular epithelial cells with HMGB1 stimulates pro-inflammatory responses through TLR4 [50], suggesting that such mediators can act in an autocrine and paracrine fashion and may contribute to further tubular cell damage. The recognition that tubular epithelial cells are actually equipped with machinery to recognize the inflammatory signal supports the hypothesis that their response may be organized and not random. In support of this, Kalakeche et al. [51] have elegantly shown that TLR4-dependent LPS recognition in the tubular epithelial cells occurs in the S1 segment of the proximal tubule, that assembly of LPS with

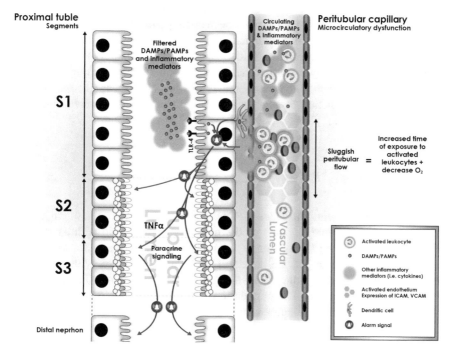

Fig. 8.1 Alterations in the Kidney During Sepsis. These alterations are characterized by increased heterogeneity of flow, as well as an increase in the proportion of capillaries with sluggish or stop flow (represented in the figure by *darker hexagons* in the peritubular capillary). We have conceptualized that these areas of sluggish peritubular flow increase the transit time of activated leukocytes and that this may set the stage for an amplification of the "danger signal" in such areas. Note that the expression of TNF receptors in the S2 segment tubular cells has led to the hypothesis that S1 cells may actually signal distal segments in a paracrine fashion through secretion of TNF. Finally, there are also data suggesting that this paracrine signal may include mediators of cell cycle arrest, namely, TIMP-2 and IGFBP-7. Source: Gomez et al. *Shock*. 2014;41:3–11

TLR-4 in the tubular epithelial cell produces internalization of LPS through fluid-filled endocytosis, and that this triggers an organized oxidative outburst in epithelial cells of the adjacent tubular segments (S2 and S3) but not in the S1 segment. These findings have led Kalakeche et al. [51] to suggest that the S1 segment of the proximal tubule may act as a sensor of danger that activates a series of events resulting in oxidative stress within distal tubular segments (S2, S3) and that could potentially explain tubular dysfunction in the setting of sepsis.

The (Adaptive) Responses of Tubular Cells to Inflammation

With the exception of T lymphocytes and intestinal epithelia, and despite multiple triggering stimuli [54], significant necrosis or apoptosis does not occur during sepsis [8, 9], which suggests that during the acute phase, regardless of the consequences at the organ level, the cellular response is successful at preventing death. This denotes a possible underlying adaptive mechanism [9, 46, 55], and an opportunity to understand the response of the tubular epithelial cells to sepsis. Accordingly, it is reasonable to think that the tubular epithelial cell response to injury may be characterized at least in part by processes that limit pro-apoptotic triggers, by (a) prioritizing energy consumption and maintaining energy homeostasis, (b) maintaining cellular organelle function through quality control processes (general autophagy and mitophagy), and (c) limiting cell cycling and DNA replication.

Repriotitization of Energy Consumption

Energy balance dysregulation and mitochondrial injury are two major triggers of apoptosis and consequently, two of the most highly regulated cellular defense mechanisms to injury [56]. Although still controversial, sepsis seems to be associated with maintenance of ATP levels in the kidney [57] albeit with a decrease in production [58, 59], suggesting a significant decrease in ATP utilization. Furthermore, analogous to the evolutionarily conserved defense response to hypoxia, where nonvital functions are limited to avoid overtaxing energy expenditure [56], sterile inflammation by administration of lipopolysaccharide has been shown to induce downregulation of renal tubular cell ion transporters [60], which account for more than 70% of ATP cellular consumption [61]. Furthermore, there is evidence that experimental sepsis induces similar effects. Gupta et al. [62] showed that, in the presence of LPS, proximal tubules of mice have a delayed uptake of low-molecular-weight dextran, a sign of reduced endocytic capacity. Good et al. [63] have shown in an LPS-induced rodent sepsis model that LPS inhibits NHE1 (Na+/H+ exchanger 1) and thus blocks bicarbonate reabsorption in the medullary thick ascending limb of the loop of Henle. Finally, Hsiao et al. have shown that sodium transport (tubular sodium reabsorption) is decreased as early as 9 h after induction of sepsis by cecal ligation and puncture [64]. Taken together this evidence suggests that during sepsis, the response of the tubular epithelial cell may be characterized by an organized, hierarchical downregulation of major energy sinks like ion transport, while only fueling processes necessary to cell survival (i.e., maintenance of membrane potential) [65]. This is a highly conserved mechanism across species that seems to frame the core strategy of cellular response to threatening circumstances. It also provides the conceptual ground to suggest that cellular metabolic downregulation and reprioritization of energy consumption are pillars of the tubular epithelial response to sepsis and furthermore explains why organ function may be sacrificed in benefit of individual cell survival [62, 63].

Mitochondrial Quality Control Processes: Mitophagy

Mitophagy is an evolutionarily conserved, quality control mechanism, by which eukaryotic cells remove and digest dysfunctional mitochondria from the cytoplasm [66, 67]. During sepsis, TLR-mediated inflammation [68], oxidative stress [69, 70], and alterations in the electron transport chain that uncouple respiration and depolarize the mitochondrial membrane are potent triggers of mitophagy [67]. This early mitochondrial uncoupling characterized by an increment in O_2 consumption (VO_2) is not to be confused with the adaptive response it triggers, which is framed by the activation of mitophagy, and is characterized by a decrement in VO_2 and conservation of energy. In the kidney, mitophagy is activated as early as 3 h after CLP-induced sepsis [64], suggesting it is part of the early response of tubular epithelial cells to injury. Importantly, insufficient activation of mitophagy has been associated with worse outcome in critically ill patients, and it has been postulated to contribute to cell and organ dysfunction [71]. On the other hand, stimulation of autophagy has been shown to be effective at protecting cells [64] and organ function [71] in the setting of experimental inflammatory insults. Furthermore, in the setting of experimental sepsis induced by CLP, decreased autophagy has been associated with increased blood urea nitrogen and creatinine levels and a decline in proximal tubular sodium transport [64]. As a protective response, mitophagy offers several advantages, namely, removal of dysfunctional mitochondria, with subsequent decrement in ROS/RNS production, energy conservation, limiting oxidative stress damage, and importantly, intercepting proapoptotic signals at the mitochondrial level impeding triggering of apoptosis [67, 72–74]. Indeed, Carchman et al. have shown that inhibition of mitophagy results in a robust apoptotic signal in hepatocytes of animals subjected to CLP [58]. It is unknown, however, what mitophagy-induced maintenance of renal function really means. The adaptive response, framed by metabolic downregulation, would most likely decrease tubular and renal function and not promote it, just as hibernation promotes the loss of function. Indeed, increased or preserved renal function in the setting of stress may result harmful in the long run. Yet, animal and human data associate acute stimulation of autophagy with preserved renal function, and its faulty activation or decline with worse outcome. It is possible that the interplay of autophagy and tubular cell function varies with time and that persistence of the initial protective response may ultimately be deleterious in the subacute or chronic phases.

Cell Cycle Arrest

There is a growing body of evidence indicating that mitochondria are intimately involved in the regulation of the cell cycle [67]. The ability of mitochondria to move within the cell, change shape, and coalesce in different ways has recently emerged as an important feature, which may influence the cell cycle [75]. Briefly, the cell cycle is the progression of cells through a number of steps in preparation for mitosis (G0, G1, S, G2, M). This preparation portrays several checkpoints in which the cell seems to evaluate whether it is prepared to advance to the next phase. Of particular interest to renal tubular injury in sepsis and the involvement of mitochondrial regulation is the G1-S checkpoint. Only at and during this stage, mitochondria have been shown to coalesce into a single, tubular network of mitochondria. This mesh seems to act as syncytia, with electrical coupling and unusual hyperpolarization [76], which fits well with prior studies showing an increase in O2 consumption during the G1-S transition of the cell cycle [77]. This also relates to the finding that a reduction in ATP production induced by specific ETC mutations produces cell cycle arrest at the G1-S checkpoint [78]. Together, these data indicate that the formation of this giant tubular network is necessary to meet the energy requirement needed to synthesize all the components for adequate cell division. It also suggests that the G1-S border is an important checkpoint of the cycle, whereby the inability to meet such energy requirements induces cell cycle arrest presumably to prevent a potentially lethal energy imbalance [75]. Yang et al. [79] recently showed in a rodent model of CLP-induced sepsis that G1-S cell cycle arrest was associated with kidney injury and that recovery of renal function paralleled cell cycle progression 48 h after CLP. These findings have become even more clinically relevant as tissue inhibitor of metalloproteinases 2 (TIMP-2) and insulin-like growth factor-binding protein 7 (IGFBP-7), two markers involved in G1-S cycle arrest, have been identified as the most sensitive and specific markers to predict risk of development of AKI in critically ill patients [80–82]. We speculate that the renal cell cycle arrest in the epithelial tubular cell may provide an advantage by avoiding replication because (a) it conserves energy and prevents triggering apoptosis or necrosis and (b) limiting replication diminishes the probability of DNA damage, reducing not only energy consumption employed in DNA repair, but also decreases the chances of triggering apoptosis.

Potential for Diagnostic and Therapeutic Targets

To date, no therapeutic measures are available to prevent or treat sepsis-induced AKI. A potential reason for this may be that often therapy is started too late in the disease process. The development of new biomarkers, which also provide insights into the pathophysiology of the disease, makes it possible to detect kidneys at risk for injury and thus enable earlier initiation of interventions [80–82].

The knowledge that inflammation, microvascular dysfunction, and adaptive responses of tubular cells are involved in the development of sepsis-induced AKI provides new diagnostic and therapeutic avenues. As these mechanisms are closely interlinked with each other, modulating one of these components simultaneously alters other components. As increased levels of pro-inflammatory mediators (e.g., IL-6) are associated with the development of AKI [40], it is tempting to speculate that eliminating these mediators or endotoxin can prevent sepsis-induced AKI. Experimentally, it has been shown that removal of such mediators by hemoadsorption completely protects against AKI in a CLP model of sepsis [7, 83, 84], and a clinical study demonstrated that reducing endotoxin by polymyxin-B hemoperfusion reduced RIFLE scores and urine tubular enzymes [7]. Along the same lines, Alkaline phosphatase (AP) is an endogenous enzyme that exerts detoxifying effects through dephosphorylation of endotoxins and pro-inflammatory extracellular ATP and is reduced during systemic inflammation. Heemskerk and colleagues [85] demonstrated that administration of AP was associated with a decreased expression of iNOS synthase in proximal tubule cells isolated from urine and that this related to an attenuated urinary excretion of glutathione S-transferase A1-1, a proximal tubule injury marker. In a small, randomized trial, Pickkers et al. showed that the administration of exogenous AP in septic patients improved endogenous creatinine clearance and reduced the requirement and duration of renal replacement therapy [86]. Modulating TNF-α signaling might be yet another therapeutic option, because a polymorphism in the promoter region of the TNFA gene is associated with markers of kidney disease severity and distant organ dysfunction [87].

To improve microcirculatory perfusion, vasodilators in the setting of sepsis are currently under investigation including nitroglycerin [17, 88], NO administration, and modulation of NO production [32, 34]. Furthermore, drugs with pleiotropic effects on the vasculature, such as statins [89] and erythropoietin [90], have the potential to prevent kidney injury by enhancing eNOS expression and decreasing vascular permeability. However, it is important to consider that regional microcirculatory autoregulation is only possible if sufficient perfusion pressure is attained, and thus early resuscitation goals still need to focus on achieving a mean arterial pressure sufficient enough to ensure perfusion. Asfar et al. have shown that such a goal must be a mean arterial pressure of 65–70 mmHg, and that higher levels of MAP only result in improved outcomes (decreased need for RRT) in the subpopulation of patients with chronic hypertension [91].

However, it is important to explore these treatment options bearing in mind that these mechanisms are part of the natural host response to sepsis, and that although known perpetrators of injury, they are also necessary for bacterial clearance, tissue protection and repair, and ultimately survival. Accordingly, the reader must not expect a single treatment modality to emerge as a magic bullet to prevention and/or treatment sepsis-induced AKI.

Conclusions

Close examination of the histology of various organs of patients dying from sepsis has dramatically changed the way we think of sepsis-induced organ dysfunction. The recognition that in the case of the kidney, sepsis-induced AKI cannot be entirely explained by the traditional concept of acute tubular necrosis, and that sepsis does not cause overt apoptosis and necrosis in failing organs, has challenged the notion that ischemia is the only mechanism explaining organ dysfunction. Importantly, it has also prompted many to suggest that the response to the septic environment may early on be adaptive in nature. In this review, we have now put forth a conceptual model that cellular energy regulation is fundamental to the adaptive response, and that such regulation is driven at least in part by metabolic down-regulation and re-prioritization of energy utilization and by mitochondrial quality control processes like mitophagy. Further work is warranted to better understand the role, timing, and reach of these multiple mechanisms in the pathogenesis of sepsis-induced AKI, and if this can be translated into novel diagnostic and therapeutic interventions to improve outcome in this patient population.

Acknowledgments The authors declare no conflicts of interest. This work was funded by NIH/NHLBI grant number 1K12HL109068-02 awarded to H.G., and research grant from the German research foundation (ZA428/10-1) and Else-Kröner Fresenius Stiftung awarded to A.Z.

References

1. Uchino S, Kellum, JA, Bellomo R, Doig GS, Morimatsu H, Morgera S, et al. Acute renal failure in critically ill patients: a multinational, multicenter study. JAMA. 2005;294(7):813–8. doi:10.1001/jama.294.7.813.
2. Thakar CV, Christianson A, Freyberg R, Almenoff P, Render ML. Incidence and outcomes of acute kidney injury in intensive care units: a Veterans Administration study. Crit Care Med. 2009;37(9):2552–8. doi:10.1097/CCM.0b013e3181a5906f.
3. Murugan R, Kellum JA. Acute kidney injury: what's the prognosis? Nat Rev Nephrol. 2011;7(4):209–17. doi:10.1038/nrneph.2011.13.
4. Langenberg C, Wan L, Egi M, May CN, Bellomo R. Renal blood flow in experimental septic acute renal failure. Kidney Int. 2006;69(11):1996–2002. doi:10.1038/sj.ki.5000440.
5. Prowle JR, Ishikawa K, May CN, Bellomo R. Renal blood flow during acute renal failure in man. Blood Purif. 2009;28(3):216–25. doi:10.1159/000230813.
6. Murugan R, Karajala-Subramanyam V, Lee M, et al. Acute kidney injury in non-severe pneumonia is associated with an increased immune response and lower survival. Kidney Int. 2010;77(6):527–35. doi:10.1038/ki.2009.502.
7. Cantaluppi V, Assenzio B, Pasero D, et al. Polymyxin-B hemoperfusion inactivates circulating proapoptotic factors. Intensive Care Med. 2008;34(9):1638–45. doi:10.1007/s00134-008-1124-6.
8. Hotchkiss RS, Swanson PE, Freeman BD, et al. Apoptotic cell death in patients with sepsis, shock, and multiple organ dysfunction. Crit Care Med. 1999;27(7):1230–51.
9. Takasu O, Gaut JP, Watanabe E, et al. Mechanisms of cardiac and renal dysfunction in patients dying of sepsis. Am J Respir Crit Care Med. 2013;187(5):509–17. doi:10.1164/rccm.201211-1983OC.
10. Wang Z, Holthoff JH, Seely KA, et al. Development of oxidative stress in the peritubular capillary microenvironment mediates sepsis-induced renal microcirculatory failure and acute kidney injury. AJPA. 2012;180(2):505–16. doi:10.1016/j.ajpath.2011.10.011.
11. Seely KA, Holthoff JH, Burns ST, et al. Hemodynamic changes in the kidney in a pediatric rat model of sepsis-induced acute kidney injury. Am J Physiol Renal Physiol. 2011;301(1):F209–17. doi:10.1152/ajprenal.00687.2010.
12. De Backer D, Creteur J, Preiser J-C, Dubois M-J, Vincent J-L. Microvascular blood flow is altered in patients with sepsis. Am J Respir Crit Care Med. 2002;166(1):98–104.
13. Singer M, De Santis V, Vitale D, Jeffcoate W. Multiorgan failure is an adaptive, endocrine-mediated, metabolic response to overwhelming systemic inflammation. Lancet. 2004;364 (9433):545–8. doi:10.1016/S0140-6736(04)16815-3.

14. KDIGO. Section 2: AKI definition. Kidney Int Suppl. 2012;2(1):19–36. doi:10.1038/kisup.2011.32.
15. Hoste EAJ, Schurgers M. Epidemiology of acute kidney injury: how big is the problem? Crit Care Med. 2008;36(4 Suppl):S146–51. doi:10.1097/CCM.0b013e318168c590.
16. Hoste EAJ, Bagshaw SM, Bellomo R, et al. Epidemiology of acute kidney injury in critically ill patients: the multinational AKI-EPI study. Intensive Care Med. 2015;41(8):1411–23. doi:10.1007/s00134-015-3934-7.
17. Spronk PE, Ince C, Gardien MJ, Mathura KR, Oudemans-van Straaten HM, Zandstra DF. Nitroglycerin in septic shock after intravascular volume resuscitation. Lancet. 2002;360(9343): 1395–6.
18. De Backer D, Donadello K, Taccone FS, Ospina-Tascon G, Salgado D, Vincent J-L. Microcirculatory alterations: potential mechanisms and implications for therapy. Ann Intensive Care. 2011;1(1):27. doi:10.1186/2110-5820-1-27.
19. Tiwari MM, Brock RW, Megyesi JK, Kaushal GP, Mayeux PR. Disruption of renal peritubular blood flow in lipopolysaccharide-induced renal failure: role of nitric oxide and caspases. Am J Physiol Renal Physiol. 2005;289(6):F1324–32. doi:10.1152/ajprenal.00124.2005.
20. Holthoff JH, Wang Z, Seely KA, Gokden N, Mayeux PR. Resveratrol improves renal microcirculation, protects the tubular epithelium, and prolongs survival in a mouse model of sepsis-induced acute kidney injury. Kidney Int. 2012;81(4):370–8. doi:10.1038/ki.2011.347.
21. Bezemer R, Legrand M, Klijn E, et al. Real-time assessment of renal cortical microvascular perfusion heterogeneities using near-infrared laser speckle imaging. Opt Express. 2010;18(14): 15054–61. doi:10.1364/OE.18.015054.
22. Dyson A, Bezemer R, Legrand M, Balestra G, Singer M, Ince C. Microvascular and interstitial oxygen tension in the renal cortex and medulla studied in a 4-h rat model of LPS-induced endotoxemia. Shock. 2011;36(1):83–9. doi:10.1097/SHK.0b013e3182169d5a.
23. Almac E, Siegemund M, Demirci C, Ince C. Microcirculatory recruitment maneuvers correct tissue CO_2 abnormalities in sepsis. Minerva Anestesiol. 2006;72(6):507–19.
24. Tyml K, Wang X, Lidington D, Ouellette Y. Lipopolysaccharide reduces intercellular coupling in vitro and arteriolar conducted response in vivo. Am J Physiol Heart Circ Physiol. 2001;281(3):H1397–406.
25. Prowle JR, Echeverri JE, Ligabo EV, Ronco C, Bellomo R. Fluid balance and acute kidney injury. Nat Rev Nephrol. 2010;6(2):107–15. doi:10.1038/nrneph.2009.213.
26. Bagshaw SM, Brophy PD, Cruz D, Ronco C. Fluid balance as a biomarker: impact of fluid overload on outcome in critically ill patients with acute kidney injury. Crit Care. 2008;12(4):169. doi:10.1186/cc6948.
27. Hollenberg SM, Ahrens TS, Annane D, et al. Practice parameters for hemodynamic support of sepsis in adult patients: 2004 update. Crit Care Med. 2004;32(9):1928–48.
28. Prowle JR, Kirwan CJ, Bellomo R. Fluid management for the prevention and attenuation of acute kidney injury. Nat Rev Nephrol. 2013;10(1):37–47. doi:10.1038/nrneph.2013.232.
29. Rajendram R, Prowle JR. Venous congestion: are we adding insult to kidney injury in sepsis? Crit Care. 2014;18(1):104. doi:10.1186/cc13709.
30. Sprague AH, Khalil RA. Inflammatory cytokines in vascular dysfunction and vascular disease. Biochem Pharmacol. 2009;78(6):539–52. doi:10.1016/j.bcp.2009.04.029.
31. Cunha FQ, Assreuy J, Moss DW, et al. Differential induction of nitric oxide synthase in various organs of the mouse during endotoxaemia: role of TNF-alpha and IL-1-beta. Immunology. 1994;81(2):211–5.
32. Trzeciak S, Cinel I, Phillip Dellinger R, et al. Resuscitating the microcirculation in sepsis: the central role of nitric oxide, emerging concepts for novel therapies, and challenges for clinical trials. Acad Emerg Med. 2008;15(5):399–413. doi:10.1111/j.1553-2712.2008.00109.x.
33. Chauhan SD, Seggara G, Vo PA, Macallister RJ, Hobbs AJ, Ahluwalia A. Protection against lipopolysaccharide-induced endothelial dysfunction in resistance and conduit vasculature of iNOS knockout mice. FASEB J. 2003;17(6):773–5. doi:10.1096/fj.02-0668fje.
34. Heemskerk S, Masereeuw R, Russel FGM, Pickkers P. Selective iNOS inhibition for the treatment of sepsis-induced acute kidney injury. Nat Rev Nephrol. 2009;5(11):629–40. doi:10.1038/nrneph.2009.155.

35. Rabelink TJ, van Zonneveld A-J. Coupling eNOS uncoupling to the innate immune response. Arterioscler Thromb Vasc Biol. 2006;26(12):2585–7. doi:10.1161/01.ATV.0000250932. 24151.50.
36. Weinbaum S, Tarbell JM, Damiano ER. The structure and function of the endothelial glycocalyx layer. Annu Rev Biomed Eng. 2007;9(1):121–67. doi:10.1146/annurev.bioeng.9.060906. 151959.
37. Goddard CM, Allard MF, Hogg JC, Herbertson MJ, Walley KR. Prolonged leukocyte transit time in coronary microcirculation of endotoxemic pigs. Am J Physiol. 1995;269(4 Pt 2):H1389–97.
38. Wu L, Tiwari MM, Messer KJ, et al. Peritubular capillary dysfunction and renal tubular epithelial cell stress following lipopolysaccharide administration in mice. Am J Physiol Renal Physiol. 2007;292(1):F261–8. doi:10.1152/ajprenal.00263.2006.
39. Wu X, Guo R, Wang Y, Cunningham PN. The role of ICAM-1 in endotoxin-induced acute renal failure. Am J Physiol Renal Physiol. 2007;293(4):F1262–71. doi:10.1152/ajprenal. 00445.2006.
40. Payen D, Lukaszewicz AC, Legrand M, et al. A multicentre study of acute kidney injury in severe sepsis and septic shock: association with inflammatory phenotype and HLA genotype. PLoS One. 2012;7(6):e35838. doi:10.1371/journal.pone.0035838.
41. Angus DC, van der Poll T. Severe sepsis and septic shock. N Engl J Med. 2013;369(9):840–51. doi:10.1056/NEJMra1208623.
42. Takeuchi O, Akira S. Pattern recognition receptors and inflammation. Cell. 2010;140(6):805–20. doi:10.1016/j.cell.2010.01.022.
43. Chan JK, Roth J, Oppenheim JJ, et al. Alarmins: awaiting a clinical response. J Clin Invest. 2012;122(8):2711–9. doi:10.1172/JCI62423.
44. Herter JM, Rossaint J, Spieker T, Zarbock A. Adhesion molecules involved in neutrophil recruitment during sepsis-induced acute kidney injury. J Innate Immun. 2014;6(5):597–606. doi:10.1159/000358238.
45. Singbartl K, Bishop JV, Wen X, et al. Differential effects of kidney-lung cross-talk during acute kidney injury and bacterial pneumonia. Kidney Int. 2011;80(6):633–44. doi:10.1038/ki.2011.201.
46. Gomez H, Ince C, De Backer D, et al. A unified theory of sepsis-induced acute kidney injury: inflammation, microcirculatory dysfunction, bioenergetics, and the tubular cell adaptation to injury. Shock. 2014;41(1):3–11. doi:10.1097/SHK.0000000000000052.
47. Brown KA, Brain SD, Pearson JD, Edgeworth JD, Lewis SM, Treacher DF. Neutrophils in development of multiple organ failure in sepsis. Lancet. 2006;368(9530):157–69. doi:10.1016/S0140-6736(06)69005-3.
48. Zarbock A, Ley K. Mechanisms and consequences of neutrophil interaction with the endothelium. AJPA. 2008;172(1):1–7. doi:10.2353/ajpath.2008.070502.
49. El-Achkar TM, Hosein M, Dagher PC. Pathways of renal injury in systemic gram-negative sepsis. Eur J Clin Invest. 2008;38:39–44. doi:10.1111/j.1365-2362.2008.02007.x.
50. Krüger B, Krick S, Dhillon N, et al. Donor Toll-like receptor 4 contributes to ischemia and reperfusion injury following human kidney transplantation. Proc Natl Acad Sci U S A. 2009;106(9):3390–5. doi:10.1073/pnas.0810169106.
51. Kalakeche R, Hato T, Rhodes G, et al. Endotoxin uptake by S1 proximal tubular segment causes oxidative stress in the downstream S2 segment. J Am Soc Nephrol. 2011;22(8):1505–16. doi:10.1681/ASN.2011020203.
52. Mudaliar H, Pollock C, Komala MG, Chadban S, Wu H, Panchapakesan U. The role of Toll-like receptor proteins (TLR) 2 and 4 in mediating inflammation in proximal tubules. Am J Physiol Renal Physiol. 2013;305(2):F143–54. doi:10.1152/ajprenal.00398.2012.
53. Lin M, Yiu WH, Wu HJ, et al. Toll-like receptor 4 promotes tubular inflammation in diabetic nephropathy. J Am Soc Nephrol. 2012;23(1):86–102. doi:10.1681/ASN.2010111210.
54. Ferraro E, Cecconi F. Autophagic and apoptotic response to stress signals in mammalian cells. Arch Biochem Biophys. 2007;462(2):210–9. doi:10.1016/j.abb.2007.02.006.

55. Singer M. The role of mitochondrial dysfunction in sepsis-induced multi-organ failure. Virulence. 2014;5(1):66–72. doi:10.4161/viru.26907.
56. Hochachka PW, Buck LT, Doll CJ, Land SC. Unifying theory of hypoxia tolerance: molecular/ metabolic defense and rescue mechanisms for surviving oxygen lack. Proc Natl Acad Sci U S A. 1996;93(18):9493–8.
57. May CN, Ishikawa K, Wan L, et al. Renal bioenergetics during early gram-negative mammalian sepsis and angiotensin II infusion. Intensive Care Med. 2012;38(5):886–93. doi:10.1007/ s00134-012-2487-2.
58. Carchman EH, Rao J, Loughran PA, Rosengart MR, Zuckerbraun BS. Heme oxygenase-1-mediated autophagy protects against hepatocyte cell death and hepatic injury from infection/ sepsis in mice. Hepatology. 2011;53(6):2053–62. doi:10.1002/hep.24324.
59. Brealey D, Karyampudi S, Jacques TS, et al. Mitochondrial dysfunction in a long-term rodent model of sepsis and organ failure. Am J Physiol Regul Integr Comp Physiol. 2004;286(3):R491–7. doi:10.1152/ajpregu.00432.2003.
60. Schmidt C, Höcherl K, Schweda F, Bucher M. Proinflammatory cytokines cause downregulation of renal chloride entry pathways during sepsis. Crit Care Med. 2007;35(9):2110–9.
61. Mandel LJ, Balaban RS. Stoichiometry and coupling of active transport to oxidative metabolism in epithelial tissues. Am J Physiol. 1981;240(5):F357–71.
62. Gupta A, Rhodes GJ, Berg DT, Gerlitz B, Molitoris BA, Grinnell BW. Activated protein C ameliorates LPS-induced acute kidney injury and downregulates renal INOS and angiotensin 2. Am J Physiol Renal Physiol. 2007;293(1):F245–54. doi:10.1152/ajprenal.00477.2006.
63. Good DW, George T, Watts BA. Lipopolysaccharide directly alters renal tubule transport through distinct TLR4-dependent pathways in basolateral and apical membranes. Am J Physiol Renal Physiol. 2009;297(4):F866–74. doi:10.1152/ajprenal.00335.2009.
64. Hsiao H-W, Tsai K-L, Wang L-F, et al. The decline of autophagy contributes to proximal tubular dysfunction during sepsis. Shock. 2012;37(3):289–96. doi:10.1097/SHK.0b013e318240b52a.
65. Carré JE, Singer M. Cellular energetic metabolism in sepsis: the need for a systems approach. Biochim Biophys Acta. 2008;1777(7–8):763–71. doi:10.1016/j.bbabio.2008.04.024.
66. Vanhorebeek I, Gunst J, Derde S, et al. Mitochondrial fusion, fission, and biogenesis in prolonged critically ill patients. J Clin Endocrinol Metab. 2012;97(1):E59–64. doi:10.1210/ jc.2011-1760.
67. Green DR, Galluzzi L, Kroemer G. Mitochondria and the autophagy-inflammation-cell death axis in organismal aging. Science. 2011;333(6046):1109–12. doi:10.1126/science.1201940.
68. Waltz P, Carchman EH, Young AC, et al. Lipopolysaccharide induces autophagic signaling in macrophages via a TLR4, heme oxygenase-1 dependent pathway. Autophagy. 2011;7(3):315–20. doi:10.4161/auto.7.3.14044.
69. Frank M, Duvezin-Caubet S, Koob S, et al. Mitophagy is triggered by mild oxidative stress in a mitochondrial fission dependent manner. Biochim Biophys Acta. 2012;1823(12):2297–310. doi:10.1016/j.bbamcr.2012.08.007.
70. Wang Y, Nartiss Y, Steipe B, McQuibban GA, Kim PK. ROS-induced mitochondrial depolarization initiates PARK2/PARKIN-dependent mitochondrial degradation by autophagy. Autophagy. 2012;8(10):1462–76. doi:10.4161/auto.21211.
71. Gunst J, Derese I, Aertgeerts A, et al. Insufficient autophagy contributes to mitochondrial dysfunction, organ failure, and adverse outcome in an animal model of critical illness. Crit Care Med. 2013;41(1):182–94. doi:10.1097/CCM.0b013e3182676657.
72. Mizushima N, Levine B, Cuervo AM, Klionsky DJ. Autophagy fights disease through cellular self-digestion. Nature. 2008;451(7182):1069–75. doi:10.1038/nature06639.
73. Levine B, Yuan J. Autophagy in cell death: an innocent convict? J Clin Invest. 2005; 115(10):2679–88. doi:10.1172/JCI26390.
74. Ciechomska IA, Goemans CG, Tolkovsky AM. Molecular links between autophagy and apoptosis. Methods Mol Biol. 2008;445(Chapter 12):175–193. doi:10.1007/978-1-59745-157-4_12.
75. Finkel T, Hwang PM. The Krebs cycle meets the cell cycle: mitochondria and the G1-S transition. Proc Natl Acad Sci U S A. 2009;106(29):11825–6. doi:10.1073/pnas.0906430106.

76. Mitra K, Wunder C, Roysam B, Lin G, Lippincott-Schwartz J. A hyperfused mitochondrial state achieved at G1-S regulates cyclin E buildup and entry into S phase. Proc Natl Acad Sci U S A. 2009;106(29):11960–5. doi:10.1073/pnas.0904875106.

77. Schieke SM, McCoy JP, Finkel T. Coordination of mitochondrial bioenergetics with G1 phase cell cycle progression. Cell Cycle. 2008;7(12):1782–7.

78. Mandal S, Guptan P, Owusu-Ansah E, Banerjee U. Mitochondrial regulation of cell cycle progression during development as revealed by the tenured mutation in Drosophila. Dev Cell. 2005;9(6):843–54. doi:10.1016/j.devcel.2005.11.006.

79. Yang Q-H, Liu D-W, Long Y, Liu H-Z, Chai W-Z, Wang X-T. Acute renal failure during sepsis: potential role of cell cycle regulation. J Infect. 2009;58(6):459–64. doi:10.1016/j.jinf.2009.04.003.

80. Meersch M, Schmidt C, Van Aken H, et al. Urinary TIMP-2 and IGFBP7 as early biomarkers of acute kidney injury and renal recovery following cardiac surgery. PLoS One. 2014;9(3): e93460. doi:10.1371/journal.pone.0093460.t005.

81. Bihorac A, Chawla LS, Shaw AD, et al. Validation of cell-cycle arrest biomarkers for acute kidney injury using clinical adjudication. Am J Respir Crit Care Med. 2014;189(8):932–9. doi:10.1164/rccm.201401-0077OC.

82. Kashani K, Al-Khafaji A, Ardiles T, et al. Discovery and validation of cell cycle arrest biomarkers in human acute kidney injury. Crit Care. 2013;17(1):R25. doi:10.1186/cc12503.

83. Kellum JA, Venkataraman R, Powner D, Elder M, Hergenroeder G, Carter M. Feasibility study of cytokine removal by hemoadsorption in brain-dead humans. Crit Care Med. 2008;36(1):268–72. doi:10.1097/01.CCM.0000291646.34815.BB.

84. Peng Z-Y, Wang H-Z, Carter MJ, et al. Acute removal of common sepsis mediators does not explain the effects of extracorporeal blood purification in experimental sepsis. Kidney Int. 2012;81(4):363–9. doi:10.1038/ki.2011.320.

85. Heemskerk S, Masereeuw R, Moesker O, et al. Alkaline phosphatase treatment improves renal function in severe sepsis or septic shock patients. Crit Care Med. 2009;37(2):417–23–e1. doi:10.1097/CCM.0b013e31819598af.

86. Pickkers P, Heemskerk S, Schouten J, et al. Alkaline phosphatase for treatment of sepsis-induced acute kidney injury: a prospective randomized double-blind placebo-controlled trial. Crit Care. 2012;16(1):R14. doi:10.1186/cc11159.

87. Susantitaphong P, Perianayagam MC, Tighiouart H, Liangos O, Bonventre JV, Jaber BL. Tumor necrosis factor alpha promoter polymorphism and severity of acute kidney injury. Nephron Clin Pract. 2013;123(1–2):67–73. doi:10.1159/000351684.

88. Boerma EC, Koopmans M, Konijn A, et al. Effects of nitroglycerin on sublingual microcirculatory blood flow in patients with severe sepsis/septic shock after a strict resuscitation protocol: a double-blind randomized placebo controlled trial. Crit Care Med. 2010;38(1):93–100. doi:10.1097/CCM.0b013e3181b02fc1.

89. Liakopoulos OJ, Choi Y-H, Haldenwang PL, et al. Impact of preoperative statin therapy on adverse postoperative outcomes in patients undergoing cardiac surgery: a meta-analysis of over 30,000 patients. Eur Heart J. 2008;29(12):1548–59. doi:10.1093/eurheartj/ehn198.

90. Song YR, Lee T, You SJ, et al. Prevention of acute kidney injury by erythropoietin in patients undergoing coronary artery bypass grafting: a pilot study. Am J Nephrol. 2009;30(3):253–60. doi:10.1159/000223229.

91. Asfar P, Meziani F, Hamel J-F, et al. High versus low blood-pressure target in patients with septic shock. N Engl J Med. 2014;370(17):1583–93. doi:10.1056/NEJMoa1312173.

Chapter 9
Sepsis and the Lung

MaryEllen Antkowiak, Lucas Mikulic, and Benjamin T. Suratt

Introduction

Infections of the lung and pleural space are frequently associated with the development of sepsis syndromes. Nearly 50% of patients with bacterial pneumonia develop severe sepsis, and around 5% develop septic shock, with consequent mortality rates as high as 50% [1]. Additionally, sepsis from any source, pulmonary or extrapulmonary, may result in additional injury to the lung, known as the acute respiratory distress syndrome (ARDS), a syndrome characterized by an over-exuberant inflammatory response in the lung leading to increased alveolar-capillary permeability and predominantly non-hydrostatic pulmonary edema and hypoxemia. Although this syndrome and its associated histopathological findings (diffuse alveolar damage) were first described in 1967 [2], the criteria for diagnosis remained loosely defined for decades. In 1994, the American-European Consensus Conference (AECC) on ARDS, comprised of members of the American Thoracic Society and the European Society of Intensive Care Medicine, published the first standardized definition of this syndrome, with the hopes that such a definition would serve to better clarify the incidence, morbidity, and mortality associated with the syndrome, and provide homogeneous criteria which could be used to enroll patients in research protocols [3]. The committee established the following criteria, all of which were required to establish a diagnosis of ARDS:

1. Acute onset
2. Hypoxemia, manifested by arterial partial pressure of oxygen to fraction of inspired oxygen ratio (PaO_2/FiO_2 ratio) < 200

M. Antkowiak, MD • L. Mikulic, MD • B.T. Suratt, MD (✉)
Division of Pulmonary and Critical Care Medicine, University of Vermont College of
Medicine, 89 Beaumont Avenue, Given E407, Burlington, VT 05405, USA
e-mail: MaryEllen.Antkowiak@vtmednet.org; Lucas.Mikulic@vtmednet.org; Benjamin.
Suratt@uvm.edu

© Springer International Publishing AG 2017
N.S. Ward, M.M. Levy (eds.), *Sepsis*, Respiratory Medicine,
DOI 10.1007/978-3-319-48470-9_9

3. Bilateral infiltrates on chest radiography
4. Pulmonary artery wedge pressure (PAWP) < 18 mmHg or no clinical evidence of left atrial hypertension

The committee also described a less severe form of injury, known as acute lung injury (ALI), which followed the same set of criteria with the exception that it encompassed patients with a PaO_2/FiO_2 ratio of <300 [3].

This definition served the clinical and research community well for more than 15 years, but throughout that period, some concerns regarding the AECC criteria were raised. The definition of acute onset was not clearly described. The clinical diagnosis of ARDS or ALI did not always correlate well with histopathologic or autopsy findings. Chest radiograph interpretation could be highly variable. PaO_2/FiO_2 ratios and PAWP could be affected by the use of varying levels of PEEP, and PAWP assessment could also be affected by a variety of clinical factors. In 2012, new set of criteria for the diagnosis of ARDS were proposed, termed the Berlin definition. This specifies that the syndrome must occur within 1 week of a known insult or new or worsening respiratory symptoms. Although chest imaging is required to show the presence of bilateral infiltrates "not fully explained by effusions, lobar/lung collapse, or nodules," PAWP measurements are no longer required. Instead, the new definition states only that respiratory failure "not be fully explained by cardiac failure or fluid overload" to be considered ARDS. Furthermore, the Berlin definition establishes three categories of severity based on PaO_2/FiO_2 ratio as measured on mechanical ventilation with a PEEP of 5 cmH_2O. Severe ARDS is defined as a PaO_2/FiO_2 ratio ≤100, moderate ARDS as a ratio >100 but ≤200, and mild ARDS as a ratio > 200 but ≤300. The term acute lung injury has been removed from the definition entirely [4]. Retrospective analysis comparing both definitions with autopsy findings demonstrates that the Berlin criteria are more sensitive but less specific than the AECC criteria for the detection of the histopathological finding of diffuse alveolar damage [5].

Epidemiology

Patients with sepsis syndromes have a markedly increased risk for the development of ARDS, with rates approaching 20%, as compared with less than 1% in inpatients without evidence of sepsis [6]. Sepsis is indeed a leading risk factor for the development of ARDS. Historically, observational studies identify sepsis as the inciting insult in over 40% of cases of ARDS [7]. More recently, a large observational studies have estimated a wide range in the incidence of ARDS, between 7.2 and 58.7/100,000 patients/year, and that pneumonia and sepsis accounted for 42.3 and 31.4% of cases of ARDS, respectively [8–11]. Additionally, the risk of ARDS is nearly three times higher in trauma patients who develop sepsis syndromes as compared with trauma patients who do not (RR = 2.94; 95% CI, 1.51–5.74) [7]. As the severity of the sepsis syndrome increases, the risk of ARDS appears to increase as well.

In one series, 100% of patients with septic shock developed ARDS, yet only 15% of septic patients without shock met criteria for ARDS [6].

Several comorbidities and patient factors have been observed to modify the risk of developing ARDS in sepsis. Interestingly, diabetes has been found to be protective against the development of ARDS. Diabetic patients with sepsis are about half as likely to develop ARDS compared to nondiabetic patients with sepsis [12]. Conversely, chronic alcohol abuse appears to increase the risk of ARDS in septic patients. In one series, more than 50% of septic patients with a history of alcohol abuse developed ARDS, while those without such history developed ARDS in only 20% of cases [13, 14].

A variety of genetic polymorphisms may also predispose patients with sepsis to the development of ARDS. Certain variants of the genes encoding angiotensin-converting enzyme (ACE) and IL-6 have been linked to increased risk for and severity of ARDS [15]. Several polymorphisms of sphingosine 1-phosphate receptor 3 appear to be strongly predictive ARDS risk in septic patients [16]. Furthermore, although our understanding of the interplay between genetics and ARDS risk is still limited, multistep genomic analyses of large databases of patients with sepsis from both pulmonary and extrapulmonary sources have identified a variety of single nucleotide polymorphisms (SNPs) that are associated with increased risk of the development of ARDS, while still others have been identified as protective [17, 18].

Regardless of etiology, patients with ARDS are at substantially increased risk for the development of further lung injury while undergoing mechanical ventilation compared to ventilated patients without ARDS (e.g., patients intubated for airway protection or respiratory failure due to neuromuscular weakness). This additional injury, referred to as ventilator-induced lung injury (VILI), has been found to occur in patients with ARDS at rates as high as 30–50% [19]. While it has been proposed that patients with ARDS secondary to a septic etiology are at higher risk for VILI than patients with ARDS of a non-septic etiology, at the time of the International Consensus Conference on Ventilator-Associated Lung Injury in ARDS, which convened in 1999, there was no definitive evidence of this phenomenon [19], and to date this association has not been more fully elucidated.

Multiple observational trials, animal models, and small controlled trials have suggested that there may be distinct differences between ARDS from "direct" pulmonary sources (e.g., pneumonia or toxic inhalation) and "indirect" extrapulmonary sources (e.g., sepsis of urinary origin or pancreatitis). Most observational studies suggest a higher incidence of ARDS in patients with pneumonia-related sepsis than in those with sepsis of an extrapulmonary source. One review of the subject found that, although several published series demonstrate increased mortality from ARDS due to pulmonary sepsis compared to extrapulmonary sepsis, others show no difference in such rates [20]. Studies aimed at identifying genetic polymorphisms associated with susceptibility to ARDS have demonstrated that polymorphisms that may confer increased risk of the development of ARDS in patients with pulmonary sepsis differ from those that may increase this risk in patients with extrapulmonary sepsis [18]. The pathophysiologic mechanisms, which are discussed in the following section, may differ. In pulmonary-related causes of ARDS, as might be expected, the inciting injury targets mostly the pulmonary epithelial cells; extrapulmonary causes of ARDS however may target the pulmonary vascular endothelium instead [20]. Mouse models have also demonstrated a significantly greater inflammatory response in pulmonary as compared to extrapulmonary ARDS [21], and both lung and chest wall mechanics may be affected differently by pulmonary and extrapulmonary ARDS [22, 23]. The remodeling that occurs in the later stages of ARDS may also differ, with higher levels of collagen deposition noted in pulmonary ARDS as compared to extrapulmonary ARDS [20, 24]. Studies have also suggested a differing response to a variety of clinical and therapeutic strategies in direct pulmonary versus indirect extrapulmonary ARDS, many of which are discussed later in this chapter [20]. While these studies were not limited to patients with sepsis and ARDS (e.g., pulmonary sources of ARDS included aspiration and pulmonary trauma), taken together, these findings suggest that ARDS of pulmonary and extrapulmonary etiologies may in fact represent different clinical entities, although to date there has been little clinical evidence to suggest the utility of differing management strategies for these two groups.

The development of ARDS carries a significant mortality risk in all patients, reported between 31 and 60% [8–11, 25], and septic patients are no exception. Septic patients who develop ARDS have an approximately 1.4-fold increase in mortality than those admitted with sepsis syndromes of similar severity who do not develop ARDS [7]. Likewise, the presence of sepsis is independently associated with mortality in patients with ARDS, with reported odds ratios of 2.8–5.6 compared to patients with ARDS from other causes [26, 27]. Chronic alcohol abuse appears to further increase mortality risk in septic patients who develop ARDS: in one series of patients with sepsis complicated by ARDS, preceding alcoholism was associated with a 25% increase in the relative risk of mortality compared to patients without a history of alcohol abuse [13, 14].

Given the substantial morbidity, mortality, and economic cost associated with ARDS in septic patients, there has been extensive interest in developing an understanding of the complex pathophysiologic mechanisms underlying sepsis-related ARDS in efforts to reduce both its incidence and severity.

Pathophysiology of Sepsis-Induced Lung Injury

As with all causes of ARDS, disruption of the alveolar-capillary membrane (ACM) plays a key role in the development of sepsis-induced ARDS (Fig. 9.1). ACM integrity is essential in preventing the uncontrolled passage of plasma blood into the airspace while maintaining alveolar-capillary gas exchange. The ACM is composed of the alveolar epithelial cells, the corresponding basement membrane, the interstitial or intramembranous space, the capillary basement membrane, and the alveolar-capillary endothelial cells. Ninety-five percent of the alveolar space is covered by type I (flat) cells and the remaining 5% by type II (cuboidal) cells [28]. The latter are responsible for the production of surfactant, and sodium and chloride ion

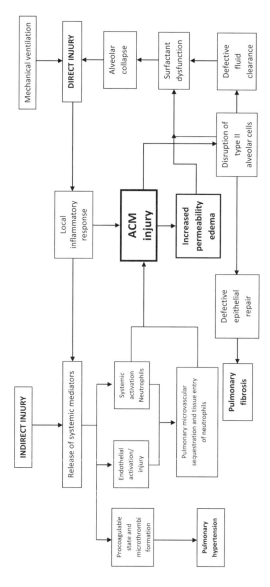

Fig. 9.1 Pathophysiologic mechanisms of the acute respiratory distress syndrome. Two main pathophysiologic pathways are believed to drive the development of ARDS. *Direct* injuries to the lung damage the alveolar-capillary membrane and initiate local and subsequently systemic inflammatory cascades. *Indirect* injuries initiate the pathophysiologic pathways of ARDS primarily through release of systemic cytokines and activation of the coagulation cascade. Following both direct and indirect initiators of ARDS, the release of systemic inflammatory mediators activates circulating neutrophils and the vascular endothelium of the lung, leading to pulmonary microvascular sequestration of neutrophils and inflammatory injury to the ACM. This results in failure of ACM barrier function and flooding of the alveoli with proteinaceous edema fluid. Both ACM injury and alveolar edema cause surfactant loss and dysfunction, which promote alveolar instability and collapse, driving further edema formation and alveolar injury, particularly in the setting of mechanical ventilation

transport, which plays a key role in removing fluid from the alveolar space. In addition, type II cells are able to proliferate and differentiate into type I cells and thus are a critical component of the response to lung injury [29, 30].

Both pulmonary and extrapulmonary sources of sepsis may lead to lung injury, with the same common end point of loss of ACM integrity, the hallmark of ARDS [3]. Disruption of this membrane results in increased permeability edema, with subsequent alveolar flooding with proteinaceous fluid (plasma) which impairs gas exchange and type II cell function. The latter leads to a decrease in surfactant production and impaired fluid removal from the alveolar spaces (Fig. 9.1). Finally, disruption of this barrier can itself lead to sepsis and septic shock due to bacterial translocation, as leading to pulmonary fibrosis due to defective epithelial repair [30, 31].

Regardless of initiating injury, two phases have been described in ARDS progression—an early inflammatory or "exudative" phase (typically lasting 5–7 days), in which both the capillary endothelium and the alveolar epithelium are affected, and a later repair phase which typically begins 7–10 days after ARDS onset and in some cases is pathologically "fibroproliferative," driven by dysregulated alveolar repair and the formation of granulation tissue and fibrosis in the airspace and interstitium [31].

Exudative Phase

As with all causes of ARDS, sepsis-associated ARDS occurring as a result of a direct pulmonary insult (e.g., severe pneumonia with sepsis) damages the ACM and initiates local and systemic inflammatory cascades. In the case of extrapulmonary sepsis, systemic release of cytokines is responsible for the cascade of events leading to ARDS, and such injury is often just one element of multi-system organ failure (Fig. 9.1).

Mediators of Humoral and Cellular Mechanisms

Neutrophils have been shown to be the predominant cell type in bronchoalveolar lavage fluid of patients who have ARDS, and these cells drive epithelial damage through the release of reactive oxygen species, proteases, and procoagulant factors [31–33]. Neutrophils are recruited to the lung and further activated by an array of soluble mediators, both endogenous (such as complement fragments or cytokines) and exogenous (such as lipopolysaccharide). The cytokine response to injury is subject to a balance between pro-inflammatory and anti-inflammatory mediators, and pathological skewing toward persistent and excessive inflammation is believed to be a major factor in ARDS pathogenesis [30, 31].

Inflammatory mediators are best characterized by the role that the innate immune system plays in the development of this cascade. The innate immune system is composed of both humoral and cellular components with the ability to recognize, via Toll-like receptors (TLRs) and other "pattern recognition receptors" (PRRs), certain highly conserved pathogen-associated molecular patterns (PAMPs), in order to provide the host with an immediate first line of defense prior to the development of a more specific adaptive immune response. TLR4 recognizes lipopolysaccharide (LPS), a component of the outer membrane of Gram-negative bacteria, and TLR2 recognizes peptidoglycan on Gram-positive bacteria. Following TLR activation (primarily on alveolar macrophages and type II epithelia), TNF-α and IL-1β are released, and these in turn induce transcription and release of additional pro-inflammatory cytokines in these and other immune cells, amplifying the immune response. Among these secondary cytokines, IL-6 and IL-8 play important roles in the activation, recruitment, and survival of neutrophils [30, 31, 34].

Once neutrophils are activated, their rheological properties are altered by the stiffening effects of intracellular actin polymerization, and these cells can no longer readily deform to pass through the small capillaries of the alveoli [35]. TNF-α- and IL-1β-mediated activation of the vascular endothelium and resulting expression of adhesion molecules (selectins and integrins) [31] furthers neutrophil pulmonary vascular sequestration and translocation to the alveolar space, thus injuring and occluding the microcirculation of the lung and exacerbating the inflammatory response. Many other inflammatory mediators have also been implicated in this early phase of ARDS, among them are the vascular endothelial growth factor (VEGF), high-mobility group box 1 protein (HMGB1), and thrombin, all of which contribute to the increased permeability edema seen in the early phase of ARDS [36]. Among the anti-inflammatory mediators present during the acute phase are the soluble TNF-α receptor and IL-1β receptor antagonists, IL-4, and IL-10, the latter playing an important role inhibiting the innate and adaptive immune system [34].

Fibrin and Platelets

Endothelial injury itself exerts an inflammatory response characterized by increased levels of circulating Von Willebrand factor [37], tissue factor, and plasminogen activator 1 inhibitor (PAI-1) [29, 31], which is responsible for the inhibition of urokinase plasminogen activator [38]. This cascade of events results in a pro-thrombotic state, leading to the formation of microthrombi in the pulmonary capillaries and fibrin-rich hyaline membranes in the alveoli. Both fibrin and thrombi may exacerbate this response by promoting the expression of adhesion molecules and further activating neutrophils, resulting in even greater permeability of the ACM [31].

Development of Pulmonary Hypertension

Several mechanisms are proposed for the often extreme pulmonary hypertension seen in ARDS. Among others, increased expression of endothelin-1 and thromboxane B2 has been reported [36]. This, together with thrombi deposition, formation of microthrombi, and vasoconstriction secondary to hypoxia, appears to drive this disorder, which not only compromises gas exchange but may also lead to additional hemodynamic instability with cardiogenic shock due to acute right heart failure.

Surfactant

Surfactant is a lipoprotein complex composed of phospholipids (90%) and four different surfactant proteins (SP) named SP-A, SP-B, SP-C, and SP-D. Surfactant's primary role appears to be the prevention of atelectasis by decreasing the alveolar surface tension and maintaining their patency, which is particularly critical in the setting of injury and plasma leakage into the airspace. During ACM disruption, flooding of the alveoli with plasma, fibrin, and other proteins results in surfactant dysfunction, alveolar collapse, impaired gas exchange, and drastically altered respiratory mechanics. Further, injury to type II cells leads to a decrease in surfactant production and worsening alveolar edema, exacerbating the process. It has also been shown that surfactant proteins SP-A and SP-D participate in the innate immune response by directly binding to antigens (such as bacteria, viruses, or fungi) and exerting both opsonizing and cidal effects, as well as helping to regulate the innate and adaptive immune responses in the lung [36, 39].

Ventilator-Induced Lung Injury

Though spatially heterogeneous, the lung in ARDS manifests three areas of alveolar ventilation: well-ventilated areas of patent alveoli (typically ventral in the supine patient), unventilated areas of fluid-filled or persistently collapsed alveoli (usually posterior), and widely spread areas of cyclically atelectatic lung which are subjected to repeated opening and closing with each respiratory cycle. Mechanical ventilation may worsen ARDS in a process termed ventilator-induced lung injury (VILI), by overdistending the patent alveoli ("volutrauma") and by shear stress injury of atelectatic areas from repeated alveolar opening, worsened by surfactant depletion and dysfunction ("atelectrauma"). These two mechanisms not only lead to direct injury but also promote the secretion of pro-inflammatory cytokines (such as TNF-α, IL-1β, and IL-6), resulting in further neutrophil recruitment, ACM damage, and impaired fluid clearance [31, 40]. Limitation of alveolar stretch in the setting of an appropriate recruitment of the lung using positive end-expiratory pressure (PEEP) decreases the release of inflammatory cytokines in both animals and humans [40]. In this context, the use of lower tidal volumes (6 mL/kg as opposed to 12 mL/kg) with scaled PEEP has been shown to decrease mortality from 40 to 31% [25].

Repair and the Fibroproliferative Phase

The regenerative phase of ARDS begins with the removal of alveolar fluid by active sodium transport. Sodium enters alveolar epithelial cells via an epithelial sodium channel, which is localized to their apical membranes, and water follows passively both via this mechanism, as well as through aquaporins, which are mostly located on type I cells. Subsequently, Na/K ATPases localized in the basolateral membrane of both type I and type II cells and are responsible for removing sodium (and accompanying water) from the cells in exchange for potassium [32]. From the interstitium, fluid is reabsorbed by lymphatics or the microcirculation or drains into the pleural space, causing effusion [32]. Soluble proteins are removed through a process of paracellular diffusion between alveolar cells [32], whereas insoluble proteins are engulfed by macrophages or alveolar epithelial cells [30]. Clearance of apoptotic neutrophils and epithelial cells by macrophages is a major mechanism of debris removal from the alveolar space [41] and has been shown to drive resolution of the inflammatory process through a mechanism called efferocytosis [42]. The delicate balance between inflammation and fluid reabsorption is a key prognostic factor in ARDS. Resolution of edema is associated with improved oxygenation, decreased mechanical ventilation days, and decreased mortality [30].

The repair of the ACM begins with the proliferation and differentiation of type II cells into type I cells, as well as by recanalization of the microcirculation and repair of damaged endothelium. Pulmonary fibroblasts play an important role during this repair process, as they secrete epithelial growth factors and basement membrane components. Although poorly understood, dysregulated repair leads to migration of the fibroblasts into the alveolar space with subsequent formation of granulation tissue and fibrosis, which impair gas exchange and may markedly decrease lung compliance [31]. The incidence of fibroproliferative ARDS varies widely by series, but may occur to some degree in more than 50% of ARDS patients based on lung biopsy data [43]. Factors influencing the progression to fibrosis are poorly understood, but its advent confers a worse prognosis for the affected patient including increased mortality, days on ventilator, and long-term respiratory impairment [44].

Clinical Considerations

To date, no effective therapy has been devised that directly addresses the underlying pathophysiology of ARDS, and treatment remains supportive. The mainstay of supportive care for patients with ARDS of any etiology, including sepsis, includes treatment of the underlying disorder and strict adherence to lung protective ventilation.

From 1996 to 1999, the ARDS Clinical Trials Network (ARDSNet) conducted the ARMA study, a randomized controlled trial of over 800 patients at ten large academic medical centers comparing low tidal volume ventilation (6 cc/kg of ideal body weight) to the standard tidal volume at the time (12 cc/kg). The protocol also sought to maintain end-inspiratory (static/plateau) pressures at 30 cmH₂O or lower and protocolized the level of positive end-expiratory pressure (PEEP) for any given level of fraction of inspired oxygen (FiO₂). Oxygen and pH goals were an arterial partial pressure of oxygen (PaO₂) of 55–80 mmHg and a pH of 7.30–7.45. With this strategy, the investigators demonstrated a reduction in 180-day mortality from nearly 40% in the standard (12 cc/kg) tidal volume group to 31% in the intervention (6 cc/kg tidal volume) group, as well as decreased days of mechanical ventilation and extrapulmonary organ injury, and a reduction in the number of patients still requiring mechanical ventilation at hospital discharge in the low tidal volume group [25]. Since the publication of these findings in 2000, low tidal volume ventilation strategies have been widely adopted in clinical practice.

Subsequently, given that morbidity and mortality in ARDS remain high despite low tidal volume ventilation, alternative ventilatory strategies have been investigated; though as of yet, none has been demonstrated to be superior to the protocol used in the original ARDSNet ARMA trial. In 2013, two randomized trials comparing early use of high-frequency oscillatory ventilation (HFOV) to usual care with low tidal volume standard ventilation in patients with moderate to severe ARDS reported no improvement in outcomes and possibly increased mortality in the patients treated with HFOV [45, 46]. Consequently, although this mode of ventilation is still considered in patients with ARDS and refractory hypoxemia, its use over standard ventilator modes early in ARDS is not recommended.

Extracorporeal membrane oxygenation (ECMO), which allows for extreme lung protective ventilation using cardiorespiratory bypass technology and "external lungs," may show promise in reducing mortality in severe cases of ARDS with refractory hypoxemia or respiratory acidosis. The use of ECMO has not been compared to low tidal volume ventilation in head-to-head randomized controlled trials. However, one randomized control trial comparing patients with severe ARDS who were referred to centers where ECMO was available to those who remained in hospitals that did not have the capacity to perform ECMO demonstrated that those patients who transferred had a 6-month survival of 63% compared to 47% survival in patients who did not transfer [47]. Although these results are promising, it should be noted that only 75% of patients transferred to centers where ECMO was available actually received the therapy, and in fact transferred patients spent more of their ventilator days on low tidal volume ventilation than those who were not transferred, suggesting better compliance with traditional ARDS protocol ventilation at the referral centers. Furthermore, the high cost, limited availability of equipment, and lack of expertise in many centers remain barriers to ECMO as a first-line therapy.

A variety of other supportive strategies aimed at reducing further lung injury and optimizing oxygenation have been evaluated in multiple trials. Traditionally, fluid resuscitation has been a mainstay of treatment of sepsis and septic shock [48], yet septic patients who develop ARDS may represent a subset in which overzealous fluid administration is detrimental. Given the increased capillary permeability seen in ARDS, it has been postulated that excessive fluid administration and volume overload may exacerbate the injury and increase the amount of total lung water, thereby worsening oxygenation and worsening lung compliance. A retrospective analysis of the ARDSNet ARMA trial compared patients whose fluid balance was more than 3.5 L positive to those who had a negative fluid balance and found a reduction in mortality in the latter ("dry") cohort, with an odds ratio of 0.50 [49]. They also noted increased ventilator and ICU-free days in the patients with a negative fluid balance. These findings were echoed in a large randomized control trial of 1000 patients which compared a conservative and liberal fluid strategy [50]. Fluids, diuretics, vasopressors, and inotropes were administered based on a study protocol assessing central venous or pulmonary capillary wedge pressures, mean arterial pressures, and other markers of hemodynamic status and organ perfusion. In the 7 days that patients remained on the protocol, the patients in the conservative fluid strategy group had an average cumulative fluid balance of −136 mL compared with the liberal fluid strategy group, who had an average cumulative fluid balance of +6992 mL. Though the conservative fluid strategy did not yield a statistically significant reduction in mortality, it was associated with fewer patient ventilator and ICU days without an increase in adverse outcomes other than electrolyte abnormalities. There was no increase in the rates of other organ failure in the conservative fluid group, including acute kidney injury and need for dialysis [50].

Since resolution of alveolar edema is an important mechanism in the resolution of ARDS and minimizing iatrogenic fluid administration has demonstrated benefit, strategies aimed at accelerating the rate of resolution of edema have also been studied. Inhaled β2-agonists have been demonstrated in vitro to stimulate cyclic AMP, leading to upregulation of sodium and chloride channels and osmotic resorption of fluid across type 1 and type 2 pneumocytes. The clinical implications of these findings were investigated in a multicenter, randomized control trial of nearly 300 patients [51]. Unfortunately, no treatment-associated reduction in mortality or days on ventilator was found, and the strategy of using β-agonists to improve alveolar edema in ARDS is not recommended [51].

Many other strategies to improve oxygenation and mitigate ongoing lung injury have been studied in patients with ARDS. Recently, several randomized controlled trials and a meta-analysis have suggested that there may be significant mortality benefit associated with the early use of both neuromuscular blocking agents and the use of "proning" or periodically ventilating patients in the prone position [52–55]. Neuromuscular blockade is thought to improve oxygenation, reduce the work of breathing, and improve patient ventilator synchrony, which may diminish the propagation of lung injury. Prone positioning improves oxygenation through improved ventilation/perfusion (V/Q) matching and may reduce ongoing lung injury as it has been shown to promote recruitment of atelectatic areas of the lung while reducing over distension in other regions. By minimizing atelectrauma and volutrauma, these maneuvers may diminish ongoing lung injury.

Strategies targeting the inflammatory response have been studied in ARDS, as well. Notably, early observational studies and a small randomized control trial suggested a potential benefit from corticosteroid therapy in ARDS. This was investigated in a larger randomized control trial of 180 patients all of whom had at least moderate ARDS for 7 days. While patients treated with corticosteroids had more ventilator-free and septic shock-free days than patients who received placebo, there was no reduction in mortality. Additionally, corticosteroid use was associated with more neuropathy and weakness, and in patients who were enrolled late in ARDS (more than 14 days after the onset of symptoms), mortality was increased [56]. Currently, corticosteroids are not recommended for routine use in patients with ARDS, although the role of steroids in very early ARDS remains controversial.

Conclusions

ARDS remains a common, serious complication in patients with sepsis of both pulmonary and extrapulmonary sources. Mortality, particularly in patients with severe ARDS, remains high, and patients who survive experience increased duration of ventilation and prolonged hospitalizations and often suffer from protracted disabilities once discharged home. While the inflammatory pathways that characterize the syndrome have been extensively described, these findings have not translated into widely available, effective therapeutic options, and much of the clinical research surrounding ARDS consists of negative trials. Treatment remains largely supportive, and although several recent therapeutic strategies show promise of mortality benefit, to date, low tidal volume ventilation and conservative fluid management remain the mainstays of clinical management.

References

1. Dremsizov T, Clermont G, Kellum JA, Kalassian KG, Fine MJ, Angus DC. Severe sepsis in community-acquired pneumonia: when does it happen, and do systemic inflammatory response syndrome criteria help predict course? Chest. 2006;129(4):968–78. doi:10.1378/chest.129.4.968.
2. Ashbaugh DG, Petty TL. Sepsis complicating the acute respiratory distress syndrome. Surg Gynecol Obstet. 1972;135(6):865–9.
3. Bernard GR, Artigas A, Brigham KL, Carlet J, Falke K, Hudson L, et al. The American-European Consensus Conference on ARDS. Definitions, mechanisms, relevant outcomes, and clinical trial coordination. Am J Respir Crit Care Med. 1994;149(3 Pt 1):818–24. doi:10.1164/ajrccm.149.3.7509706.
4. Ferguson ND, Fan E, Camporota L, Antonelli M, Anzueto A, Beale R, et al. The Berlin definition of ARDS: an expanded rationale, justification, and supplementary material. Intensive Care Med. 2012;38(10):1573–82. doi:10.1007/s00134-012-2682-1.
5. Thille AW, Esteban A, Fernandez-Segoviano P, Rodriguez JM, Aramburu JA, Penuelas O, et al. Comparison of the Berlin definition for acute respiratory distress syndrome with autopsy. Am J Respir Crit Care Med. 2013;187(7):761–7. doi:10.1164/rccm.201211-1981OC.
6. Fein AM, Lippmann M, Holtzman H, Eliraz A, Goldberg SK. The risk factors, incidence, and prognosis of ARDS following septicemia. Chest. 1983;83(1):40–2.
7. Hudson LD, Milberg JA, Anardi D, Maunder RJ. Clinical risks for development of the acute respiratory distress syndrome. Am J Respir Crit Care Med. 1995;151(2 Pt 1):293–301. doi:10.1164/ajrccm.151.2.7842182.
8. Li G, Malinchoc M, Cartin-Ceba R, Venkata CV, Kor DJ, Peters SG, et al. Eight-year trend of acute respiratory distress syndrome: a population-based study in Olmsted County, Minnesota. Am J Respir Crit Care Med. 2011;183(1):59–66. doi:10.1164/rccm.201003-0436OC.

9. Rubenfeld GD, Caldwell E, Peabody E, Weaver J, Martin DP, Neff M, et al. Incidence and outcomes of acute lung injury. N Engl J Med. 2005;353(16):1685–93. doi:10.1056/NEJMoa050333.
10. Rubenfeld GD, Herridge MS. Epidemiology and outcomes of acute lung injury. Chest. 2007;131(2):554–62. doi:10.1378/chest.06-1976.
11. Villar J, Blanco J, Anon JM, Santos-Bouza A, Blanch L, Ambros A, et al. The ALIEN study: incidence and outcome of acute respiratory distress syndrome in the era of lung protective ventilation. Intensive Care Med. 2011;37(12):1932–41. doi:10.1007/s00134-011-2380-4.
12. Moss M, Guidot DM, Steinberg KP, Duhon GF, Treece P, Wolken R, et al. Diabetic patients have a decreased incidence of acute respiratory distress syndrome. Crit Care Med. 2000;28(7):2187–92.
13. Moss M, Bucher B, Moore FA, Moore EE, Parsons PE. The role of chronic alcohol abuse in the development of acute respiratory distress syndrome in adults. JAMA. 1996;275(1):50–4.
14. Moss M, Burnham EL. Chronic alcohol abuse, acute respiratory distress syndrome, and multiple organ dysfunction. Crit Care Med. 2003;31(4 Suppl):S207–12. doi:10.1097/01.CCM.0000057845.77458.25.
15. Marshall RP, Webb S, Hill MR, Humphries SE, Laurent GJ. Genetic polymorphisms associated with susceptibility and outcome in ARDS. Chest. 2002;121(3 Suppl):68S–9S.
16. Sun X, Ma SF, Wade MS, Acosta-Herrera M, Villar J, Pino-Yanes M, et al. Functional promoter variants in sphingosine 1-phosphate receptor 3 associate with susceptibility to sepsis-associated acute respiratory distress syndrome. Am J Physiol Lung Cell Mol Physiol. 2013;305(7):L467–77. doi:10.1152/ajplung.00010.2013.
17. Bajwa EK, Cremer PC, Gong MN, Zhai R, Su L, Thompson BT, et al. An NFKB1 promoter insertion/deletion polymorphism influences risk and outcome in acute respiratory distress syndrome among Caucasians. PLoS One. 2011;6(5):e19469. doi:10.1371/journal.pone.0019469.
18. Tejera P, Meyer NJ, Chen F, Feng R, Zhao Y, O'Mahony DS, et al. Distinct and replicable genetic risk factors for acute respiratory distress syndrome of pulmonary or extrapulmonary origin. J Med Genet. 2012;49(11):671–80. doi:10.1136/jmedgenet-2012-100972.
19. American Thoracic Society, The European Society of Intensive Care Medicine, and The Societe de Reanimation de Langue Francaise, and was approved by the ATS Board of Directors, July 1999, International consensus conferences in intensive care medicine: ventilator-associated Lung Injury in ARDS. Am J Respir Crit Care Med. 1999;160(6):2118–24. doi:10.1164/ajrccm.160.6.ats16060.
20. Rocco PR, Pelosi P. Pulmonary and extrapulmonary acute respiratory distress syndrome: myth or reality? Curr Opin Crit Care. 2008;14(1):50–5. doi:10.1097/MCC.0b013e3282f2405b.
21. Menezes SL, Bozza PT, Neto HC, Laranjeira AP, Negri EM, Capelozzi VL, et al. Pulmonary and extrapulmonary acute lung injury: inflammatory and ultrastructural analyses. J Appl Physiol (1985). 2005;98(5):1777–83. doi:10.1152/japplphysiol.01182.2004.
22. Albaiceta GM, Taboada F, Parra D, Blanco A, Escudero D, Otero J. Differences in the deflation limb of the pressure-volume curves in acute respiratory distress syndrome from pulmonary and extrapulmonary origin. Intensive Care Med. 2003;29(11):1943–9. doi:10.1007/s00134-003-1965-y.
23. Gattinoni L, Pelosi P, Suter PM, Pedoto A, Vercesi P, Lissoni A. Acute respiratory distress syndrome caused by pulmonary and extrapulmonary disease. Different syndromes? Am J Respir Crit Care Med. 1998;158(1):3–11. doi:10.1164/ajrccm.158.1.9708031.
24. Negri EM, Hoelz C, Barbas CS, Montes GS, Saldiva PH, Capelozzi VL. Acute remodeling of parenchyma in pulmonary and extrapulmonary ARDS. An autopsy study of collagen-elastic system fibers. Pathol Res Pract. 2002;198(5):355–61. doi:10.1078/0344-0338-00266.
25. The Acute Respiratory Distress Syndrome Network. Ventilation with lower tidal volumes as compared with traditional tidal volumes for acute lung injury and the acute respiratory distress syndrome. N Engl J Med. 2000;342(18):1301–8. doi:10.1056/NEJM200005043421801.
26. Doyle RL, Szaflarski N, Modin GW, Wiener-Kronish JP, Matthay MA. Identification of patients with acute lung injury. Predictors of mortality. Am J Respir Crit Care Med. 1995;152(6 Pt 1):1818–24. doi:10.1164/ajrccm.152.6.8520742.

27. TenHoor T, Mannino DM, Moss M. Risk factors for ARDS in the United States: analysis of the 1993 National Mortality Followback Study. Chest. 2001;119(4):1179–84.
28. Divertie MB, Brown Jr AL. The fine structure of the normal human alveolocapillary membrane. JAMA. 1964;187:938–41.
29. Adeniji K, Steel AC. The pathophysiology of perioperative lung injury. Anesthesiol Clin. 2012;30(4):573–90. doi:10.1016/j.anclin.2012.08.011.
30. Ware LB, Matthay MA. The acute respiratory distress syndrome. N Engl J Med. 2000; 342(18):1334–49. doi:10.1056/NEJM200005043421806.
31. Suratt BT, Parsons PE. Mechanisms of acute lung injury/acute respiratory distress syndrome. Clin Chest Med. 2006;27(4):579–89. abstract viii doi:10.1016/j.ccm.2006.06.005.
32. Matthay MA, Zimmerman GA. Acute lung injury and the acute respiratory distress syndrome: four decades of inquiry into pathogenesis and rational management. Am J Respir Cell Mol Biol. 2005;33(4):319–27. doi:10.1165/rcmb.F305.
33. Pierrakos C, Karanikolas M, Scolletta S, Karamouzos V, Velissaris D. Acute respiratory distress syndrome: pathophysiology and therapeutic options. J Clin Med Res. 2012;4(1):7–16. doi:10.4021/jocmr761w.
34. Strieter RM, Belperio JA, Keane MP. Cytokines in innate host defense in the lung. J Clin Invest. 2002;109(6):699–705. doi:10.1172/JCI15277.
35. Skoutelis AT, Kaleridis V, Athanassiou GM, Kokkinis KI, Missirlis YF, Bassaris HP. Neutrophil deformability in patients with sepsis, septic shock, and adult respiratory distress syndrome. Crit Care Med. 2000;28(7):2355–9.
36. Bellingan GJ. The pulmonary physician in critical care * 6: the pathogenesis of ALI/ARDS. Thorax. 2002;57(6):540–6.
37. Ware LB, Eisner MD, Thompson BT, Parsons PE, Matthay MA. Significance of von Willebrand factor in septic and nonseptic patients with acute lung injury. Am J Respir Crit Care Med. 2004;170(7):766–72. doi:10.1164/rccm.200310-1434OC.
38. Idell S. Endothelium and disordered fibrin turnover in the injured lung: newly recognized pathways. Crit Care Med. 2002;30(5 Suppl):S274–80.
39. Wright JR. Immunoregulatory functions of surfactant proteins. Nat Rev Immunol. 2005; 5(1):58–68. doi:10.1038/nri1528.
40. Michaud G, Cardinal P. Mechanisms of ventilator-induced lung injury: the clinician's perspective. Crit Care. 2003;7(3):209–10. doi:10.1186/cc1874.
41. Galani V, Tatsaki E, Bai M, Kitsoulis P, Lekka M, Nakos G, et al. The role of apoptosis in the pathophysiology of acute respiratory distress syndrome (ARDS): an up-to-date cell-specific review. Pathol Res Pract. 2010;206(3):145–50. doi:10.1016/j.prp.2009.12.002.
42. Korns D, Frasch SC, Fernandez-Boyanapalli R, Henson PM, Bratton DL. Modulation of macrophage efferocytosis in inflammation. Front Immunol. 2011;2:57. doi:10.3389/fimmu.2011.00057.
43. Papazian L, Doddoli C, Chetaille B, Gernez Y, Thirion X, Roch A, et al. A contributive result of open-lung biopsy improves survival in acute respiratory distress syndrome patients. Crit Care Med. 2007;35(3):755–62. doi:10.1097/01.CCM.0000257325.88144.30.
44. Burnham EL, Janssen WJ, Riches DW, Moss M, Downey GP. The fibroproliferative response in acute respiratory distress syndrome: mechanisms and clinical significance. Eur Respir J. 2014;43(1):276–85. doi:10.1183/09031936.00196412.
45. Ferguson ND, Cook DJ, Guyatt GH, Mehta S, Hand L, Austin P, et al. High-frequency oscillation in early acute respiratory distress syndrome. N Engl J Med. 2013;368(9):795–805. doi:10.1056/NEJMoa1215554.
46. Young D, Lamb SE, Shah S, MacKenzie I, Tunnicliffe W, Lall R, et al. High-frequency oscillation for acute respiratory distress syndrome. N Engl J Med. 2013;368(9):806–13. doi:10.1056/NEJMoa1215716.
47. Peek GJ, Mugford M, Tiruvoipati R, Wilson A, Allen E, Thalanany MM, et al. Efficacy and economic assessment of conventional ventilatory support versus extracorporeal membrane oxygenation for severe adult respiratory failure (CESAR): a multicentre randomised controlled trial. Lancet. 2009;374(9698):1351–63. doi:10.1016/S0140-6736(09)61069-2.

48. Rivers E, Nguyen B, Havstad S, Ressler J, Muzzin A, Knoblich B, et al. Early goal-directed therapy in the treatment of severe sepsis and septic shock. N Engl J Med. 2001;345(19):1368–77. doi:10.1056/NEJMoa010307.
49. Rosenberg AL, Dechert RE, Park PK, Bartlett RH, Network NNA. Review of a large clinical series: association of cumulative fluid balance on outcome in acute lung injury: a retrospective review of the ARDSnet tidal volume study cohort. J Intensive Care Med. 2009;24(1):35–46. doi:10.1177/0885066608329850.
50. National Heart, Lung, and Blood Institute Acute Respiratory Distress Syndrome (ARDS) Clinical Trials Network, Wiedemann HP, Wheeler AP, Bernard GR, Thompson BT, Hayden D, et al. Comparison of two fluid-management strategies in acute lung injury. N Engl J Med. 2006;354(24):2564–75. doi:10.1056/NEJMoa062200.
51. National Heart, Lung, and Blood Institute Acute Respiratory Distress Syndrome (ARDS) Clinical Trials Network, Matthay MA, Brower RG, Carson S, Douglas IS, Eisner M, et al. Randomized, placebo-controlled clinical trial of an aerosolized beta(2)-agonist for treatment of acute lung injury. Am J Respir Crit Care Med. 2011;184(5):561–8. doi:10.1164/rccm.201012-2090OC.
52. Alhazzani W, Alshahrani M, Jaeschke R, Forel JM, Papazian L, Sevransky J, et al. Neuromuscular blocking agents in acute respiratory distress syndrome: a systematic review and meta-analysis of randomized controlled trials. Crit Care. 2013;17(2):R43. doi:10.1186/cc12557.
53. Beitler JR, Shaefi S, Montesi SB, Devlin A, Loring SH, Talmor D, et al. Prone positioning reduces mortality from acute respiratory distress syndrome in the low tidal volume era: a meta-analysis. Intensive Care Med. 2014;40(3):332–41. doi:10.1007/s00134-013-3194-3.
54. Guerin C, Reignier J, Richard JC, Beuret P, Gacouin A, Boulain T, et al. Prone positioning in severe acute respiratory distress syndrome. N Engl J Med. 2013;368(23):2159–68. doi:10.1056/NEJMoa1214103.
55. Papazian L, Forel JM, Gacouin A, Penot-Ragon C, Perrin G, Loundou A, et al. Neuromuscular blockers in early acute respiratory distress syndrome. N Engl J Med. 2010;363(12):1107–16. doi:10.1056/NEJMoa1005372.
56. Steinberg KP, Hudson LD, Goodman RB, Hough CL, Lanken PN, Hyzy R, et al. Efficacy and safety of corticosteroids for persistent acute respiratory distress syndrome. N Engl J Med. 2006;354(16):1671–84. doi:10.1056/NEJMoa051693.

Chapter 10
Organ Dysfunction in Sepsis: Brain, Neuromuscular, Cardiovascular, and Gastrointestinal

Brian J. Anderson and Mark E. Mikkelsen

Introduction

Sepsis-related organ dysfunction is common, complex, and associated with significant morbidity and mortality. Its presence defines sepsis, in addition to sepsis-related hypotension and sepsis-related hypoperfusion [1], and it has utility as a risk stratification tool to identify those at increased risk of death. Organ failure manifests in myriad ways in sepsis, mediated by a complex interplay between preexisting organ function and acute inflammation and endothelial and coagulation dysfunction incited by the infectious insult. Given the pathophysiology of sepsis-associated organ dysfunction, each organ in the body is known to manifest tissue injury in response to sepsis that is clinically apparent to various degrees (Table 10.1).

Using readily available diagnostic criteria to define organ dysfunction, a number of scoring systems have been validated to define sepsis and predict outcomes [1–3]. Given the prevalence and frequent need for life support in the setting of sepsis-related respiratory and renal failure, lung injury and kidney injury are covered in separate chapters. In this chapter, we focus on non-pulmonary, non-renal sepsis-associated organ dysfunction. We begin by examining neurologic complications of sepsis, followed by examination of cardiovascular and gastrointestinal organ dysfunction.

B.J. Anderson, MD, MSCE
Pulmonary, Allergy and Critical Care Division, Perelman School of Medicine at the University of Pennsylvania, Gibson 05002, 3400 Spruce Street, Philadelphia, PA 19104, USA
e-mail: brian.anderson@uphs.upenn.edu

M.E. Mikkelsen, MD, MSCE (✉)
Pulmonary, Allergy and Critical Care Division, Perelman School of Medicine at the University of Pennsylvania, Gates 05042, 3400 Spruce Street, Philadelphia, PA 19104, USA
e-mail: mark.mikkelsen@uphs.upenn.edu

© Springer International Publishing AG 2017
N.S. Ward, M.M. Levy (eds.), *Sepsis*, Respiratory Medicine,
DOI 10.1007/978-3-319-48470-9_10

Table 10.1 Clinically apparent organ dysfunction related to sepsis and criteria established to define sepsis [1–3]

Organ system	Clinical manifestation	Diagnostic criteria
Neurologic	Altered mental status Consciousness level Delirium	Glasgow Coma Scale Richmond Agitation-Sedation Scale (RASS) Sedation-Agitation Scale (SAS) Confusion Assessment Method for the ICU (CAM-ICU)
Neuromuscular	Myopathy Neuropathy Neuromyopathy Functional impairment	Medical Research Council (MRC) score Electrophysiology testing Barthel Index Functional Status Score for the ICU
Cardiovascular	Cardiomyopathy Arrythmia Myocardial ischemia Myocardial injury Hypotension	Echocardiogram Electrocardiogram Cardiac biomarkers Systolic blood pressure Mean arterial pressure
Respiratory	Tachypnea Hypoxemia	Use of mechanical ventilation Respiratory rate $PaO_2:FiO_2$
Gastrointestinal	Hepatocellular injury Biliary Intestinal	Alanine aminotransferase Aspartate aminotransferase Bilirubin Ileus
Renal	Acute kidney injury	Serum creatinine Urine output
Hematologic	Thrombocytopenia Coagulopathy Disseminated intravascular coagulopathy	Platelet count Protime Activated partial thromboplastin time Fibrinogen
Skin	Reduced capillary refill Mottling Livedo reticularis	Physical examination

Brain Dysfunction

Introduction

One of the initial signs of sepsis is often a change in mental status, one of many clinical manifestations that define its presence. In the literature, this clinical manifestation is known as sepsis-associated encephalopathy or septic encephalopathy, in addition to the more general terms of coma or delirium. Acute brain dysfunction, defined as coma and/or delirium during the critical illness state, is common and is associated with short- and long-term morbidity and mortality.

Diagnosis

Sepsis-associated encephalopathy is defined variably in the literature, ranging from objective measures such as an abnormal Glasgow Coma Score (GCS) to subjective measures such as an abnormal mental status according to a health provider [4–9]. Many studies now use coma and delirium as outcomes to describe brain dysfunction in critical illness because they utilize reliable and valid measurements to define these states. However, as GCS is included in many well-accepted illness severity scores, it remains an important measure of neurologic function that is routinely used in clinical practice.

At the bedside, an objective evaluation of consciousness is a vital initial step in the neurologic examination. Two of the more commonly used scales to assess consciousness are the Richmond Agitation-Sedation Scale (RASS) [10] and the Riker Sedation-Agitation Scale (SAS) [11], both of which can be used to screen for eligibility for delirium assessment. The RASS is a 10-point scale ranging from −5 to +4 (Fig. 10.1). A score of 0 corresponds to an alert and calm state, increasingly negative values correspond to deeper degrees of sedation, and increasingly positive values correspond to an increasingly agitated state [10]. The RASS has been validated against a variety of neurologic measures including neuropsychiatric evaluation, GCS, and electroencephalography [10]. In addition, the RASS has excellent inter-rater reliability that is superior to GCS [10]. Most studies define coma as a RASS of −4 or −5 and define deep sedation as a RASS of −3, −4, or −5 [12–40].

The most frequently cited method for diagnosing delirium in critically ill patients is the Confusion Assessment Method for the Intensive Care Unit (CAM-ICU) (Fig. 10.2) [12–37, 39–44]. The CAM-ICU is a well-validated screen for delirium with high sensitivity and specificity when compared to expert evaluation using the Diagnostic and Statistical Manual of Mental Disorders (DSM) criteria, has excellent inter-rater reliability, and can be administered to the nonverbal mechanically ventilated patient [43, 44]. Other strategies to identify delirium include the Intensive Care Delirium Screening Checklist (ICDSC) [38, 45–49], the Neelon and Champagne Confusion Scale [50], and the DSM criteria [45, 51, 52]. Strategies to measure delirium severity appear promising [53], but require further investigation before implementation in the clinical setting.

Ancillary neurologic testing, including EEG and brain imaging, frequently reveals nonspecific findings. Recent evidence suggests that certain malignant EEG patterns (e.g., triphasic spikes) correlate with abnormal brain MRI findings in sepsis (e.g., ischemic lesions, leukoencephalopathy) [54]. While these strategies have the potential to enhance our understanding of the neuropathology of sepsis-associated brain dysfunction [55–57], the clinical utility of these diagnostic studies remains uncertain.

From: **Monitoring Sedation Status Over Time in ICU Patients: Reliability and Validity of the Richmond Agitation-Sedation Scale (RASS) JAMA. 2003:289(22):2983-2991. doi:10.1001/jama.289.22.2983**

Table 1. The Richmond Agitation-Sedation Scale (RASS)

Score	Term	Description	
+4	Combative	Overtly combative, violent, immediate danger to staff	
+3	Very agitated	Pulls or removes tube(s) or catheter(s); aggressive	
+2	Agitated	Frequent nonpurposeful movement, fights ventilator	
+1	Restless	Anxious but movements not aggressive or vigorous	
0	Alert and calm		
−1	Drowsy	Not fully alert, but has sustained awakening (eye opening/eye contact) to voice (>10 seconds)	Verbal stimulation
−2	Light sedation	Briefly awakens with eye contact to voice (<10 seconds)	
−3	Moderate sedation	Movement or eye opening to voice (but no eye contact)	
−4	Deep sedation	No response to voice, but movement or eye opening to physical stimulation	Physical stimulation
−5	Unarousable	No response to voice or physical stimulation	

Procedure for RASS Assessment

1. Observe patient
   - Patient is alert, restless, or agitated.   Score 0 to +4
2. If not alert, state patient's name and say to open eyes and look at speaker.
   - Patient awakens with sustained eye opening and eye contact.   Score −1
   - Patient awakens with eye opening and eye contact, but not sustained.   Score −2
   - Patient has any movement in response to voice but no eye contact.   Score −3
3. When no response to verbal stimulation, physically stimulate patient by shaking shoulder and/or rubbing sternum.
   - Patient has any movement to physical stimulation.   Score −4
   - Patient has no response to any stimulation.   Score −5

Adapted with permission.[29]

Fig. 10.1 Consciousness assessment: Richmond Agitation-Sedation Scale as an example. From: Monitoring Sedation Status Over Time in ICU Patients: Reliability and Validity of the Richmond Agitation-Sedation Scale (RASS) JAMA. 2003;289(22):2983–2991 doi:10.1001/jama.289.22.2983

Epidemiology

Acute brain dysfunction occurs in the majority of critically ill septic patients. Early studies of sepsis-associated encephalopathy reported an incidence as high as 62 % [4–8]. The incidence of coma and delirium among patients with sepsis is difficult to know with certainty because most studies have enrolled critically ill patients with a variety of diagnoses, and the rates may vary by disease process. Although few studies have evaluated coma as a distinct outcome from delirium, an incidence of coma between 56 and 92 % [14, 15, 23, 38] with a median duration of approximately 2–3 days has been reported [12–14, 23]. However, many studies exclude patients

Fig. 10.2 Delirium assessment according to the Confusion Assessment Method for the ICU (CAM-ICU). From: Ely EW, Inouye SK, Bernard GR, Gordon S, Francis J, May L, et al. Delirium in mechanically ventilated patients: Validity and reliability of the confusion assessment method for the intensive care unit (CAM-ICU). JAMA. 2001;286(21):2703–10

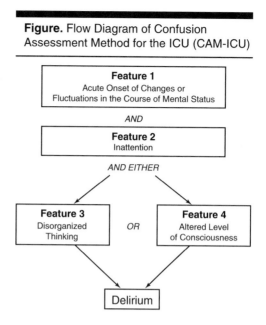

with persistent coma, accounting for roughly 2–18 % of patients, so the true burden of coma may be underestimated [13, 20–22, 33–36, 40, 41, 46]. As many as 75–90 % of critically ill patients suffer delirium during their illness [12–21, 33–38, 41, 42, 45–47, 50–52]. Delirium occurs early in the ICU course, with an onset usually within the first 1–4 days [20, 41, 45, 51, 52], and lasts for an average of approximately 2–5 days [12–14, 17, 18, 20–22, 33, 35, 41, 51, 52] representing approximately 50 % of all ICU days in one study [21].

Risk Factors

Studies evaluating risk factors for delirium have not exclusively enrolled patients with sepsis but provide some important findings. Observational studies in a variety of critically ill populations have reported that age [40], severity of illness [24, 40, 41, 46, 50], dementia or preexisting cognitive impairment [16, 41, 50], hypertension [45, 46], current smoking [45, 50], alcoholism [46, 50], and the use of restraints [58] are all risk factors for delirium. Sedative medications have also been identified as risk factors for delirium. While studies have reported conflicting results demonstrating a relationship between opiates and delirium [33–35, 38, 40, 41, 45, 50], in part due to the association between pain and delirium, benzodiazepines have more consistently been identified as a risk factor [13, 24, 33–35, 38, 40, 41, 45, 46, 50]. Of interest, a genetic predisposition to delirium may exist, as apolipoprotein E epsilon 4 genotype has been associated with increased risk and/or duration of delirium [36, 59–64].

Although the pathophysiology of sepsis-associated delirium remains unclear, inflammation, microglial activation, and disruption of the blood-brain barrier are frequently implicated [55–57]. Based on the inflammatory hypothesis, a number of studies have investigated statins as an intervention that may mitigate the risk of delirium development or severity. While the effect of prehospital statin use remains unclear in the surgical patient population [65–68], recent evidence suggests that continuing statins in prehospital statin users may reduce the risk of delirium, and this relationship may be of greatest benefit early in the course of critical illness in patients with sepsis [32, 42].

Prognosis

Acute brain dysfunction during sepsis is associated with worse outcomes. Early studies of sepsis-associated encephalopathy demonstrated an association with a longer duration of mechanical ventilation [7], longer ICU and hospital length of stay [7], and higher mortality [4–9]. Early deep sedation (RASS < 2) has also been shown to be associated with longer duration of mechanical ventilation and mortality [37]. Delirium, more specifically, is associated with myriad sequelae including longer duration of mechanical ventilation [13, 34, 39], longer ICU and hospital length of stay [19, 21, 24, 34, 39, 46, 51, 52], and mortality [13, 20, 24, 39, 46]. Furthermore, there appears to be a dose-response relationship, with longer duration of delirium (i.e., higher dose) being associated with future functional disability [12] and both short- and long-term mortality [13, 21, 22, 39].

Patients who experience delirium are also at higher risk of long-term cognitive impairment (LTCI) [13, 14, 17, 18]. LTCI has been reported in as many as 78 % of critical illness survivors at 1 year depending on the type of cognitive test used [14, 15, 17, 69, 70]. In the largest study to date, which enrolled patients with shock or respiratory failure, 34 % of patients had cognitive impairment at 1 year similar in severity to patients with moderate traumatic brain injury [14]. Radiographic studies in critical illness survivors have revealed an association between delirium and volume loss in specific brain regions, as well as disruption of the white matter tract integrity, providing further evidence for a link between delirium and LTCI [71, 72].

Prevention and Treatment

Several clinical trials in a variety of critically ill populations have evaluated interventions aimed at preventing or treating coma and/or delirium. Interventions have included pharmacological and non-pharmacological interventions, as well as different sedation regimens.

The most successful strategies to date have prioritized daily sedation interruption, sedation protocols, and early mobilization. Daily sedation interruption has been shown to reduce the duration of mechanical ventilation, the number of diagnostic tests ordered to assess changes in mental status [73], and to reduce duration of coma [30], but an effect on the incidence or duration of delirium has not been demonstrated consistently [30, 47]. Implementation of a protocol for de-escalation of excess sedation was associated with reduced odds of developing delirium in one before and after study in a trauma-surgical ICU [31]. Finally, interruption of sedation, paired with early mobilization, has been shown to reduce the duration of delirium [27].

Pharmacological interventions have included the use of antipsychotics, anticholinergics, and different sedation regimens. Antipsychotics may reduce the duration of delirium [48], but additional studies are still ongoing [26]. In the absence of demonstrative data to suggest the benefit of antipsychotic use to prevent or reduce the duration of delirium, and given potential harm [74–76], current guidelines do not recommend their routine use until additional data is available [77]. Rivastigmine, a cholinesterase inhibitor, was associated with longer duration of delirium and higher mortality in one study [25]. Several randomized clinical trials have suggested that dexmedetomidine may be the preferred sedative in treatment of coma and/or delirium [23, 28, 29, 78]. Sedation with dexmedetomidine is associated with lower rates of coma and more coma/delirium-free days when compared to lorazepam [23, 78] and with lower rates of delirium when compared to midazolam [29]. Ultimately, further research is needed to identify preventive and treatment options aimed at reducing rates and duration of acute brain dysfunction in order to potentially improve outcomes.

Neuromuscular Dysfunction

Introduction

Neuromuscular dysfunction in sepsis has been defined by a variety of terms including ICU-acquired weakness, ICU-acquired paresis, critical illness polyneuropathy, critical illness myopathy, or critical illness neuromyopathy. Its development is associated with functional disability that frequently endures and an increased risk of long-term mortality [79].

Diagnosis

Neuromuscular dysfunction in critical illness has been variably defined with some studies using clinical parameters such as muscle strength testing, others using electrophysiological testing, and some using a combination of the two. In the literature, the terms used to describe neuromuscular dysfunction are often used interchangeably prompting the proposal for uniform nomenclature and diagnostic criteria [80].

Table 10.2 Strength testing for ICUAW[a]

Muscle strength	Score
No movement is observed	0
Fasciculation or trace movement observed	1
Movement if the resistance of gravity is removed	2
Movement against gravity	3
Movement against some resistance	4
Movement against full resistance	5

Adapted from Medical Research Council (MRC) Scale for Muscle Strength [81]

[a]Testing for ICUAW involves bilateral evaluation using the above scale of six muscles: shoulder abduction, elbow flexion, wrist extension, hip flexion, knee extension, and ankle dorsiflexion

For the purposes of this review, we refer to this complication as ICU-acquired weakness (ICUAW). ICUAW describes clinically detectable weakness in the setting of critical illness with no other identifiable causes [80]. Critical illness polyneuropathy (CIP) refers to patients with ICUAW and evidence of axonal polyneuropathy on electrophysiological testing [80]. Critical illness myopathy (CIM) describes patients with ICUAW and either electrophysiological or histological myopathy [80]. Critical illness neuromyopathy (CINM) refers to patients who have ICUAW and evidence of both neuropathy and myopathy based on electrophysiological and/or histological testing [80].

The most commonly published method for identifying clinical muscle weakness is use of the Medical Research Council (MRC) muscle strength scale, which rates the strength of 12 muscles on a scale from 0 to 5 (Table 10.2) [81]. Most studies define ICUAW as a MRC sum score of <48 [82–89]. While the MRC scale has been shown to have good inter-rater reliability [82, 83, 86, 88, 90], it requires an interactive patient and is often not feasible to use early in critical illness given the frequency of coma and/or delirium [82]. A less commonly used measure of strength is the Function Disability Score [91, 92]. Some more recent studies have evaluated the use of ultrasonography, handgrip strength [83, 90, 93, 94], or portable dynamometry [94] as diagnostic tools or measures of clinical strength but additional studies are necessary.

Epidemiology

The true incidence of neuromuscular dysfunction in sepsis is uncertain because most studies enrolled patients with a variety of ICU diagnoses, evaluated patients at different times across studies, and focused on the most severely ill (e.g., prolonged ICU length of stay). In studies that enrolled septic patients, the incidence of abnormal electrophysiological testing ranged from 50 to 76 % [95–97], supporting that neuromuscular dysfunction is common after sepsis.

Additional estimates of the incidence of neuromuscular dysfunction come from studies enrolling all intensive care unit patients regardless of diagnosis or duration of illness. In these studies, ICUAW was diagnosed in 11–18 % based on MRC criteria [89, 98] and 21–57 % based on abnormal electrophysiological testing alone [99, 100]. Among patients admitted with acute respiratory distress syndrome, the incidence of ICUAW appears higher, estimated at 54 % [101]. The rate of neuromuscular dysfunction is higher in critically ill patients who remain in the ICU for at least 3–7 days, with an incidence of ICUAW based on MRC score of approximately 25 % [83, 84]. In this population, the combined incidence of CIP, CIM, or CINM ranges from 33 to 57 % [91, 102, 103], and the incidence of abnormal electrophysiological testing is 32–79 % [104–107]. Additional studies evaluating patients who required at least 10–14 days of mechanical ventilation demonstrated an incidence of ICUAW of 24 % by MRC criteria [98] and an incidence of neuromuscular dysfunction diagnosed by electrophysiological testing alone of 63–75 % [108, 109].

Risk Factors

A multitude of risk factors have been suggested to be associated with the development of neuromuscular dysfunction in critical illness. Risk factors include age [85], gender [84, 98], severity of illness [98], number of organ failures [84, 99], duration of mechanical ventilation [84], renal replacement therapy [98], gram-negative bacteremia [98], sepsis [107], hyperglycemia [98], aminoglycosides [98], and corticosteroid use [84, 110, 111].

Prognosis

Patients with neuromuscular dysfunction in critical illness have longer ICU and hospital lengths of stay [83, 84, 101, 107, 108], longer duration of mechanical ventilation [83, 84, 91, 99, 101, 107, 108, 112, 113], higher ICU readmission rates [83, 114], and higher mortality [79, 83, 96, 105, 108]. In addition, muscle weakness in long-term ventilated patients is associated with pharyngeal dysfunction and symptomatic aspiration [87]. Although patients with ICUAW can improve over time [84, 85], additional evidence demonstrates that critical illness results in prolonged neuromuscular dysfunction and decreased long-term physical function. Survivors of the acute respiratory distress syndrome, which is frequently the result of sepsis, have reduced exercise capacity [15, 85, 115, 116] and report subjective muscle weakness up to 2 years after their illness [85, 115, 116]. In addition, approximately one third of critically ill patients report a disability with their activities of daily living (ADL) 1 year out from critical illness [12]. Finally, studies evaluating quality of life in ICU survivors show low physical function domain scores lasting for several years [117].

Treatment and Prevention

Several studies have evaluated treatments and/or preventive strategies for neuromuscular dysfunction in critically ill patients, although these studies did not specifically enroll patients with ICUAW, CIP, CIM, or CINM. Early mobilization results in improved neuromuscular outcomes including an increased proportion of patients achieving functional independence at the time of hospital discharge [27], shorter time for patients to reach specific milestones such as getting out of bed or walking [27, 118], shorter ICU length of stay [118], shorter duration of mechanical ventilation [27], and a trend toward lower rates of ICUAW [27]. Intensive insulin therapy is associated with a reduced incidence of neuromuscular dysfunction diagnosed based on electrophysiological testing [119–121]; however, additional studies have reported higher risks of adverse events and mortality with intensive insulin therapy [122–124]. Given recent evidence showing that early mobilization promotes euglycemia, the preferred approach at present is to pair sedative interruption, spontaneous breathing trials, and early mobilization with a less intensive insulin therapy protocol [125, 126]. Transcutaneous neuromuscular electrical stimulation may lead to improvement in muscle strength and reduce the incidence of ICUAW, but confirmatory trials are warranted before this technology can be recommended [127]. Recent evidence also suggests that post-discharge rehabilitation after sepsis may reduce long-term mortality, but further investigation is needed [128].

Cardiovascular Dysfunction

Introduction

Cardiovascular dysfunction in sepsis includes myocardial dysfunction, arrhythmias, and reduced systemic vascular resistance that typifies sepsis and frequently requires the use of vasoactive agents to support adequate perfusion pressures. In this chapter, we focus on myocardial dysfunction and arrhythmias.

Myocardial Dysfunction

Myocardial dysfunction can include left ventricular (LV) systolic or diastolic dysfunction as well as right ventricular (RV) systolic dysfunction and is most commonly diagnosed by echocardiography [129–141]. Some reports in the literature have used direct hemodynamic measurements [134, 142–149] to evaluate cardiac function in sepsis, but this is challenging as sepsis is often characterized by a high-output state, and the use of invasive hemodynamic monitoring has declined in recent years. By echocardiogram, approximately 29–67% of patients with sepsis or septic shock have left ventricular (LV) systolic dysfunction (ejection fraction less than 45–55 %) [129–134], and approximately 15 % have severe LV systolic dysfunction (ejection fraction <30 %) [140]. Using direct hemodynamics or radionucleotide studies, as many as 56 % of septic ICU patients have LV systolic dysfunction [142, 143, 147]. LV diastolic dysfunction is also common [135, 139, 150], occurring in as many as 57 % of patients with sepsis [130]. Few studies have specifically evaluated right ventricular (RV) systolic dysfunction in sepsis, but it has been reported in as many as 32–52 % of patients [129, 142, 145]. Biventricular systolic impairment has been reported to occur in as many as 32 % of patients [142].

The presence of LV or RV systolic dysfunction in sepsis may be associated with higher rates of mortality, although results have been inconsistent [129–131, 147–149, 151, 152] across studies as the relationship may be modified by age and preexisting comorbid conditions [129–131, 147–149, 151, 152]. LV diastolic dysfunction in sepsis, however, has been shown to be associated with mortality in several studies [129, 130, 135, 141].

More recently, cardiac biomarkers have been evaluated as measures of myocardial dysfunction and/or subclinical myocardial ischemia [130–132, 135–138, 153–160]. Brain natriuretic peptide (BNP) and the N-terminal fragment of its prohormone (NT-proBNP), markers of left ventricular filling pressure and myocardial wall stretch, have been evaluated as markers of sepsis-associated myocardial dysfunction. BNP is elevated in approximately 71 % of patients with sepsis [130] but is not specific and may signify either LV systolic or diastolic dysfunction [131, 135, 159, 160]. Elevated BNP levels may be associated with mortality in septic patients, although the data are not conclusive [130, 131, 135, 159]. NT-proBNP has also been shown to be elevated in a wide range of 28–98 % of septic patients [130, 153, 161] and similarly may also be associated with mortality [130, 161]. Both troponin-I and troponin-T, markers of myocardial ischemia, are elevated in patients with sepsis. Elevations in troponin-I have been reported in 41–85 % of patients with sepsis [136–138, 154–158], while troponin-T has been reported to be elevated in 36–67 % of patients with sepsis [130, 138]. Both troponin-I and troponin-T have been proposed as markers of myocardial dysfunction [131, 136, 137] but are not specific and may signify LV systolic or diastolic dysfunction [131, 136, 137]. Elevated troponin in sepsis may be associated with longer ICU length of stay [137, 156] and increased mortality [130, 131, 136, 137, 155–157], although the clinical utility of these measures remains controversial.

Arrhythmias

The incidence of new-onset arrhythmias in critically patients is approximately 12 % [162]. The majority of new-onset arrhythmias are supraventricular tachycardias, most commonly atrial fibrillation [162]. New-onset ventricular arrhythmias are rare with an incidence of approximately 2 % [162]. Additional studies specifically in patients with sepsis report new-onset atrial fibrillation develops in approximately

6–8 % of patients [8, 162–169]. Sepsis appears to be a risk factor for atrial fibrillation and other tachyarrhythmias in both medical and surgical critically ill patients [167, 168, 170–174]. Atrial fibrillation during sepsis occurs within the first 3 days in the majority of patients [168, 169].

Risk factors for the development of arrhythmias in critical illness include age [162, 165, 166, 168, 169], history of paroxysmal atrial fibrillation [165, 169], history of coronary bypass [166], higher severity of illness [165], higher organ failure score [162, 168], lower left ventricular ejection fraction [165], need for mechanical ventilation [166], use of vasopressors [162], and presence of at least one episode of shock [163]. In addition, a recent clinical trial comparing low versus high blood pressure targets in septic shock demonstrated an increased incidence of new-onset atrial fibrillation in the high blood pressure target group presumably due to higher doses of vasopressors [175].

Several studies of noncardiac ICU patients (not exclusive to sepsis) demonstrate that patients with new-onset atrial fibrillation have longer ICU length of stay [163, 164, 168, 172, 173], a greater need for mechanical ventilation [163], and higher mortality rates [163–165, 171–173]. Additional studies evaluating new-onset atrial fibrillation specifically in patients with sepsis demonstrate an increased risk of inhospital stroke and inhospital mortality [167].

To our knowledge, no randomized controlled trials have been performed evaluating treatment of arrhythmias during sepsis nor have studies examined the optimal duration of therapy after developing new-onset atrial fibrillation related to sepsis. One open-label randomized trial of esmolol in patients with septic shock requiring vasopressor therapy with persistent tachycardia but not necessarily with an arrhythmia demonstrated an improvement in heart rate and mortality, but further studies are needed to confirm these findings [176].

Gastrointestinal Dysfunction

Introduction

Gastrointestinal dysfunction associated with sepsis includes liver dysfunction, ischemic hepatitis, and gastrointestinal hemorrhage. In addition, a common manifestation of sepsis that defines sepsis is the development of an ileus.

Hepatobiliary Dysfunction

Hepatobiliary dysfunction is generally identified by lab abnormalities including hyperbilirubinemia, elevated transaminases, and coagulopathy. See Chap. 10 for a detailed discussion of coagulopathy and hematologic dysfunction (e.g., thrombocytopenia) associated with sepsis.

The incidence of cholestasis is approximately 11 % in patients with sepsis [177], with studies in patients with bacteremia or endocarditis with or without sepsis reporting an incidence of hyperbilirubinemia ranging from 20 % when using a cutoff of serum bilirubin level ≥ 2 mg/dL up to 53 % when using a cutoff of serum bilirubin level ≥ 1.2 mg/dL [178–182]. Several other studies enrolling critically ill patients with a wide variety of ICU diagnoses report an incidence of hyperbilirubinemia ranging from 8 to 31 % when defined as a total bilirubin level ≥ 2 mg/dL [183–189]. Finally, in a large cohort of critically ill patients requiring mechanical ventilation, the incidence of hepatic failure was 6.3 % when defined as a total bilirubin ≥ 2 mg/dL in addition to elevated aminotransferase or lactate dehydrogenase levels [190].

Ischemic hepatitis can also complicate critical illness. To our knowledge, no study has evaluated the incidence of ischemic hepatitis specifically in patients with sepsis. However, in a study of 984 critically ill patients, the incidence of ischemic hepatitis defined as a ≥ 20-fold elevation of aminotransferase levels was 12 % [191]. In this study as well as other series of ischemic hepatitis, sepsis was identified as the inciting factor in 13–32 % of the cases [191–195]. Clinically relevant sequelae resulting from ischemic hepatitis include vascular changes consistent with hepatopulmonary syndrome [196], as well as an increased risk for both hypoglycemia and death [191, 197]. Patients with ischemic hepatitis who develop hyperbilirubinemia concomitantly appear to be at even higher risk for adverse outcomes, including nosocomial infections and death [194]. Fulminant hepatic failure is a rare complication of sepsis [198].

Risk factors for hepatobiliary dysfunction in critical illness include age [177, 179, 183, 189], male gender [188], severity of illness [177], degree of organ failure [177, 199], sepsis [184, 185, 199], presence of shock [183–185, 189], major surgery [184], use of positive end-expiratory pressure (PEEP) ventilation [184], gram-negative infection [177, 179, 184], number of blood transfusions [183, 185], and use of total parenteral nutrition [199].

Critical illness associated with hepatobiliary dysfunction is associated with a multitude of poor outcomes including longer ICU and hospital length of stay [177, 183, 186, 189], increased risk for acute respiratory distress syndrome [188], longer duration of mechanical ventilation [183], increased risk of gastrointestinal bleeding [183], and increased mortality [177, 181, 183, 185–190, 200]. Importantly, given the role of biliary transport in drug clearance and the frequency with which renal and hepatic dysfunction coexist in sepsis, impaired drug (e.g., antibiotic) clearance resulting in toxicity likely contributes to the adverse outcomes associated with multisystem organ failure. No specific therapies are currently available for treatment of hepatobiliary dysfunction outside of supportive care.

Gastrointestinal Hemorrhage

Gastrointestinal (GI) bleeding, usually the result of what has been termed stress ulcers, is another feared gastrointestinal complication of critical illness. Several studies have evaluated the incidence of GI bleeding in general critically ill patients, and estimates range from 8 to 20 % [201–206] down to 0.2–1.5 % [207, 208] depending on the population studied, the definition used, and the frequency of prophylaxis. Risk factors for the development of GI hemorrhage include age [207], respiratory failure requiring mechanical ventilation [201, 204, 206, 208, 209], shock [202, 209], sepsis [207, 209], postsurgical infection [202, 210], renal failure [206, 209], and thrombocytopenia or coagulopathy [201, 204, 206, 208, 211]. The source of hemorrhage is most commonly ulceration of the stomach followed by the duodenum, with esophageal being the least common [202, 206, 208, 210, 211]. GI bleeding in critically ill patients is associated with a higher need for mechanical ventilation [201], longer duration of mechanical ventilation [201], longer ICU length of stay [207], and mortality [201, 206]. Although there have been no randomized controlled trials of stress ulcer prophylaxis specifically in patients with sepsis, a significant number of patients enrolled in the stress ulcer prophylaxis trials had a diagnosis of sepsis. As a result, current recommendations include stress ulcer prophylaxis, using proton pump inhibitors or H2-receptor antagonists, for patients with sepsis or septic shock who have bleeding risk factors [125].

Conclusion

In summary, sepsis-associated organ dysfunction is common and its development is associated with significant morbidity and mortality. In sepsis survivors, the consequences of sepsis-related organ dysfunction frequently endure, which highlights the importance of evaluation and identification of impairment and the timely use of interventions and rehabilitation to restore function.

References

1. Levy MM, Fink MP, Marshall JC, Abraham E, Angus D, Cook D, et al. 2001 SCCM/ESICM/ACCP/ATS/SIS international sepsis definitions conference. Intensive Care Med. 2003;29(4):530–8.
2. Ferreira FL, Bota DP, Bross A, Melot C, Vincent JL. Serial evaluation of the SOFA score to predict outcome in critically ill patients. JAMA. 2001;286(14):1754–8.
3. Marshall JC, Cook DJ, Christou NV, Bernard GR, Sprung CL, Sibbald WJ. Multiple organ dysfunction score: a reliable descriptor of a complex clinical outcome. Crit Care Med. 1995;23(10):1638–52.
4. Eidelman LA, Putterman D, Putterman C, Sprung CL. The spectrum of septic encephalopathy. definitions, etiologies, and mortalities. JAMA. 1996;275(6):470–3.
5. Sprung CL, Peduzzi PN, Shatney CH, Schein RM, Wilson MF, Sheagren JN, et al. Impact of encephalopathy on mortality in the sepsis syndrome. the veterans administration systemic sepsis cooperative study group. Crit Care Med. 1990;18(8):801–6.
6. Pine RW, Wertz MJ, Lennard ES, Dellinger EP, Carrico CJ, Minshew BH. Determinants of organ malfunction or death in patients with intra-abdominal sepsis. A discriminant analysis. Arch Surg. 1983;118(2):242–9.

7. Zhang L, Wang X, Ai Y, Guo Q, Huang L, Liu Z, et al. Epidemiological features and risk factors of sepsis-associated encephalopathy in intensive care unit patients: 2008–2011. Chin Med J (English Edn). 2012;125(5):828–31.
8. Ledingham IM, McArdle CS. Prospective study of the treatment of septic shock. Lancet. 1978;1(8075):1194–7.
9. Tran DD, Groeneveld AB, van der Meulen J, Nauta JJ, Strack van Schijndel RJ, Thijs LG. Age, chronic disease, sepsis, organ system failure, and mortality in a medical intensive care unit. Crit Care Med. 1990;18(5):474–9.
10. Ely EW, Truman B, Shintani A, Thomason JW, Wheeler AP, Gordon S, et al. Monitoring sedation status over time in ICU patients: reliability and validity of the richmond agitation-sedation scale (RASS). JAMA. 2003;289(22):2983–91.
11. Khan BA, Guzman O, Campbell NL, Walroth T, Tricker J, Hui SL, et al. Comparison and agreement between the richmond agitation-sedation scale and the riker sedation-agitation scale in evaluating patients' eligibility for delirium assessment in the ICU. Chest. 2012;142(1):48–54.
12. Brummel NE, Jackson JC, Pandharipande PP, Thompson JL, Shintani AK, Dittus RS, et al. Delirium in the ICU and subsequent long-term disability among survivors of mechanical ventilation. Crit Care Med. 42(2):369–77.
13. Ely EW, Shintani A, Truman B, Speroff T, Gordon SM, Harrell Jr FE, et al. Delirium as a predictor of mortality in mechanically ventilated patients in the intensive care unit. JAMA. 2004;291(14):1753–62.
14. Pandharipande PP, Girard TD, Jackson JC, Morandi A, Thompson JL, Pun BT, et al. Long-term cognitive impairment after critical illness. N Engl J Med. 2013;369(14):1306–16.
15. Needham DM, Dinglas VD, Morris PE, Jackson JC, Hough CL, Mendez-Tellez PA, et al. Physical and cognitive performance of patients with acute lung injury 1 year after initial trophic versus full enteral feeding. EDEN trial follow-up. Am J Respir Crit Care Med. 2013;188(5):567–76.
16. McNicoll L, Pisani MA, Zhang Y, Ely EW, Siegel MD, Inouye SK. Delirium in the intensive care unit: occurrence and clinical course in older patients. J Am Geriatr Soc. 2003;51(5):591–8.
17. Girard TD, Jackson JC, Pandharipande PP, Pun BT, Thompson JL, Shintani AK, et al. Delirium as a predictor of long-term cognitive impairment in survivors of critical illness. Crit Care Med. 2010;38(7):1513–20.
18. van den Boogaard M, Schoonhoven L, Evers AW, van der Hoeven JG, van Achterberg T, Pickkers P. Delirium in critically ill patients: impact on long-term health-related quality of life and cognitive functioning. Crit Care Med. 2012;40(1):112–8.
19. Thomason JW, Shintani A, Peterson JF, Pun BT, Jackson JC, Ely EW. Intensive care unit delirium is an independent predictor of longer hospital stay: a prospective analysis of 261 non-ventilated patients. Crit Care. 2005;9(4):R375–81.
20. Lin SM, Liu CY, Wang CH, Lin HC, Huang CD, Huang PY, et al. The impact of delirium on the survival of mechanically ventilated patients. Crit Care Med. 2004;32(11):2254–9.
21. Patel SB, Poston JT, Pohlman A, Hall JB, Kress JP. Rapidly reversible, sedation-related delirium versus persistent delirium in the intensive care unit. Am J Respir Crit Care Med. 2014;189(6):658–65.
22. Pisani MA, Kong SY, Kasl SV, Murphy TE, Araujo KL, Van Ness PH. Days of delirium are associated with 1-year mortality in an older intensive care unit population. Am J Respir Crit Care Med. 2009;180(11):1092–7.
23. Pandharipande PP, Pun BT, Herr DL, Maze M, Girard TD, Miller RR, et al. Effect of sedation with dexmedetomidine vs lorazepam on acute brain dysfunction in mechanically ventilated patients: the MENDS randomized controlled trial. JAMA. 2007;298(22):2644–53.
24. Salluh JI, Soares M, Teles JM, Ceraso D, Raimondi N, Nava VS, et al. Delirium epidemiology in critical care (DECCA): an international study. Crit Care. 2010;14(6):R210.
25. van Eijk MM, Roes KC, Honing ML, Kuiper MA, Karakus A, van der Jagt M, et al. Effect of rivastigmine as an adjunct to usual care with haloperidol on duration of delirium and mortal-

ity in critically ill patients: a multicentre, double-blind, placebo-controlled randomised trial. Lancet. 2010;376(9755):1829–37.

26. Girard TD, Pandharipande PP, Carson SS, Schmidt GA, Wright PE, Canonico AE, et al. Feasibility, efficacy, and safety of antipsychotics for intensive care unit delirium: the MIND randomized, placebo-controlled trial. Crit Care Med. 2010;38(2):428–37.

27. Schweickert WD, Pohlman MC, Pohlman AS, Nigos C, Pawlik AJ, Esbrook CL, et al. Early physical and occupational therapy in mechanically ventilated, critically ill patients: a randomised controlled trial. Lancet. 2009;373(9678):1874–82.

28. Ruokonen E, Parviainen I, Jakob SM, Nunes S, Kaukonen M, Shepherd ST, et al. "Dexmedetomidine for Continuous Sedation" Investigators. Dexmedetomidine versus propofol/midazolam for long-term sedation during mechanical ventilation. Intensive Care Med. 2009;35(2):282–90.

29. Riker RR, Shehabi Y, Bokesch PM, Ceraso D, Wisemandle W, Koura F, et al. SEDCOM (safety and efficacy of dexmedetomidine compared with midazolam) study group. Dexmedetomidine vs midazolam for sedation of critically ill patients: a randomized trial. JAMA. 2009;301(5):489–99.

30. Girard TD, Kress JP, Fuchs BD, Thomason JW, Schweickert WD, Pun BT, et al. Efficacy and safety of a paired sedation and ventilator weaning protocol for mechanically ventilated patients in intensive care (awakening and breathing controlled trial): a randomised controlled trial. Lancet. 2008;371(9607):126–34.

31. Dale CR, Kannas DA, Fan VS, Daniel SL, Deem S, Yanez III ND, et al. Improved analgesia, sedation, and delirium protocol associated with decreased duration of delirium and mechanical ventilation. Ann Am Thorac Soc. 2014;11(3):367–74.

32. Page VJ, Davis D, Zhao XB, Norton S, Casarin A, Brown T, et al. Statin use and risk of delirium in the critically ill. Am J Respir Crit Care Med. 2014;189(6):666–73.

33. Agarwal V, O'Neill PJ, Cotton BA, Pun BT, Haney S, Thompson J, et al. Prevalence and risk factors for development of delirium in burn intensive care unit patients. J Burn Care Res. 2010;31(5):706–15.

34. Lat I, McMillian W, Taylor S, Janzen JM, Papadopoulos S, Korth L, et al. The impact of delirium on clinical outcomes in mechanically ventilated surgical and trauma patients. Crit Care Med. 2009;37(6):1898–905.

35. Pandharipande P, Cotton BA, Shintani A, Thompson J, Pun BT, Morris Jr JA, et al. Prevalence and risk factors for development of delirium in surgical and trauma intensive care unit patients. J Trauma Injury Infect Crit Care. 2008;65(1):34–41.

36. Ely EW, Girard TD, Shintani AK, Jackson JC, Gordon SM, Thomason JW, et al. Apolipoprotein E4 polymorphism as a genetic predisposition to delirium in critically ill patients. Crit Care Med. 2007;35(1):112–7.

37. Shehabi Y, Bellomo R, Reade MC, Bailey M, Bass F, Howe B, et al. Sedation Practice in Intensive Care Evaluation (SPICE) Study Investigators. ANZICS Clinical Trials Group. Early intensive care sedation predicts long-term mortality in ventilated critically ill patients. Am J Respir Crit Care Med. 2012;186(8):724–31.

38. Skrobik Y, Leger C, Cossette M, Michaud V, Turgeon J. Factors predisposing to coma and delirium: fentanyl and midazolam exposure; CYP3A5, ABCB1, and ABCG2 genetic polymorphisms; and inflammatory factors. Crit Care Med. 2013;41(4):999–1008.

39. Shehabi Y, Riker RR, Bokesch PM, Wisemandle W, Shintani A, Ely EW. SEDCOM (Safety and Efficacy of Dexmedetomidine Compared With Midazolam) Study Group. Delirium duration and mortality in lightly sedated, mechanically ventilated intensive care patients. Crit Care Med. 2010;38(12):2311–8.

40. Pandharipande P, Shintani A, Peterson J, Pun BT, Wilkinson GR, Dittus RS, et al. Lorazepam is an independent risk factor for transitioning to delirium in intensive care unit patients. Anesthesiology. 2006;104(1):21–6.

41. Pisani MA, Murphy TE, Araujo KL, Slattum P, Van Ness PH, Inouye SK. Benzodiazepine and opioid use and the duration of intensive care unit delirium in an older population. Crit Care Med. 2009;37(1):177–83.

42. Morandi A, Hughes CG, Thompson JL, Pandharipande PP, Shintani AK, Vasilevskis EE, et al. Statins and delirium during critical illness: a multicenter, prospective cohort study*. Crit Care Med. 2014;42(8):1899–909.
43. Ely EW, Margolin R, Francis J, May L, Truman B, Dittus R, et al. Evaluation of delirium in critically ill patients: validation of the confusion assessment method for the intensive care unit (CAM-ICU). Crit Care Med. 2001;29(7):1370–9.
44. Ely EW, Inouye SK, Bernard GR, Gordon S, Francis J, May L, et al. Delirium in mechanically ventilated patients: validity and reliability of the confusion assessment method for the intensive care unit (CAM-ICU). JAMA. 2001;286(21):2703–10.
45. Dubois MJ, Bergeron N, Dumont M, Dial S, Skrobik Y. Delirium in an intensive care unit: a study of risk factors. Intensive Care Med. 2001;27(8):1297–304.
46. Ouimet S, Kavanagh BP, Gottfried SB, Skrobik Y. Incidence, risk factors and consequences of ICU delirium. Intensive Care Med. 2007;33(1):66–73.
47. Mehta S, Burry L, Cook D, Fergusson D, Steinberg M, Granton J, et al. Daily sedation interruption in mechanically ventilated critically ill patients cared for with a sedation protocol: a randomized controlled trial. JAMA. 2012;308(19):1985–92.
48. Devlin JW, Roberts RJ, Fong JJ, Skrobik Y, Riker RR, Hill NS, et al. Efficacy and safety of quetiapine in critically ill patients with delirium: a prospective, multicenter, randomized, double-blind, placebo-controlled pilot study. Crit Care Med. 2010;38(2):419–27.
49. Reade MC, O'Sullivan K, Bates S, Goldsmith D, Ainslie WR, Bellomo R. Dexmedetomidine vs. haloperidol in delirious, agitated, intubated patients: a randomised open-label trial. Crit Care. 2009;13(3):R75.
50. Van Rompaey B, Elseviers MM, Schuurmans MJ, Shortridge-Baggett LM, Truijen S, Bossaert L. Risk factors for delirium in intensive care patients: a prospective cohort study. Crit Care. 2009;13(3):R77.
51. Kishi Y, Iwasaki Y, Takezawa K, Kurosawa H, Endo S. Delirium in critical care unit patients admitted through an emergency room. Gen Hosp Psychiatry. 1995;17(5):371–9.
52. Ely EW, Gautam S, Margolin R, Francis J, May L, Speroff T, et al. The impact of delirium in the intensive care unit on hospital length of stay. Intensive Care Med. 2001;27(12):1892–900.
53. Inouye SK, Kosar CM, Tommet D, Schmitt EM, Puelle MR, Saczynski JS, et al. The CAM-S: development and validation of a new scoring system for delirium severity in 2 cohorts. Ann Intern Med. 2014;160(8):526–33.
54. Polito A, Eischwald F, Maho AL, Polito A, Azabou E, Annane D, et al. Pattern of brain injury in the acute setting of human septic shock. Crit Care. 2013;17(5):R204.
55. Sharshar T, Annane D, de la Grandmaison GL, Brouland JP, Hopkinson NS, Francoise G. The neuropathology of septic shock. Brain Pathol. 2004;14(1):21–33.
56. Sharshar T, Hopkinson NS, Orlikowski D, Annane D. Science review: the brain in sepsis—culprit and victim. Crit Care. 2005;9(1):37–44.
57. Sonneville R, Verdonk F, Rauturier C, Klein IF, Wolff M, Annane D, et al. Understanding brain dysfunction in sepsis. Ann Intensive Care. 2013;3(1):15.
58. Inouye SK. Prevention of delirium in hospitalized older patients: risk factors and targeted intervention strategies. Ann Med. 2000;32(4):257–63.
59. Bryson GL, Wyand A, Wozny D, Rees L, Taljaard M, Nathan H. A prospective cohort study evaluating associations among delirium, postoperative cognitive dysfunction, and apolipoprotein E genotype following open aortic repair. Can J Anaesth. 2011;58(3):246–55.
60. van Munster BC, Korevaar JC, Zwinderman AH, Leeflang MM, de Rooij SE. The association between delirium and the apolipoprotein E epsilon 4 allele: new study results and a meta-analysis. Am J Geriatr Psychiatry. 2009;17(10):856–62.
61. van Munster BC, Korevaar JC, de Rooij SE, Levi M, Zwinderman AH. The association between delirium and the apolipoprotein E epsilon4 allele in the elderly. Psychiatr Genet. 2007;17(5):261–6.
62. Leung JM, Sands LP, Wang Y, Poon A, Kwok PY, Kane JP, et al. Apolipoprotein E e4 allele increases the risk of early postoperative delirium in older patients undergoing noncardiac surgery. Anesthesiology. 2007;107(3):406–11.

63. Adamis D, Treloar A, Martin FC, Gregson N, Hamilton G, Macdonald AJ. APOE and cytokines as biological markers for recovery of prevalent delirium in elderly medical inpatients. Int J Geriatr Psychiatry. 2007;22(7):688–94.

64. Tagarakis GI, Tsolaki-Tagaraki F, Tsolaki M, Diegeler A, Tsilimingas NB, Papassotiropoulos A. The role of apolipoprotein E in cognitive decline and delirium after bypass heart operations. Am J Alzheimer Dis Other Dement. 2007;22(3):223–8.

65. Katznelson R, Djaiani GN, Borger MA, Friedman Z, Abbey SE, Fedorko L, et al. Preoperative use of statins is associated with reduced early delirium rates after cardiac surgery. Anesthesiology. 2009;110(1):67–73.

66. Katznelson R, Djaiani G, Mitsakakis N, Lindsay TF, Tait G, Friedman Z, et al. Delirium following vascular surgery: increased incidence with preoperative beta-blocker administration. Can J Anaesth. 2009;56(11):793–801.

67. Mariscalco G, Cottini M, Zanobini M, Salis S, Dominici C, Banach M, et al. Preoperative statin therapy is not associated with a decrease in the incidence of delirium after cardiac operations. Ann Thorac Surg. 2012;93(5):1439–47.

68. Redelmeier DA, Thiruchelvam D, Daneman N. Delirium after elective surgery among elderly patients taking statins. CMAJ. 2008;179(7):645–52.

69. Hopkins RO, Weaver LK, Pope D, Orme JF, Bigler ED, Larson-LOHR V. Neuropsychological sequelae and impaired health status in survivors of severe acute respiratory distress syndrome. Am J Respir Crit Care Med. 1999;160(1):50–6.

70. Hopkins RO, Jackson JC. Long-term neurocognitive function after critical illness. Chest. 2006;130(3):869–78.

71. Gunther ML, Morandi A, Krauskopf E, Pandharipande P, Girard TD, Jackson JC, et al. The association between brain volumes, delirium duration, and cognitive outcomes in intensive care unit survivors: the VISIONS cohort magnetic resonance imaging study*. Crit Care Med. 2012;40(7):2022–2032.

72. Morandi A, Rogers BP, Gunther ML, Merkle K, Pandharipande P, Girard TD, et al. The relationship between delirium duration, white matter integrity, and cognitive impairment in intensive care unit survivors as determined by diffusion tensor imaging: the VISIONS prospective cohort magnetic resonance imaging study*. Crit Care Med. 2012;40(7):2182–9.

73. Kress JP, Pohlman AS, O'Connor MF, Hall JB. Daily interruption of sedative infusions in critically ill patients undergoing mechanical ventilation. N Engl J Med. 2000;342(20):1471–7.

74. Hwang YJ, Dixon SN, Reiss JP, Wald R, Parikh CR, Gandhi S, et al. Atypical antipsychotic drugs and the risk for acute kidney injury and other adverse outcomes in older adults: a population-based cohort study. Ann Intern Med. 2014;161(4):242–8.

75. Gill SS, Bronskill SE, Normand SL, Anderson GM, Sykora K, Lam K, et al. Antipsychotic drug use and mortality in older adults with dementia. Ann Intern Med. 2007;146(11):775–86.

76. Wang PS, Schneeweiss S, Avorn J, Fischer MA, Mogun H, Solomon DH, et al. Risk of death in elderly users of conventional vs. atypical antipsychotic medications. N Engl J Med. 2005;353(22):2335–41.

77. Barr J, Fraser GL, Puntillo K, Ely EW, Gelinas C, Dasta JF, et al. Clinical practice guidelines for the management of pain, agitation, and delirium in adult patients in the intensive care unit. Crit Care Med. 2013;41(1):263–306.

78. Pandharipande PP, Sanders RD, Girard TD, McGrane S, Thompson JL, Shintani AK, et al. Effect of dexmedetomidine versus lorazepam on outcome in patients with sepsis: an a priori-designed analysis of the MENDS randomized controlled trial. Crit Care. 2010;14(2):R38.

79. Hermans G, Van Mechelen H, Clerckx B, Vanhullebusch T, Mesotten D, Wilmer A, et al. Acute outcomes and 1-year mortality of intensive care unit-acquired weakness. A cohort study and propensity-matched analysis. Am J Respir Crit Care Med. 2014;190(4):410–20.

80. Stevens RD, Marshall SA, Cornblath DR, Hoke A, Needham DM, de Jonghe B, et al. A framework for diagnosing and classifying intensive care unit-acquired weakness. Crit Care Med. 2009;37(10 Suppl):S299–308.

81. Medical Research Council. Aids to the examination of the peripheral nervous system, memorandum no. 45. London: Her Majesty's Stationery Office; 1981.

82. Hough CL, Lieu BK, Caldwell ES. Manual muscle strength testing of critically ill patients: feasibility and interobserver agreement. Crit Care. 2011;15(1):R43.

83. Ali NA, O'Brien Jr JM, Hoffmann SP, Phillips G, Garland A, Finley JC, et al. Acquired weakness, handgrip strength, and mortality in critically ill patients. Am J Respir Crit Care Med. 2008;178(3):261–8.

84. De Jonghe B, Sharshar T, Lefaucheur JP, Authier FJ, Durand-Zaleski I, Boussarsar M, et al. Paresis acquired in the intensive care unit: a prospective multicenter study. JAMA. 2002;288(22):2859–67.

85. Fan E. Critical illness neuromyopathy and the role of physical therapy and rehabilitation in critically ill patients (discussion 944–6). Respir Care. 2012;57(6):933–44.

86. Hermans G, Clerckx B, Vanhullebusch T, Segers J, Vanpee G, Robbeets C, et al. Interobserver agreement of medical research council sum-score and handgrip strength in the intensive care unit. Muscle Nerve. 2012;45(1):18–25.

87. Mirzakhani H, Williams JN, Mello J, Joseph S, Meyer MJ, Waak K, et al. Muscle weakness predicts pharyngeal dysfunction and symptomatic aspiration in long-term ventilated patients. Anesthesiology. 2013;119(2):389–97.

88. Fan E, Ciesla ND, Truong AD, Bhoopathi V, Zeger SL, Needham DM. Inter-rater reliability of manual muscle strength testing in ICU survivors and simulated patients. Intensive Care Med. 2010;36(6):1038–43.

89. Wieske L, Chan Pin Yin DR, Verhamme C, Schultz MJ, van Schaik IN, Horn J. Autonomic dysfunction in ICU-acquired weakness: a prospective observational pilot study. Intensive Care Med. 2013;39(9):1610–7.

90. Vanpee G, Hermans G, Segers J, Gosselink R. Assessment of limb muscle strength in critically ill patients: a systematic review. Crit Care Med. 2014;42(3):701–11.

91. Druschky A, Herkert M, Radespiel-Troger M, Druschky K, Hund E, Becker CM, et al. Critical illness polyneuropathy: clinical findings and cell culture assay of neurotoxicity assessed by a prospective study. Intensive Care Med. 2001;27(4):686–93.

92. Berek K, Margreiter J, Willeit J, Berek A, Schmutzhard E, Mutz NJ. Polyneuropathies in critically ill patients: a prospective evaluation. Intensive Care Med. 1996;22(9):849–55.

93. Vanpee G, Segers J, Van Mechelen H, Wouters P, Van den Berghe G, Hermans G, et al. The interobserver agreement of handheld dynamometry for muscle strength assessment in critically ill patients. Crit Care Med. 2011;39(8):1929–34.

94. Baldwin CE, Paratz JD, Bersten AD. Muscle strength assessment in critically ill patients with handheld dynamometry: an investigation of reliability, minimal detectable change, and time to peak force generation. J Crit Care. 2013;28(1):77–86.

95. Hund E, Genzwurker H, Bohrer H, Jakob H, Thiele R, Hacke W. Predominant involvement of motor fibres in patients with critical illness polyneuropathy. Br J Anaesth. 1997;78(3):274–8.

96. Khan J, Harrison TB, Rich MM, Moss M. Early development of critical illness myopathy and neuropathy in patients with severe sepsis. Neurology. 2006;67(8):1421–5.

97. Tepper M, Rakic S, Haas JA, Woittiez AJ. Incidence and onset of critical illness polyneuropathy in patients with septic shock. Neth J Med. 2000;56(6):211–4.

98. Nanas S, Kritikos K, Angelopoulos E, Siafaka A, Tsikriki S, Poriazi M, et al. Predisposing factors for critical illness polyneuromyopathy in a multidisciplinary intensive care unit. Acta Neurol Scand. 2008;118(3):175–81.

99. Bednarik J, Lukas Z, Vondracek P. Critical illness polyneuromyopathy: the electrophysiological components of a complex entity. Intensive Care Med. 2003;29(9):1505–14.

100. Mohr M, Englisch L, Roth A, Burchardi H, Zielmann S. Effects of early treatment with immunoglobulin on critical illness polyneuropathy following multiple organ failure and gram-negative sepsis. Intensive Care Med. 1997;23(11):1144–9.

101. Bercker S, Weber-Carstens S, Deja M, Grimm C, Wolf S, Behse F, et al. Critical illness polyneuropathy and myopathy in patients with acute respiratory distress syndrome. Crit Care Med. 2005;33(4):711–5.

102. de Letter MA, Schmitz PI, Visser LH, Verheul FA, Schellens RL, Op de Coul DA, et al. Risk factors for the development of polyneuropathy and myopathy in critically ill patients. Crit Care Med. 2001;29(12):2281–6.
103. De Letter MA, van Doorn PA, Savelkoul HF, Laman JD, Schmitz PI, Op de Coul DA, et al. Critical illness polyneuropathy and myopathy (CIPNM): evidence for local immune activation by cytokine-expression in the muscle tissue. J Neuroimmunol. 2000;106(1–2):206–13.
104. Coakley JH, Nagendran K, Yarwood GD, Honavar M, Hinds CJ. Patterns of neurophysiological abnormality in prolonged critical illness. Intensive Care Med. 1998;24(8):801–7.
105. Leijten FS, Harinck-de Weerd JE, Poortvliet DC, de Weerd AW. The role of polyneuropathy in motor convalescence after prolonged mechanical ventilation. JAMA. 1995;274(15):1221–5.
106. Witt NJ, Zochodne DW, Bolton CF, Grand'Maison F, Wells G, Young GB, et al. Peripheral nerve function in sepsis and multiple organ failure. Chest. 1991;99(1):176–84.
107. Thiele RI, Jakob H, Hund E, Tantzky S, Keller S, Kamler M, et al. Sepsis and catecholamine support are the major risk factors for critical illness polyneuropathy after open heart surgery. Thorac Cardiovasc Surg. 2000;48(3):145–50.
108. Garnacho-Montero J, Madrazo-Osuna J, Garcia-Garmendia JL, Ortiz-Leyba C, Jimenez-Jimenez FJ, Barrero-Almodovar A, et al. Critical illness polyneuropathy: risk factors and clinical consequences. A cohort study in septic patients. Intensive Care Med. 2001;27(8):1288–96.
109. Santos PD, Teixeira C, Savi A, Maccari JG, Neres FS, Machado AS, et al. The critical illness polyneuropathy in septic patients with prolonged weaning from mechanical ventilation: is the diaphragm also affected? A pilot study. Respir Care. 2012;57(10):1594–601.
110. Steinberg KP, Hudson LD, Goodman RB, Hough CL, Lanken PN, Hyzy R, et al. National Heart, Lung, and Blood Institute Acute Respiratory Distress Syndrome (ARDS) Clinical Trials Network. Efficacy and safety of corticosteroids for persistent acute respiratory distress syndrome. N Engl J Med. 2006;354(16):1671–84.
111. de Jonghe B, Lacherade JC, Sharshar T, Outin H. Intensive care unit-acquired weakness: risk factors and prevention. Crit Care Med. 2009;37(10 Suppl):S309–15.
112. De Jonghe B, Bastuji-Garin S, Sharshar T, Outin H, Brochard L. Does ICU-acquired paresis lengthen weaning from mechanical ventilation? Intensive Care Med. 2004;30(6):1117–21.
113. Leijten FS, De Weerd AW, Poortvliet DC, De Ridder VA, Ulrich C, Harink-De Weerd JE. Critical illness polyneuropathy in multiple organ dysfunction syndrome and weaning from the ventilator. Intensive Care Med. 1996;22(9):856–61.
114. Paratz J, Thomas P, Adsett J. Re-admission to intensive care: identification of risk factors. Physiother Res Int. 2005;10(3):154–63.
115. Herridge MS, Cheung AM, Tansey CM, Matte-Martyn A, Diaz-Granados N, Al-Saidi F, et al. One-year outcomes in survivors of the acute respiratory distress syndrome. N Engl J Med. 2003;348(8):683–93.
116. Cheung AM, Tansey CM, Tomlinson G, Diaz-Granados N, Matte A, Barr A, et al. Two-year outcomes, health care use, and costs of survivors of acute respiratory distress syndrome. Am J Respir Crit Care Med. 2006;174(5):538–44.
117. Dowdy DW, Eid MP, Sedrakyan A, Mendez-Tellez PA, Pronovost PJ, Herridge MS, et al. Quality of life in adult survivors of critical illness: a systematic review of the literature. Intensive Care Med. 2005;31(5):611–20.
118. Morris PE, Goad A, Thompson C, Taylor K, Harry B, Passmore L, et al. Early intensive care unit mobility therapy in the treatment of acute respiratory failure. Crit Care Med. 2008;36(8):2238–43.
119. Hermans G, Wilmer A, Meersseman W, Milants I, Wouters PJ, Bobbaers H, et al. Impact of intensive insulin therapy on neuromuscular complications and ventilator dependency in the medical intensive care unit. Am J Respir Crit Care Med. 2007;175(5):480–9.
120. van den Berghe G, Wouters P, Weekers F, Verwaest C, Bruyninckx F, Schetz M, et al. Intensive insulin therapy in critically ill patients. N Engl J Med. 2001;345(19):1359–67.
121. Van den Berghe G, Schoonheydt K, Becx P, Bruyninckx F, Wouters PJ. Insulin therapy protects the central and peripheral nervous system of intensive care patients. Neurology. 2005;64(8):1348–53.

122. NICE-SUGAR Study Investigators, Finfer S, Chittock DR, Su SY, Blair D, Foster D, et al. Intensive versus conventional glucose control in critically ill patients. N Engl J Med. 2009;360(13):1283–97.

123. NICE-SUGAR Study Investigators, Finfer S, Liu B, Chittock DR, Norton R, Myburgh JA, et al. Hypoglycemia and risk of death in critically ill patients. N Engl J Med. 2012;367(12):1108–18.

124. Brunkhorst FM, Engel C, Bloos F, Meier-Hellmann A, Ragaller M, Weiler N, et al. Intensive insulin therapy and pentastarch resuscitation in severe sepsis. N Engl J Med. 2008;358(2):125–39.

125. Dellinger RP, Levy MM, Rhodes A, Annane D, Gerlach H, Opal SM, et al. Surviving sepsis campaign: international guidelines for management of severe sepsis and septic shock, 2012. Intensive Care Med. 2013;39(2):165–228.

126. Patel BK, Pohlman AS, Hall JB, Kress JP. Impact of early mobilization on glycemic control and ICU-acquired weakness in critically ill patients who are mechanically ventilated. Chest. 2014;146(3):583–9.

127. Rodriguez PO, Setten M, Maskin LP, Bonelli I, Vidomlansky SR, Attie S, et al. Muscle weakness in septic patients requiring mechanical ventilation: protective effect of transcutaneous neuromuscular electrical stimulation. J Crit Care. 2012;27(3):319.e1–8.

128. Chao P, Shih C, Lee Y, Tseng C, Kuo S, Shih Y, et al. Association of post-discharge rehabilitation with mortality in intensive care unit survivors of sepsis. Am J Respir Crit Care Med. 2014;190(9):1003–11.

129. Furian T, Aguiar C, Prado K, Ribeiro RV, Becker L, Martinelli N, et al. Ventricular dysfunction and dilation in severe sepsis and septic shock: relation to endothelial function and mortality. J Crit Care. 2012;27(3):319.e9–15.

130. Sturgess DJ, Marwick TH, Joyce C, Jenkins C, Jones M, Masci P, et al. Prediction of hospital outcome in septic shock: a prospective comparison of tissue doppler and cardiac biomarkers. Crit Care. 2010;14(2):R44.

131. Charpentier J, Luyt CE, Fulla Y, Vinsonneau C, Cariou A, Grabar S, et al. Brain natriuretic peptide: a marker of myocardial dysfunction and prognosis during severe sepsis. Crit Care Med. 2004;32(3):660–5.

132. Fernandes Jr CJ, Akamine N, Knobel E. Cardiac troponin: a new serum marker of myocardial injury in sepsis. Intensive Care Med. 1999;25(10):1165–8.

133. Vieillard-Baron A, Caille V, Charron C, Belliard G, Page B, Jardin F. Actual incidence of global left ventricular hypokinesia in adult septic shock. Crit Care Med. 2008;36(6):1701–6.

134. Jardin F, Brun-Ney D, Auvert B, Beauchet A, Bourdarias JP. Sepsis-related cardiogenic shock. Crit Care Med. 1990;18(10):1055–60.

135. Ikonomidis I, Nikolaou M, Dimopoulou I, Paraskevaidis I, Lekakis J, Mavrou I, et al. Association of left ventricular diastolic dysfunction with elevated NT-pro-BNP in general intensive care unit patients with preserved ejection fraction: a complementary role of tissue doppler imaging parameters and NT-pro-BNP levels for adverse outcome. Shock. 2010;33(2):141–8.

136. Bouhemad B, Nicolas-Robin A, Arbelot C, Arthaud M, Feger F, Rouby JJ. Isolated and reversible impairment of ventricular relaxation in patients with septic shock. Crit Care Med. 2008;36(3):766–74.

137. Mehta NJ, Khan IA, Gupta V, Jani K, Gowda RM, Smith PR. Cardiac troponin I predicts myocardial dysfunction and adverse outcome in septic shock. Int J Cardiol. 2004;95(1):13–7.

138. ver Elst KM, Spapen HD, Nguyen DN, Garbar C, Huyghens LP, Gorus FK. Cardiac troponins I and T are biological markers of left ventricular dysfunction in septic shock. Clin Chem. 2000;46(5):650–7.

139. Jafri SM, Lavine S, Field BE, Bahorozian MT, Carlson RW. Left ventricular diastolic function in sepsis. Crit Care Med. 1990;18(7):709–14.

140. Jardin F, Fourme T, Page B, Loubieres Y, Vieillard-Baron A, Beauchet A, et al. Persistent preload defect in severe sepsis despite fluid loading: a longitudinal echocardiographic study in patients with septic shock. Chest. 1999;116(5):1354–9.

141. Munt B, Jue J, Gin K, Fenwick J, Tweeddale M. Diastolic filling in human severe sepsis: an echocardiographic study. Crit Care Med. 1998;26(11):1829–33.

142. Kimchi A, Ellrodt AG, Berman DS, Riedinger MS, Swan HJ, Murata GH. Right ventricular performance in septic shock: a combined radionuclide and hemodynamic study. J Am Coll Cardiol. 1984;4(5):945–51.

143. Parker MM, Shelhamer JH, Bacharach SL, Green MV, Natanson C, Frederick TM, et al. Profound but reversible myocardial depression in patients with septic shock. Ann Intern Med. 1984;100(4):483–90.

144. Schneider AJ, Teule GJ, Groeneveld AB, Nauta J, Heidendal GA, Thijs LG. Biventricular performance during volume loading in patients with early septic shock, with emphasis on the right ventricle: a combined hemodynamic and radionuclide study. Am Heart J. 1988;116(1 Pt 1):103–12.

145. Parker MM, McCarthy KE, Ognibene FP, Parrillo JE. Right ventricular dysfunction and dilatation, similar to left ventricular changes, characterize the cardiac depression of septic shock in humans. Chest. 1990;97(1):126–31.

146. Parker MM, Ognibene FP, Parrillo JE. Peak systolic pressure/end-systolic volume ratio, a load-independent measure of ventricular function, is reversibly decreased in human septic shock. Crit Care Med. 1994;22(12):1955–9.

147. Ellrodt AG, Riedinger MS, Kimchi A, Berman DS, Maddahi J, Swan HJ, et al. Left ventricular performance in septic shock: reversible segmental and global abnormalities. Am Heart J. 1985;110(2):402–9.

148. Parker MM, Shelhamer JH, Natanson C, Alling DW, Parrillo JE. Serial cardiovascular variables in survivors and nonsurvivors of human septic shock: heart rate as an early predictor of prognosis. Crit Care Med. 1987;15(10):923–9.

149. Werdan K, Oelke A, Hettwer S, Nuding S, Bubel S, Hoke R, et al. Septic cardiomyopathy: hemodynamic quantification, occurrence, and prognostic implications. Clin Res Cardiol. 2011;100(8):661–8.

150. Poelaert J, Declerck C, Vogelaers D, Colardyn F, Visser CA. Left ventricular systolic and diastolic function in septic shock. Intensive Care Med. 1997;23(5):553–60.

151. Artucio H, Digenio A, Pereyra M. Left ventricular function during sepsis. Crit Care Med. 1989;17(4):323–7.

152. Wilhelm J, Hettwer S, Schuermann M, Bagger S, Gerhardt F, Mundt S, et al. Severity of cardiac impairment in the early stage of community-acquired sepsis determines worse prognosis. Clin Res Cardiol. 2013;102(10):735–44.

153. Chua G, Kang-Hoe L. Marked elevations in N-terminal brain natriuretic peptide levels in septic shock. Crit Care. 2004;8(4):R248–50.

154. Ammann P, Fehr T, Minder EI, Gunter C, Bertel O. Elevation of troponin I in sepsis and septic shock. Intensive Care Med. 2001;27(6):965–9.

155. Arlati S, Brenna S, Prencipe L, Marocchi A, Casella GP, Lanzani M, et al. Myocardial necrosis in ICU patients with acute non-cardiac disease: a prospective study. Intensive Care Med. 2000;26(1):31–7.

156. Spies C, Haude V, Fitzner R, Schroder K, Overbeck M, Runkel N, et al. Serum cardiac troponin T as a prognostic marker in early sepsis. Chest. 1998;113(4):1055–63.

157. Tiruvoipati R, Sultana N, Lewis D. Cardiac troponin I does not independently predict mortality in critically ill patients with severe sepsis. Emerg Med Australas. 2012;24(2):151–8.

158. Turner A, Tsamitros M, Bellomo R. Myocardial cell injury in septic shock. Crit Care Med. 1999;27(9):1775–80.

159. Post F, Weilemann LS, Messow CM, Sinning C, Munzel T. B-type natriuretic peptide as a marker for sepsis-induced myocardial depression in intensive care patients. Crit Care Med. 2008;36(11):3030–7.

160. Witthaut R, Busch C, Fraunberger P, Walli A, Seidel D, Pilz G, et al. Plasma atrial natriuretic peptide and brain natriuretic peptide are increased in septic shock: impact of interleukin-6 and sepsis-associated left ventricular dysfunction. Intensive Care Med. 2003;29(10):1696–702.

161. Varpula M, Pulkki K, Karlsson S, Ruokonen E, Pettila V, FINNSEPSIS Study Group. Predictive value of N-terminal pro-brain natriuretic peptide in severe sepsis and septic shock. Crit Care Med. 2007;35(5):1277–83.

162. Annane D, Sebille V, Duboc D, Le Heuzey JY, Sadoul N, Bouvier E, et al. Incidence and prognosis of sustained arrhythmias in critically ill patients. Am J Respir Crit Care Med. 2008;178(1):20–5.

163. Christian SA, Schorr C, Ferchau L, Jarbrink ME, Parrillo JE, Gerber DR. Clinical character-istics and outcomes of septic patients with new-onset atrial fibrillation. J Crit Care. 2008;23(4):532–6.

164. Lee-Iannotti JK, Capampangan DJ, Hoffman-Snyder C, Wellik KE, Patel B, Tondato F, et al. New-onset atrial fibrillation in severe sepsis and risk of stroke and death: a critically appraised topic. Neurologist. 2012;18(4):239–43.

165. Salman S, Bajwa A, Gajic O, Afessa B. Paroxysmal atrial fibrillation in critically ill patients with sepsis. J Intensive Care Med. 2008;23(3):178–83.

166. Walkey AJ, Greiner MA, Heckbert SR, Jensen PN, Piccini JP, Sinner MF, et al. Atrial fibril-lation among medicare beneficiaries hospitalized with sepsis: incidence and risk factors. Am Heart J. 2013;165(6):949–955.e3.

167. Walkey AJ, Wiener RS, Ghobrial JM, Curtis LH, Benjamin EJ. Incident stroke and mortality associated with new-onset atrial fibrillation in patients hospitalized with severe sepsis. JAMA. 2011;306(20):2248–54.

168. Meierhenrich R, Steinhilber E, Eggermann C, Weiss M, Voglic S, Bogelein D, et al. Incidence and prognostic impact of new-onset atrial fibrillation in patients with septic shock: a prospec-tive observational study. Crit Care. 2010;14(3):R108.

169. Kindem IA, Reindal EK, Wester AL, Blaasaas KG, Atar D. New-onset atrial fibrillation in bacteremia is not associated with C-reactive protein, but is an indicator of increased mortality during hospitalization. Cardiology. 2008;111(3):171–80.

170. Knotzer H, Mayr A, Ulmer H, Lederer W, Schobersberger W, Mutz N, et al. Tachyarrhythmias in a surgical intensive care unit: a case-controlled epidemiologic study. Intensive Care Med. 2000;26(7):908–14.

171. Goodman S, Shirov T, Weissman C. Supraventricular arrhythmias in intensive care unit patients: short and long-term consequences. Anesth Analg. 2007;104(4):880–6.

172. Arora S, Lang I, Nayyar V, Stachowski E, Ross DL. Atrial fibrillation in a tertiary care multidisciplinary intensive care unit—incidence and risk factors. Anaesth Intensive Care. 2007;35(5):707–13.

173. Seguin P, Signouret T, Laviolle B, Branger B, Malledant Y. Incidence and risk factors of atrial fibrillation in a surgical intensive care unit. Crit Care Med. 2004;32(3):722–6.

174. Bender JS. Supraventricular tachyarrhythmias in the surgical intensive care unit: an under-recognized event. Am Surg. 1996;62(1):73–5.

175. Asfar P, Meziani F, Hamel JF, Grelon F, Megarbane B, Anguel N, et al. High versus low blood-pressure target in patients with septic shock. N Engl J Med. 2014;370(17):1583–93.

176. Morelli A, Ertmer C, Westphal M, Rehberg S, Kampmeier T, Ligges S, et al. Effect of heart rate control with esmolol on hemodynamic and clinical outcomes in patients with septic shock: a randomized clinical trial. JAMA. 2013;310(16):1683–91.

177. Fan HB, Yang DL, Chen AS, Li Z, Xu LT, Ma XJ, et al. Sepsis-associated cholestasis in adult patients: a prospective study. Am J Med Sci. 2013;346(6):462–6.

178. Chow AW, Guze LB. Bacteroidaceae bacteremia: clinical experience with 112 patients. Medicine (Baltimore). 1974;53(2):93–126.

179. Franson TR, Hierholzer Jr WJ, LaBrecque DR. Frequency and characteristics of hyperbiliru-binemia associated with bacteremia. Rev Infect Dis. 1985;7(1):1–9.

180. Henry S, DeMaria Jr A, McCabe WR. Bacteremia due to fusobacterium species. Am J Med. 1983;75(2):225–31.

181. Quale JM, Mandel LJ, Bergasa NV, Straus EW. Clinical significance and pathogenesis of hyperbilirubinemia associated with *Staphylococcus aureus* septicemia. Am J Med. 1988;85(5):615–8.

182. Torres JM, Cardenas O, Vasquez A, Schlossberg D. Streptococcus pneumoniae bacteremia in a community hospital. Chest. 1998;113(2):387–90.

183. Harbrecht BG, Zenati MS, Doyle HR, McMichael J, Townsend RN, Clancy KD, et al. Hepatic dysfunction increases length of stay and risk of death after injury. J Trauma. 2002;53(3):517–23.

184. Brienza N, Dalfino L, Cinnella G, Diele C, Bruno F, Fiore T. Jaundice in critical illness: promoting factors of a concealed reality. Intensive Care Med. 2006;32(2):267–74.

185. Helftenbein A, Windolf J, Sanger P, Hanisch E. Incidence and prognosis of postoperative jaundice in surgical intensive care patients. Chirurg. 1997;68(12):1292–6.

186. Kramer L, Jordan B, Druml W, Bauer P, Metnitz PG, Austrian Epidemiologic Study on Intensive Care, ASDI Study Group, Incidence and prognosis of early hepatic dysfunction in critically ill patients—a prospective multicenter study. Crit Care Med 2007;35(4):1099–1104.

187. Schwartz DB, Bone RC, Balk RA, Szidon JP. Hepatic dysfunction in the adult respiratory distress syndrome. Chest. 1989;95(4):871–5.

188. Zhai R, Sheu CC, Su L, Gong MN, Tejera P, Chen F, et al. Serum bilirubin levels on ICU admission are associated with ARDS development and mortality in sepsis. Thorax. 2009;64(9):784–90.

189. Harbrecht BG, Doyle HR, Clancy KD, Townsend RN, Billiar TR, Peitzman AB. The impact of liver dysfunction on outcome in patients with multiple injuries. Am Surg. 2001;67(2):122–6.

190. Esteban A, Anzueto A, Frutos F, Alia I, Brochard L, Stewart TE, et al. Characteristics and outcomes in adult patients receiving mechanical ventilation: a 28-day international study. JAMA. 2002;287(3):345–55.

191. Fuhrmann V, Kneidinger N, Herkner H, Heinz G, Nikfardjam M, Bojic A, et al. Hypoxic hepatitis: underlying conditions and risk factors for mortality in critically ill patients. Intensive Care Med. 2009;35(8):1397–405.

192. Henrion J, Schapira M, Luwaert R, Colin L, Delannoy A, Heller FR. Hypoxic hepatitis: clinical and hemodynamic study in 142 consecutive cases. Medicine. 2003;82(6):392–406.

193. Birrer R, Takuda Y, Takara T. Hypoxic hepatopathy: pathophysiology and prognosis. Intern Med. 2007;46(14):1063–70.

194. Jager B, Drolz A, Michl B, Schellongowski P, Bojic A, Nikfardjam M, et al. Jaundice increases the rate of complications and one-year mortality in patients with hypoxic hepatitis. Hepatology. 2012;56(6):2297–304.

195. Johnson RD, O'Connor ML, Kerr RM. Extreme serum elevations of aspartate aminotransferase. Am J Gastroenterol. 1995;90(8):1244–5.

196. Fuhrmann V, Madl C, Mueller C, Holzinger U, Kitzberger R, Funk GC, et al. Hepatopulmonary syndrome in patients with hypoxic hepatitis. Gastroenterology. 2006;131(1):69–75.

197. Fuchs S, Bogomolski-Yahalom V, Paltiel O, Ackerman Z. Ischemic hepatitis: clinical and laboratory observations of 34 patients. J Clin Gastroenterol. 1998;26(3):183–6.

198. Silvestre JP, Coelho LM, Povoa PM. Impact of fulminant hepatic failure in C-reactive protein? J Crit Care. 2010;25(4):657.e7–12.

199. Grau T, Bonet A, Rubio M, Mateo D, Farre M, Acosta JA, et al. Liver dysfunction associated with artificial nutrition in critically ill patients. Crit Care. 2007;11(1):R10.

200. Watanakunakorn C, Chan SJ, Demarco DG, Palmer JA. Staphylococcus aureus bacteremia: significance of hyperbilirubinemia. Scand J Infect Dis. 1987;19(2):195–203.

201. Schuster DP, Rowley H, Feinstein S, McGue MK, Zuckerman GR. Prospective evaluation of the risk of upper gastrointestinal bleeding after admission to a medical intensive care unit. Am J Med. 1984;76(4):623–30.

202. Fusamoto H, Hagiwara H, Meren H, Kasahara A, Hayashi N, Kawano S, et al. A clinical study of acute gastrointestinal hemorrhage associated with various shock states. Am J Gastroenterol. 1991;86(4):429–33.

203. Khan F, Parekh A, Patel S, Chitkara R, Rehman M, Goyal R. Results of gastric neutralization with hourly antacids and cimetidine in 320 intubated patients with respiratory failure. Chest. 1981;79(4):409–12.

204. Harris SK, Bone RC, Ruth WE. Gastrointestinal hemorrhage in patients in a respiratory intensive care unit. Chest. 1977;72(3):301–4.
205. Groll A, Simon JB, Wigle RD, Taguchi K, Todd RJ, Depew WT. Cimetidine prophylaxis for gastrointestinal bleeding in an intensive care unit. Gut. 1986;27(2):135–40.
206. Brown RB, Klar J, Teres D, Lemeshow S, Sands M. Prospective study of clinical bleeding in intensive care unit patients. Crit Care Med. 1988;16(12):1171–6.
207. Pimentel M, Roberts DE, Bernstein CN, Hoppensack M, Duerksen DR. Clinically significant gastrointestinal bleeding in critically ill patients in an era of prophylaxis. Am J Gastroenterol. 2000;95(10):2801–6.
208. Cook DJ, Fuller HD, Guyatt GH, Marshall JC, Leasa D, Hall R, et al. Risk factors for gastrointestinal bleeding in critically ill patients. canadian critical care trials group. N Engl J Med. 1994;330(6):377–81.
209. Hastings PR, Skillman JJ, Bushnell LS, Silen W. Antacid titration in the prevention of acute gastrointestinal bleeding: a controlled, randomized trial in 100 critically ill patients. N Engl J Med. 1978;298(19):1041–5.
210. Garvey JM, Fogelman MJ. Septic peptic ulceration. J Trauma. 1966;6(5):644–65.
211. Altemeier WA, Fullen WD, McDonough JJ. Sepsis and gastrointestinal bleeding. Ann Surg. 1972;175(5):759–70.

Part IV

Chapter 11
Diagnosis of Sepsis: Clinical Findings and the Role of Biomarkers

Daithi S. Heffernan

Introduction

The concept of "sepsis" is derived from the ancient Greek understanding of the decomposition and putrefaction of tissue. The word sepsis is derived from the Greek meaning decomposition of organic matter and a derivative of the verb *sepo* meaning "to rot" [1]. Sepsis is an increasingly common diagnosis among hospitalized and critically ill patients. Despite significant advances in diagnosis and management, mortality remains high. Severe sepsis and septic shock account for approximately 50% of ICU-related deaths [2, 3]. Reduction in sepsis-related morbidity and mortality starts with a rapid and accurate diagnosis. It has been clearly demonstrated through the Surviving Sepsis Campaign (SSC) that a delay in diagnosis of sepsis is associated with increasing morbidity and mortality [2]. However, inappropriate antimicrobial usage can lead to complications such as secondary infections and the emergence of multidrug-resistant organisms. Diagnosing sepsis can be especially challenging in critically ill and immunocompromised patients, and many of the clinical findings related to sepsis often overlap with those found in patients with severe inflammation from noninfectious etiologies. Fortunately, several new biomarkers have the potential for rapid and accurate identification of patients with infections. Nevertheless, it is clear that significant progress in reducing the morbidity and mortality from sepsis must begin with improvements in the diagnosis of sepsis.

D.S. Heffernan, MD, FACS, AFRCSI (✉)
Division of Surgical Research, Department of Surgery, Rhode Island Hospital/Brown University, Room 205, Aldrich Building, Providence, RI, 02093, USA
e-mail: DHeffernan@Brown.edu

© Springer International Publishing AG 2017
N.S. Ward, M.M. Levy (eds.), *Sepsis*, Respiratory Medicine,
DOI 10.1007/978-3-319-48470-9_11

Defining Sepsis

Sepsis is defined as the systemic inflammatory response syndrome (SIRS) in the presence of an infection [4]. This classic approach to diagnosis is based on clinical findings such as tachycardia and fevers and laboratory findings including leukocytosis in the presence of relevant microbiological data. The sensitivity and specificity of any one feature for the diagnosis of sepsis is very low, however. Furthermore, there is considerable overlap in the clinical features of patients with SIRS from sterile inflammation and patients with inflammation from infection (sepsis). Over the years, lack of a unified definition has led to multiple problems from study design to clinical practice. Additionally, this lack of a standardized definition led to remarkable discrepancies between studies with respect to incidence of sepsis and mortality rates from sepsis.

Bone et al. laid the foundations for our current definition of sepsis, wherein a series of readily available noninvasive clinical parameters was set that could easily define the early and progressive phases of a patient's reaction to an infection [5]. The term "sepsis syndrome" was coined for patients with an infection, as well as temperature and cardiopulmonary alterations in response to the infection, and was used to stratify patients in a double-blind study of methylprednisolone for patients with inflammation (SIRS) with or without shock [6]. The hope was to identify when an infection occurred early in patients with systemic inflammation (SIRS), thereby offering an early therapeutic intervention and thus preventing the progression to the later stages of sepsis with multiple organ failure wherein the mortality was considerably higher.

The "sepsis syndrome" described by Bone was noted to also include at least one end organ with dysfunction and failed to capture the true clinical spectrum of the septic cascade. In an attempt to form a unified approach to sepsis, a combined statement was issued from the American College of Chest Physicians and Critical Care Consensus Conference in 1992. Herein, diagnostic guidelines were issued for SIRS, sepsis, severe sepsis, and septic shock [7]. SIRS is the inflammatory response to a sterile insult such as traumatic or sterile injuries. SIRS was defined as the presence of two or more of the four following criteria: hypo- or hyperthermia, tachycardia, leukocytosis or leukopenia, and respiratory distress with either tachypnea or hypocapnia. Sepsis was defined as SIRS triggered by an infectious etiology. An infection was defined as "a pathological process caused by invasion of normally sterile tissue, fluid or body cavity by pathogenic or potentially pathogenic micro-organisms." Severe sepsis was defined as sepsis with the inclusion of multiple organ failure. Septic shock was defined as the sepsis with the presence of hypotension unresponsive to fluid resuscitation (Table 11.1). Thus, the term sepsis syndrome, which encompassed infection, systemic manifestations, and end-organ failure, has since been replaced by the term severe sepsis. The presence of viable bacteria in the bloodstream was defined as bacteremia. The term septicemia, although often used by clinicians, adds nothing to the understanding of the progression of sepsis and is considered too ambiguous and imprecise, and the use of this term is discouraged.

Table 11.1 Systemic inflammatory response syndrome (SIRS), sepsis, severe sepsis, and septic shock

SIRS is the presence of at least two of the following four criteria
• Temperature greater than 38.3 °C or less than 36 °C
• Heart rate greater than 90 beats per minute
• Respiratory rate greater than 20 breaths per minute, or $PaCO_2$ less than 32 mmHg
• White cell count greater than 12,000 cells/µL or less than 4000 cells/µL or the presence of greater than 10% of immature neutrophils (bands)
Sepsis
• Sepsis is SIRS with an infection source
Severe sepsis
• Sepsis with evidence of organ dysfunction, hypoperfusion, or multiple organ failure
Septic shock
• Sepsis with shock (hypotension) with blood pressure less than 90 mmHg

In defining these broad and nonspecific criteria, several features were considered critical. The definitions should not be overly complicated, which would potentially limit their usage. The criteria should be useful both at the bedside for daily care and in the design of trials for sepsis treatment. The inclusion of any laboratory-based criteria needed to be easily available across a wide spectrum or treating centers and countries. Finally, all criteria should be applicable across multiple patient populations.

In the years following those initial definitions, it was felt that the criteria for SIRS were overly sensitive and nonspecific and often failed to capture other evidence of inflammatory dysfunction and organ perfusion anomalies. The concept of sepsis as being SIRS plus any source of infection was felt to be too simplistic. By that definition over 90% of ICU patients fulfill sepsis criteria, and yet many ICU admissions are for reasons other than infection related [8]. Furthermore, these criteria did not factor the degree of physiologic response and failed to give weight to the paradoxical inflammatory signs like leucopenia or hypothermia which may, in fact, portend worse prognosis.

The 1992 definitions were updated and revised in 2003 to include other signs and symptoms noted in critically ill patients based on a better understanding of the pathophysiology of sepsis [4]. Although the basis remained the same, these definitions considerably expanded clinical and biochemical criteria [4], recognizing the wide diversity of the body's response to an infection (Table 11.2). For example, altered mental status was added to the general parameters, a finding that is very common in elderly patients who may either have few systemic manifestations or who are more likely to exhibit the hypoinflammatory response to an infection such as leukopenia and hypothermia [9]. A large fluid resuscitation may denote a significant neutrophil-mediated capillary and endothelial barrier dysfunction in response to the infection. This neutrophil/endothelial interaction is often related to the nature of the infection (primary versus nosocomial) and underlying patient characteristics [10]. It was recognized that the absolute value of the white cell count failed to capture subtleties of the immune response to sepsis.

Table 11.2 Generalized criteria for the diagnosis of sepsis

Sepsis diagnosed by the combination of documented or suspected infection, coupled with some of the following

General variables

Fever (>38.3 °C)

Hypothermia (core temperature <36 °C)

Heart rate >90 min^{-1} or more than 2 s.d. above the normal value for age

Tachypnea

Altered mental status

Significant edema or positive fluid balance (>20 mL/kg over 24 h)

Hyperglycemia (plasma glucose >140 mg/dL or 7.7 mmol/L) in the absence of diabetes

Inflammatory variables

Leukocytosis (WBC count >12,000/μL)

Leukopenia (WBC count < 4000/μL)

Normal WBC count with greater than 10% immature forms

Plasma C-reactive protein more than two standard deviations above the normal value

Plasma procalcitonin more than two standard deviations above the normal value

Hemodynamic variables

Arterial hypotension (SBP <90 mm Hg, MAP < 70 mm Hg, or an SBP decrease >40 mmHg in adults or less than two standard deviations below normal for age)

Organ dysfunction variables

Arterial hypoxemia (Pao_2/Fio_2 < 300)

Acute oliguria (urine output < 0.5 mL/kg/hour for at least 2 h despite adequate fluid resuscitation)

Creatinine increase > 0.5 mg/dL or 44.2 μmol/L

Coagulation abnormalities (INR > 1.5 or aPTT > 60 s)

Ileus (absent bowel sounds)

Thrombocytopenia (platelet count < 100,000 μL^{-1})

Hyperbilirubinemia (plasma total bilirubin > 4 mg/dL or 70 μmol/L)

Tissue perfusion variables

Hyperlactatemia (> 1 mmol/L)

Decreased capillary refill or mottling

Table—adapted from Levy MM, Fink MP, Marshall JC et al. 2001 SCCM/ESICM/ACCP/ATS/SIS International Sepsis Definitions Conference. Crit Care Med 2003; 31: 1250–1256 [4]

Given the nonspecific nature of a reactive leukocytosis, the selection of available criteria included several biomarkers which may be more indicative of an infectious etiology. These included procalcitonin (PCT) which was shown to be released from the tissues in response to bacterial products. This expansion of the diagnostic criteria also included specific defining criteria for acute lung injury (ALI/ARDS), acute kidney injury, potential bowel or hepatic dysfunction, as well as anomalies of the hematologic system. Defining tissue perfusion deficits as being a minor elevation of lactic acid level (lactate >1 mmol/L) is a reflection of the need for early diagnosis rather than waiting for overt tissue ischemia from hypoperfusion, as well as a reflection of the detrimental effects of even mild hypoperfusion on the, often elderly, septic patient. In essence many authorities try to move beyond the mere "host

Table 11.3 Definition of severe sepsis

Sepsis-induced hypotension
Lactate above upper limits of laboratory normal values
Urine output < 0.5 mL/kg/h for more than 2 h despite adequate fluid resuscitation
Acute lung injury with Pao2/Fio2 < 250 in the absence of pneumonia as infection source
Acute lung injury with Pao2/Fio2 < 200 in the presence of pneumonia as infection source
Creatinine > 2.0 mg/dL (176.8 μmol/L)
Bilirubin > 2 mg/dL (34.2 μmol/L)
Platelet count < 100,000 μL
Coagulopathy (international normalized ratio > 1.5)

Severe sepsis is defined as sepsis-induced tissue hypoperfusion or organ dysfunction as defined by the presence of any of the following believed to be related to the infection
Adapted from Levy MM, Fink MP, Marshall JC, et al.: 2001 SCCM/ESICM/ACCP/ATS/SIS International Sepsis Definitions Conference. Crit Care Med 2003; 31: 1250–1256 [4]

response to an infection" as the definition of sepsis and rather aim to describe a patient with cellular and organ dysfunction as a result of an infection. In a recent International Sepsis Forum, a call was made to consider sepsis as a "life threatening condition that arises when the body's response to an infection injuries its own tissues and organs" [11]. To echo this sentiment, Vincent et al. strongly contended that sepsis be defined as "a systemic response to infection with the presence of some degree of organ dysfunction" [12].

While the consensus panel felt that the basic categories continued to prove useful and should remain, it was accepted that the criteria outlined failed to offer any disease stratification or prognostication. Thus the authors developed a classification system they designated PIRO—the *Predisposing* conditions, the nature and extent of the *Insult*, the magnitude of the host *Response*, and the degree of *Organ* failure/dysfunction [4]. Predisposing factors would address both currently known features such as comorbid diseases as well as laying ground for potentially uncovering future genetic predispositions to an inappropriate inflammatory response to a pathogen. For example, an overexuberant immune or inflammatory response may rapidly clear microbes but in so doing may lead to considerable organ destruction. The nature of the infection has been shown to carry significant prognostic value such that a nosocomial infection is associated with higher mortality rates than a primary infection [13]. Although the literature vacillates on whether gram-positive or gram-negative infections carry a worse prognosis, the degree of organ failure induced by a specific organism is more prognostic of outcome. It has been clearly demonstrated across a number of well-validated scoring systems that with each failed organ, survival from sepsis declines. The combination of the spectrum of virulence among organisms, the susceptibility of the affected organ system, and the, as yet not fully defined, genetic predisposition to an altered inflammatory response drive the morbidity and mortality of sepsis. Understanding the immune response to infection still remains elusive but continues to grow and will likely to be incorporated into future iterations of the definition of sepsis.

Many of the key principles used in diagnosing sepsis were utilized in the Surviving Sepsis Campaign (SSC) which aimed to decrease sepsis mortality by increasing awareness of the rising incidence of sepsis, as well as aimed to establish easily applicable diagnosis and management guidelines which would improve survival from sepsis. Key to the SSC campaign was early and aggressive fluid resuscitation and antibiotic administration. However, a cornerstone to this concept was early recognition and establishing a diagnosis of sepsis. The SSC adopted and has continued to refine the definitions of sepsis as outlined by Levy et al. [4] (Table 11.3). Through early diagnosis of sepsis, aggressive treatment, and compliance with sepsis bundles, a 25% relative risk reduction in mortality rate has been observed with the SSC [14, 15].

Several infection scoring systems have been described to try to predict the presence of an infection in a patient with acute inflammation (SIRS) in whom their clinical and biochemical features cover both SIRS and sepsis. One such prediction model is the Infection Probability Score (IPS) described by Peres-Bota [16]. Rather than being a yes or no as in the consensus definition, the IPS gives variable weighted points to clinical features including heart rate and temperature, basic laboratory test including white cell count, biomarkers including C-reactive protein (CRP), and organ failure. The IPS is scored on a range of 0–26. Peres-Bota et al. noted that a score of 13 as a cutoff value led to a positive predictive value of 72% and negative predictive value of 96% for the presence of an infection. Patients with a score of less than 13 were noted to have a 10% risk of having an infection [16]. Scoring systems continue to be proposed, but often fail to achieve a better sensitivity or specificity. Establishing the presence of an infection and proving that this infection is the cause to the profound physiological disturbance can remain elusive in a considerable number of critically ill patients. Advances in medical care have led to increasing numbers of sicker or older patients among the in-hospital population, including patients who have undergone organ transplantation, chemotherapy, and high-dose steroids or the super-elderly patient. Despite the myriad of diagnostic criteria and scoring systems, the greatest impact on sepsis-related morbidity and mortality remains with clinical vigilance and a heightened index of suspicion.

Identification of Bacteria

Diagnosis of sepsis is traditionally predicated upon detection of an infecting organism. Microbial culture has remained the gold standard for the detection of bacteria. However, such techniques are time-consuming and remain with significant false-negative rates, especially in regard to fastidious or slow-growing organism or in patients with ongoing antimicrobial exposure. Conventional blood culture techniques have been reported to detect organisms in as few as 30% of patients with known infectious sources [17]. Culture-negative patients are believed to potentially comprise up to 25% of patients with sepsis [18]. Further, the time-consuming nature of conventional culture techniques may leave septic patients with inappropriate or no antimicrobial cover for extended periods of time. Following the onset of shock from sepsis, an approximate 8% decrease in survival has been reported for every hour of delay in administering effective antimicrobial therapy [19]. Several technologies have emerged as potential alternatives to culture techniques.

Polymerase chain reaction (PCR), first described for diagnosing infections in 1987 [20], has been employed across the spectrum of screening for MRSA carriage [21] to rapid detection of *Clostridium difficile* infection. Universal PCR amplifies nucleic acids, specifically the 16S ribosomal RNA present in all bacteria, followed by DNA sequencing of the amplification products. Specific PCR works via primers complementary to known DNA sequences of specific bacteria. Specificity and time to diagnosis are continuing to improve.

Microarray analysis detects and analyzes large numbers of microbial genes including virulence and resistance genes. Oligonucleotide probes are bound to a microchip in a defined array. Nucleic acids from a pathogen are labeled and then hybridized to the complementary probe bound to the chip. A fluorescent scanner or cytometer then measures this hybridization. Microbial microarrays have characterized *E. coli*, *S. aureus*, and *P. aeruginosa* [22] as well as identifying genes for toxin production, resistance, and virulence [23, 24], as well as *Staphylococcus aureus* coagulase profile differences [25].

Bacteriophages, or bacterial viruses, recognize and inject their genetic material into their target host bacteria. The bacteriophage then rapidly reproduces within the host bacteria. This kills the host bacteria releasing later numbers of bacteriophage progeny. The presence of large quantities of rapidly produced bacteriophage is thus a marker of the presence of a live offending bacterium. Bacteriophages rely upon the presence of live organism which offers an advantage over PCR which may detect already killed organisms. Further, in patients already undergoing antimicrobial therapy, bacteriophage production and detection is only possible if the bacterium is resistant to the patient's current therapeutic regime. Bacteriophage technology is being employed to detect multidrug-resistant *S. aureus* (KeyPath assay, MicroPhage) and multidrug-resistant TB [26, 27]. MicroPhage technology yields diagnostic results more than 30 h faster than conventional culture techniques.

Microfluidics involves analysis of droplets of fluid employing techniques including microscale PCR [28], flow cytometry, and immunoassays [29]. This technology is especially useful for difficult to culture microbes including *M. pneumoniae*, often in half the time of conventional PCR methods. Advances in microfluidics technology have improved infection detection in developing countries with limited resources [29].

Advances are currently being made with respect to implantable devices, such as central venous catheters, being capable of diagnosing infections. These "smart venous catheters" use a microelectrode to detect electrical impedance characteristics of bacterial biofilm formation [30]. Such devices are capable of detecting bioimpedance changes related to the biofilm formation with hours of the presence of bacteria in the bloodstream. Furthermore, once bacteria have been detected or diagnosed by a "smart device," further advances have been proposed to allow the device to locally release antimicrobial agents capable of neutralizing the bacterial biofilm production. However such devices may potentially be oversensitive, being capable of detecting very low levels of bacteria. Redefining new thresholds for detection of bacteria and potentially triggering antimicrobial release will be essential to future developments.

Special Populations

Individual immune responses vary based on age, gender, comorbidities, location of the septic focus, and underlying immune status. However, there remain certain populations in whom diagnosis of sepsis is difficult. The causes of an immunocompromised state are diverse, ranging from age, underlying infections such as HIV, transplant recipients, and medication induced including steroids and cancer-related chemotherapeutic regimes. Infections are an increasingly common complication faced by immunocompromised patients as well as those at the extremes of age. Common infectious presentations still include community-acquired pneumonia, CNS infections, appendicitis, cholecystitis, and cellulitis. Further etiologies often include implantable devices such as central venous catheters. Mortality from sepsis among immunocompromised patients requiring ICU admission is noted to approximate 90%. As with all patients with sepsis, early diagnosis is critical to improving survival. However, many of the classic clinical features of sepsis may not present in patients who are immunocompromised. We herein focus on three patient groups—neutropenic, geriatric, and neonatal patients.

Neutropenic Patients

Neutropenia is defined as having <1500 neutrophils/mm^3. However, a cutoff of <500 neutrophils/mm^3 is generally considered as the cut point for the increased risk of development of sepsis. The risk of infection is related to the speed of the decline of the neutrophil count as well as the duration of neutropenia. Although neutropenic patients often lack many of the cardinal symptoms of sepsis, a persistently elevated unexplained fever is often considered diagnostic of an infection and should prompt early initiation of antimicrobial agents. Clinicians must perform a meticulous and detailed physical examination, noting even minor or subtle findings. Daily examinations should focus on any minor changes from the prior day since the lack of an adequate immune response will dampen the physical manifestations of an infection. A consensus statement on the definition of sepsis in neutropenic patients concurred with the already accepted expanded criteria for diagnosing sepsis [Table 11.2] [4] with the caveat that alterations in white cell count or components thereof cannot be used.

Geriatric Patients

Geriatric patients are the largest growing patient population at risk of both developing sepsis and dying from the sepsis. Geriatric patients often exhibit atypical clinical manifestations of infections. The most common of these atypical findings include confusion, agitation, or increasing somnolence, decline in mobility, and overall lethargy. Elderly patients are more likely to demonstrate the hypoinflammatory components of the SIRS response. A lack of a febrile response to an infection may often be due to the fact that the average core body temperature of an older patient is almost 1 °C lower than that of younger patient. It has been proposed that for patients aged over 75 years, a temperature over 37.5 °C should be considered to be a febrile response [31]. Given the changes in the cardiac and circulatory systems associated with aging, as well as the incidence of cardiac disease such as hypertension and CHF, a better appreciation for "normal" vital signs in the elderly is essential [32]. Geriatric patients may not manifest tachycardia, and clinicians often fail to recognize hypotension (greater than 40 mmHg change from baseline systolic blood pressure).

The aging immune system displays immunosenescence, marked by a decline in number and function or key aspects of the inflammatory and immune systems, including a dampened cytokine and chemokine production and profound changes in the lymphocyte populations [33, 34]. This decline also contributes to the lack of systemic manifestations to an invading pathogen. This contributes to both the difficulty in diagnosing infections and predisposes geriatric patients to secondary infections. Overtly this is often manifested by either a normal leukocyte count despite the presence of a clinically evident infection or leukopenia which portends a worse prognosis. Biomarkers, especially C-reactive protein (CRP) and procalcitonin (PCT), may play a role when other indicators of infections are not supportive of the clinician's suspicion of an infection. In a meta-analysis of PCT in elderly patients, Lee et al. noted no marked difference in the applicability when compared with non-elderly adults. However, it remains a more useful tool for potentially ruling out bacterial infections rather than diagnosing infections [35].

Neonatal Sepsis

Preterm neonates or very low birth weight (VLBW) infants, especially those with comorbidities, are most at risk for both development of sepsis and succumbing to the effects of the sepsis. Early-onset neonatal sepsis (EOS) is defined as infection occurring within 72 h of life and occurs in approximately 2% of VLBW infants. Late-onset neonatal sepsis (LOS) is defined as occurring after 72 h of life and is noted to have a prevalence of approximately 20% of VLBW neonates. The findings of sepsis in the neonate are often nonspecific and may include lethargy or irritability, icterus, bulging or sunken fontanels, difficulty with feeding, abdominal

Table 11.4 Characteristics
of an ideal biomarker

Cost-efficient
Accurate reference standards
Applicable across a broad spectrum of patient populations
Able to offer outcome prognosis
Well-known kinetics

distention, respiratory difficulties, or unexplained bleeding. Thus, a heightened index of suspicion is essential, and early changes in behavior need prompt attention. Preterm infants are more likely to develop a hypoinflammatory response than SIRS, namely, hypothermia and leukopenia, as well as bradycardia [36]. Although the diagnosis of sepsis is often dependent upon identifying an infecting organism, there are significant limitations with current culture techniques. Neonates often have low levels of bacteremia, and the optimal volume of 6 ml of blood is not feasible to be obtained from low-weight neonates. Thus, a heavy emphasis is placed on both clinical suspicion and potential biomarkers indicative of the presence of an infection [37].

Biomarkers

Despite advances in techniques to identify microbes, a microbiological diagnosis of sepsis cannot be made in almost one third of patients with overt clinical manifestations of sepsis. To this end, several biomarkers have emerged in guiding the early diagnosis of sepsis. A biomarker is a measurable entity denoting the presence or progression of a disease. The NIH Biomarkers Definitions Working Group defined a biomarker as "a characteristic that is objectively measured and evaluated as an indicator of normal biological processes, pathogenic processes or pharmacologic responses to a therapeutic intervention" [38]. The ideal characteristics of a biomarker should include ease of reproducibility, cost-effective, able to be objectively measured, as well as capable of clearly distinguishing between infection and other causes of critical illness (Table 11.4). Ideal biomarkers can aid in both the early diagnosis and risk stratification and prognosis. Almost 200 biomarkers have been studied in the evaluation of sepsis [39]. The updated criteria for the diagnosis of sepsis (Table 11.2) now include two biomarkers, C-reactive protein (CRP) and procalcitonin (PCT), as part of the inflammatory variables.

Cytokine analysis. Many cytokines including TNF-α, IL-6, IL-8, and IL-1β have been demonstrated to be elevated early in the septic response [40]. They are often elevated in response to microbial products and can produce fevers and cardiovascular collapse. These pro-inflammatory cytokines activate and alter many immune cells. IL-6 has been the most studied cytokine for the diagnosis of sepsis and other critical illnesses. IL-6 enhances production of CRP and other acute-phase reactants from the liver. It has become evident that the degree of IL-6 elevation correlates with risk of mortality from sepsis [41, 42].

Gram-negative endotoxin-related sepsis leads to elevation of TNF and IL-1β. However, the usefulness of specific cytokines as sepsis biomarkers is rather limited as such cytokines are also noted to be markedly elevated in patients with traumatic injuries, complex elective surgical procedures, or stroke. The major role of cytokines as biomarkers appears to be for prognostic rather than diagnostic value [43]. A specific cytokine profile does not correlate to any specific diagnosis. Recent work has begun to focus on developing a potential panel of cytokines that might distinguish sepsis from other inflammatory conditions, but to date results have proven to be limited [44–46].

C-reactive protein (CRP) is an acute-phase reactant synthesized in the liver in response to infection and inflammation that was first identified in 1930 [47]. Despite that, it is still commonly used both for acute diagnosis of sepsis and following chronic courses of infections such as osteomyelitis. It is believed that CRP may bind the phospholipid components of bacteria, thereby facilitating bacterial removal by macrophages. However CRP is a very nonspecific marker of inflammation, noted to increase after elective surgical procedures, traumatic injuries, burns, or myocardial infarction. The sensitivity and specificity of CRP as a marker for bacterial infections are 68–92% and 40–67%, respectively [48]. CRP remains useful for sepsis prognosis and treatment progression. CRP levels correlate with degree of illness and severity of infection, and declining CRP levels correlate with clinical resolution and response to antimicrobial therapy [49, 50]. The widespread availability of CRP makes it a useful adjunct for diagnostic criteria; however, the very nonspecific nature of CRP greatly limits its specificity.

Procalcitonin (PCT) is often increased during systemic bacterial infection and sepsis.

PCT is a precursor of calcitonin, a calcium-regulatory hormone secreted at low levels by the C cells of the thyroid gland in healthy individuals. Healthy individuals have a circulating level of PCT less than 0.05 ng/ml. However, in patients with infections, PCT is noted to be released from a number of tissues and organs. PCT has increasingly proven effective as a diagnostic marker of bacterial infection; the use of which has been supported by both IDSA and the American College of Critical Care Medicine [51]. However, unlike bacterial or fungal infections, in patients with viral infections, PCT levels are noted to be low or normal. In response to either injury or infection, PCT is noted to rapidly rise within 2–4 h [52, 53]. This is in distinction to CRP which takes up to 24 h to rise. Furthermore, PCT levels are unaffected by immunocompromised states, neutropenia, or use of immune-altering drugs such as steroids. PCT levels have been shown to be associated with the severity of illness in septic patients, correlating with severity scores such as APACHE or SOFA scores.

PCT levels have been noted to decline with bacterial clearance, with some investigators noting a halving of PCT levels within 24 h of controlling an infection. Thus, several authors have advocated using PCT levels to guide and potentially shorten duration of antimicrobial agents. Both a Cochrane review and a meta-analysis of PCT-directed duration of antimicrobial agents noted markedly reduced total antibiotic exposure with no adverse effect upon mortality or treatment failure [54].

Although specific cutoffs for the diagnosis of sepsis or for the guidance of antimicrobial usage have yet to be full elucidated, Schuetz et al. contended that antibiotics may be withheld in patients with PCT levels <0.25 ng/mL [55]. Meta-analyses of PCT for diagnosing sepsis from bacterial infections were noted to have a sensitivity and specificity of 75 and 80%, respectively [48, 56]. PCT does not have equal predictive value across all infection types. In a meta-analysis of six studies, it was noted that although CRP outperformed PCT for the diagnosis of endocarditis [57], the authors contended that neither CRP nor PCT be used to rule out endocarditis.

PCT clearly can distinguish patients with infection from healthy controls. However, PCT has limitations in critically ill patients with severe inflammation, especially seen in surgical and trauma patients. Products of tissue damage which may be released in noninfected patients with SIRS, traumatic injuries, or immediately after an operation are also noted to stimulate PCT release as well as activate other biomarkers. Several meta-analyses and reviews have been performed looking at the role of PCT for sepsis diagnosis as well as comparing PCT to CRP. Although early reports were encouraging in believing that PCT was superior to CRP and could distinguish SIRS from sepsis, the subsequent studies and meta-analyses have revealed conflicting data [37, 58–60].

Uzzan et al. reviewed 33 studies of exclusively surgical and trauma patients for the ability of PCT to aid in diagnosis of an infection in these critically ill patients [59]. For comparing septic patients to noninfected patients with SIRS, PCT fared better than CRP and was noted to have a global diagnostic accuracy odds ratio of 15.7 (95% CI 9.1–27.1). However the overall specificity and sensitivity remained low. Yu et al. noted that the overall accuracy of PCT was better than CRP, but this was attributed to the timing of testing and the fact that PCT rises sooner than CRP. A limitation to this work was the inclusion of neonates and the fact that a significant number of studies reviewed mandating documentation of infection [37]. A similar comparison of CRP to PCT in burn patients also failed to show superiority of either test for diagnosis of infection [60].

Tang et al. undertook a review of a broader group of critically ill patients [58]. This included surgical and medical patients and excluded studies in which the diagnoses were considered "too narrow" such as exclusively abdominal sources of critical illness. The authors concluded that the addition of PCT to pretest probability was insufficient to justify altering clinical care and should not influence either administering or withholding antimicrobial agents. A significant finding from the analysis of Tang et al. was that small studies tended to overestimate the ability of PCT to add to diagnostic decision-making. Overall, Tang et al. noted a pooled diagnostic OR of 7.8 which implies that PCT would be very unlikely to clinically aid in accurately diagnosing or excluding sepsis in critically ill patients with SIRS. A significant limitation of the analysis was the inclusion of studies that only demonstrated proof of infection [58]. Since it is now accepted that bacteremia is not an absolute prerequisite for diagnosing sepsis, the conclusions of the analysis are limited.

Overall, these meta-analyses have demonstrated several important points about biomarkers in general and specifically PCT. Patients with critical illness from surgical or traumatic causes may need a higher cutoff point for the diagnosis of sepsis may be needed. Many of the studies assessed the association between PCT levels drawn early in the course, but it has been demonstrated that PCT, CRP, or other biomarkers may vary in their onset, peak, and duration in the early phase. Repeat PCT testing has been advocated, with guidelines advocating that repeatedly normal PCT levels be used to exclude an infectious etiology. Further, initially elevated levels of PCT that rapidly normalize may not reflect infection but rather a transient inflammatory response. The Procalcitonin and Survival Study (PASS), a large randomized trial, assessed the value and clinical applicability of following repeated PCT levels over time [61]. Interestingly, patients in the PCT group were noted to have a longer hospital length of stay as well as a greater degree of impaired renal function. The authors speculated that PCT patients were more likely to be exposed to a greater duration of broader-spectrum antibiotics which may have been harmful. A significant, but obvious, conclusion from the study was to reaffirm that PCT should not be used exclusively to diagnose sepsis or to determine the need for antimicrobial agents. Rather, as with any individual clinical finding or test, PCT should guide judgment in the broader context of the compendium of the patient's clinical presentation and laboratory investigations.

High-mobility group box 1 protein (HMGB-1) is a cytoplasmic and nuclear protein that is normally undetectable in normal individuals. Although there are multiple sources of HMGB-1, it is released from monocytes following activation during infection. The HMGB-1is rapidly released following the onset of infection. Plasma levels of HMGB-1 have been shown to correlate with the degree of sepsis as well as organ failure in septic patients [62, 63]. As early as day 3 following presentation with sepsis, plasma HMGB-1 levels were notably different between ultimate survivors and non-survivors. Plasma levels of HMGB-1 exceeding 4 ng/ml on day 3 were associated with over a fivefold increase risk of death [64]. Although a useful tool in patients with sepsis, HMGB-1 can also be released in response to sterile necrosis, thereby limiting its usefulness.

The *soluble form of the receptor for advanced glycation end products (sRAGE)* is a useful marker for the activation of monocytes and has been considered a potential biomarker of sepsis. RAGE is DAMP receptor capable of binding several pattern recognition molecules. HMGB-1 is capable of signaling through RAGE. However RAGE activation is also signaled by necrotic cells. RAGE activation by ligands results in pro-inflammatory gene expression. Elevated RAGE levels are predictive of survival in patients with pneumonia [65]. However, since lung alveolar cells are capable of normally expressing high levels of RAGE, it is possible that pulmonary inflammation from causes other than infection may induce high levels of sRAGE, thus limiting the utility of this biomarker for the diagnosis of sepsis.

sTREM-1—the triggering receptor expressed on myeloid cells-1 (TREM-1)—is a member of the immunoglobulin super family. TREM-1 expression on phagocytosis is upregulated in the presence of bacteria and fungi [66, 67]. The soluble fraction of sTREM-1 has been studied as a predictive tool for sepsis, septic shock, and death in adults [68]. The sensitivity and specificity of sTREM-1 for distinguishing infection were similar to those of CRP or PCT. However, unlike many of the studies involving PCT, it was noted that sTREM-1 upon admission correlated with survival from sepsis [43, 69], noting that a rapid decline in sTREM-1 levels after initiation of therapy correlates with better odds of survival [67]. sTREM-1 has not shown promise in helping diagnose infection in patients with SIRS.

Neutrophil surface receptor expression. The Fc receptor (FcR) is a protein expressed on the surface of many immune cells. FcRs mediate immune cell response to a variety of antigenic stimuli. In the setting of infection, FcRs enable immune cells to bind to antibodies attached to microbial surfaces or microbe-infected cells, leading to elimination of microbes. Fc-gamma receptor-1 (FcγR1) (also known as CD64) is an integral membrane glycoprotein constitutively expressed on macrophages and monocytes. CD64 is only expressed at low levels of neutrophils in healthy individuals [70]. However, following inflammation or in the setting of active infection, there is a significant elevation of CD64 expression on neutrophils. Davis et al. [71] reported a sensitivity of 88% and specificity of 77% for the presence of infection. Neutrophil CD64 (nCD64) expression has been shown to correlate with the presence of infection versus SIRS [72], as well as the degree of sepsis (sepsis versus severe sepsis versus septic shock) [73]. nCD64 has also shown correlation with prognosis and survival from sepsis [40, 73]. nCD64, while predicting infection, was unable to distinguish bacterial from viral infections [74]. When nCD64 was simultaneously measured with neutrophil CD35 (complement receptor-1) expression, distinct pattern was noted that could distinguish viral infections from bacterial infection and sterile inflammation (SIRS) [75]. FcRIIIb (CD16b) is noted to be shed from the cell surface following trauma and infection, leading to decreased neutrophil surface expression of CD16b and increased soluble CD16b. Levels of soluble CD16b correlate with sepsis disease severity [76]. Interestingly, Hsu et al. noted that CD64 and CD64/CD16 ratio had better abilities than PCT in distinguishing sepsis from SIRS in critically ill patients. Further, it was noted that CD64 expression and the CD64/CD16 ratio predicted survival from sepsis, whereas neither PCT nor CD16 were significantly different between sepsis survivors and non-survivors [73]. CD64 is proving a potentially valuable resource in sepsis diagnosis in neonates.

Other Biomarkers

Mid-regional pro-adrenomedullin (MR-proADM) is a fragment of adrenomedullin, a peptide produced by the adrenal gland in response to physiological stress. ProADM modulates vasodilation and demonstrates bactericidal activity. MR-proADM was noted to be significantly higher in patients with infections when compared to patients with sterile inflammation (SIRS) [77]. ProADM showed a dose response for predicting mortality. When proADM was combined with PCT, the posttest probability was noted to be 0.99 [78]. *Soluble urokinase plasminogen activator receptor (suPAR)* plays a role in migration of immune cells from the bloodstream into tissues during an infection. It was first reported in 1990 to be elevated in patients with sepsis as well as other inflammatory conditions. The correlation between suPAR and sepsis is inferior to PCT or CRP [79]; however, suPAR levels do associate with severity of sepsis as well as 30- and 90-day mortalities [80]. *Angiopoietin (Ang)-1 and Ang-2* are endothelial-derived vascular growth factors that play modulating roles in the inflammatory and immune responses to sepsis. Ang-1 is noted to stabilize the endothelium, whereas Ang-2 induces loss of endothelial integrity and vascular leakage. Both Ang-1 and Ang-2 mediate their action through the transmembrane endothelial tyrosine kinase Tie2. Elevated levels of Ang-2 were noted in severe sepsis. Elevated Ang-1 and lower levels of Ang-2 were noted in sepsis survivors [81]. Plasma *macrophage migration inhibitory factor (MIF)* levels are noted to elevate in response to sepsis and septic shock, and MIF levels have been noted to potentially correlate with sepsis prognosis [82, 83]. *Beta-d-glucan* has been used for atypical infections and has been proven to be an effective adjunct in the diagnosis of invasive candidiasis.

Biomarker combinations and panels. Given the redundancy in the immune and inflammatory systems, several authors have contended that combinations or panels of biomarkers [79, 84, 85] may be more useful in distinguishing sepsis from SIRS. The diagnostic criteria already reflect this understanding that sepsis is not based on a single criterion or laboratory test (Table 11.2). As mentioned previously, some biomarkers may be used in combination with clinical indicators to develop scoring systems such as the IPS [16]. Combining PCT and MR-proADM was shown to have a posttest probability of 0.998 for diagnosing septic patients. The combination of as many as six pro-inflammatory biomarkers more accurately identifies sepsis. Shapiro et al. narrowed down over 150 biomarkers to three reported as a "sepsis score" [85]. Interestingly this panel does not include previously mentioned biomarkers but included IL-1 receptor antagonist (IL-1ra), protein c, and neutrophil gelatinase-associated lipocalin (NAGL). Gibot et al. described a "bioscore" for the combination of multiple biomarkers [84]. The bioscore combined sTREM-1, PCT, and CD64. The most predictive of these three was the neutrophil CD64 index; however, combining all three offered a superior ability to diagnose sepsis in critically ill patients. Future directions appear to be aimed at a better understanding of gene expression profiles of septic versus noninfected critically ill patients. However, this work remains hampered by many of the issues with the abovementioned clinical or laboratory findings, namely, the remarkable overlap in the immune and inflammatory cascades in patients with an acute illness whether it's from a sterile inflammation or related to a septic event.

Conclusions

Sepsis remains a leading cause of death among hospitalized patients, and early and accurate diagnosis is critical to improving sepsis-related outcomes. Standard definitions of sepsis and severe sepsis are critical to effective communication among providers as well as to frame future sepsis-related studies. The clinical manifestations of severe infections often mimic other, noninfectious, processes. An oversimplified set of diagnostic criteria for the diagnosis of sepsis leads to potentially inappropriate antimicrobial exposure. Thus, the current set of criteria includes an expansion of markers of organ dysfunction and offers potential biomarkers. The gold standard for diagnosing sepsis has always been considered the demonstration of an infecting organism. However, it has become evident that current culture-based techniques have severe limitations and advances in methods for routine detection of bacterial, fungal, and other atypical organisms are needed. Although many biomarkers have been described over the years, there remains no current consensus regarding the optimal biomarker or combination of biomarkers. Advances in the care of septic patients are predicated upon effective, timely, and efficient diagnosis of sepsis.

References

1. Geroulanos S, Douka E. Historical perspective of the word "sepsis". Intensive Care Med. 2006;32(12):2077.
2. Dellinger R, Levy M, Rhodes A, Annane D, Gerlach H, Opal S, et al. Surviving sepsis campaign: international guidelines for management of severe sepsis and septic shock. Crit Care Med. 2013;41(2):580–637.
3. Mayr F, Yende S, Angus D. Epidemiology of severe sepsis. Virulence. 2014;5(1):4–11.
4. Levy M, Fink M, Marshall J, Abraham E, Angus D, Cook D, et al. Ramsay and The international sepsis definition conference. 2001 SCCM/ESICM/ACCP/ATS/SIS International sepsis definitions conference. Intensive Care Med. 2003;29(4):530–8.
5. Bone R, Fisher C, Clemmer T, Slotman G, Metz C, Balk P. Sepsis syndrome A valid clinical entity methylprednoslone severe sepsis study group. Crit Care Med. 1989;17(5):389–93.
6. Bone R, Fisher C, Clemmer T, Slotman G, Metz C, Balk R, et al. A controlled clinical trial of high dose methylprednisolone in the treatment of severe sepsis and septic shock. N Engl J Med. 1987;317(11):353–8.
7. Bone R, Balk R, Cerra F, Dellinger R, Fein A, Knaus W, et al. Definitions for sepsis and organ failure and guidelines for the use of innovative therapies in sepsis. The ACCP/SCCM consensus conference committee. American College of Chest Physicians/Society of Critical Care Medicine. Chest. 1992;101(6):1644–55.
8. Sprung C, Sakr Y, Vincent J, Gall J, Reinhart K, Ranieri V, et al. An evaluation of systemic inflammatory response syndrome signs in the Sepsis Occurrence in Acutely Ill Patients (SOAP) study. Intensive Care Med. 2006;32(3):421–7.
9. Heppner H, Cornel S, Peter W, Philipp B, Katrin S. Infections in the elderly. Crit Care Clin. 2013;29(3):757–74.
10. Fox E, Heffernan D, Cioffi W, Reichner J. Neutrophils from critically ill septic patients mediate profound loss of endothelial barrier integrity. Crit Care. 2013;17(5):R226.
11. Czura C. Merinoff symposium 2010: sepsis – speaking with one voice. Mol Med. 2011; 17:2–3.
12. Vincent J, Opal S, Marshall J, Tracey K. Sepsis definitions: time for change. Lancet. 2013; 381:774–5.
13. Renaud B, Brun-Buisson C, ICU-Bacteremia Study Group. Outcomes of primary and catheter related bacteremia. A cohort and case control study in critically ill patients. Am J Respir Crit Care Med. 2001;163:1584–90.
14. Levy M, Rhodes A, Phillips G, Townsend S, Schorr C, Beale R, et al. Surviving sepsis campaign: association between performance metrics and outcomes in a 7.5 year study. Crit Care Med. 2015;43(1):3–12.

15. Marshall J, Dellinger R, Levy M. The surviving sepsis campaign: a history and a perspective. Surg Infect (Larchmt). 2011;11(3):275–81.
16. Peres-Bota D, Melot C, Lopes Ferreira F, Vincent J. Infection probability score (IPS): a method to help assess the probability of infection in critically ill patients. Crit Care Med. 2003;31:2579–84.
17. Calandra T, Cohen J. The international sepsis forum consensus conference on definitions of infection in the intensive care unit. Crit Care Med. 2005;33:1538–48.
18. Phua J, Ngerng W, See K, Tay C, Kiong T, Lim H, et al. Characteristics and outcomes of culture negative versus culture positive severe sepsis. Crit Care. 2013;17(5):R202.
19. Kumar A, Roberts D, Wood K, Light B, Parrillo J, Sharma S, et al. Duration of hypotension before initiation of effective antimicrobial therapy is the critical determinant of survival in human septic shock. Crit Care Med. 2006;34(6):1589–96.
20. Mullins K, Faloona F. Specific synthesis of DNA in vitro via a polymerase catalyzed chain reaction. Methods. 1987;155:335–50.
21. Aydiner A, Lusebrink J, Schildgen V, Winterfeld I, Knuver O, Schwarz K, et al. Comparison of two commercial PCR methods for methicillin-resistant *Staphylococcus aureus* (MRSA) screening in a tertiary care hospital. PLoS One. 2012;7(9):e43935.
22. Snyder L, Loman N, Faraj L, Levi K, Weinstock G, Boswell T, et al. Epidemiological investigation of Pseudomonas aeruginosa isolates from a six-year long hospital outbreak using high-throughput whole genome screening. Euro Surveill. 2013;18(42):20611.
23. Schrenzel J. Clinical relevance of new diagnostic methods for blood stream infections. Int J Antimicrob Agents. 2007;21(3):161–70.
24. Strommenger B, Schmidt C, Werner G, Roessie-Lorch B, Bachmann T, Witte W. DNA microarray for the detection of therapeutically relevant antibiotic resistance determinants in clinical isolates of *Staphylococcus aureus*. Mol Cell Probes. 2007;21(3):161–70.
25. Otsuka J, Kondoh Y, Amemiya T, Kitamura A, Ito T, Baba S, et al. Development and validation of microarray based assay for epidemiological study of MRSA. Mol Cell Probes. 2008; 22(1):1–13.
26. Bhowmick T, Mirrett S, Reller L, Price C, Qi C, Weinstein M, et al. Controlled multicenter evaluation of a bacteriophage-based method for rapid detection of *Staphylococcus aureus* in positive blood cultures. J Clin Microbiol. 2013;51(4):1226–30.
27. Sullivan K, Turner N, Roundtree S, McGowan K. Rapid detection of methicillin-resistant *Staphylococcus aureus* (MRSA) and methicillin-susceptible *Staphylococcus aureus* (MSSA) using the KeyPath MRSA/MSSA blood cultre test and the BacT/ALERT system in a pediatric population. Arch Pathol Lab Med. 2013;137(8):1103–5.
28. Park S, Zhang Y, Lin S, Wang T, Yang S. Advances in microfluidic PCR for point-of-care infectious disease diagnostics. Biotechnol Adv. 2011;29(6):830–9.
29. Lee W, Kim Y, Chung B, Demirci U, Khademhosseini A. Nano/Microfluidics for diagnosis of infectious diseases in developing countries. Adv Drug Deliv Rev. 2010;62(4–5):449–57.
30. Paredes J, Alonso-Arce M, Schmidt C, Valderas D, Sedano B, Legarda J, et al. Smart central venous port for early detection of bacterial biofilm related infections. Biomed Microdevices. 2014;16(3):365–74.
31. Blatteis C. Age dependent changes in temperature regulation—a mini review. Gerontology. 2012;58:289–95.
32. Heffernan D, Thakkar R, Monaghan S, Ravindran R, Adams C, Kozloff M, et al. Normal presenting vital signs are unreliable in geriatric blunt trauma victims. J Trauma. 2010;69(4): 813–20.
33. Ottinger M, Monaghan S, Gravenstein S, Cioffi W, Ayala A, Heffernan D. The geriatric cytokine response to trauma: time to consider a new threshold. Surg Infect (Larchmt). 2014; 15(6):800–5.
34. Boraschi D, Aguado M, Dutel C, Goronzy J, Louis J, Grubeck-Lobenstein B, et al. The gracefully aging immune system. Sci Transl Med. 2013;5(185):185ps8.

35. Lee S, Chan R, Wu J, Chen H, Chang S, Lee C. Diagnostic value of procalcitonin for bacterial infection in elderly patients—a systemic review and meta-analysis. Int J Clin Pract. 2013; 67(12):1350–7.
36. Gerdes J. Clinicopathologic approach to the diagnosis of neonatal sepsis. Clin Perinatol. 1991;18:361–81.
37. Yu Z, Liu J, Sun Q, Qui Y, Han S, Guo X. The accuracy of the procalcitonin test for the diagnosis of neonatal sepsis: a meta-analysis. Scand J Infect Dis. 2010;42(10):723–33.
38. Biomarkers Definition Working Group. Biomarkers and surrogate endopoints: preferred definitions and conceptual framework. Clin Pharmacol Ther. 2001;69(3):89–95.
39. Pierrakos C, Vincent J. Sepsis biomarkers: a review. Crit Care. 2010;14:R15.
40. Livaditi O, Kotanidou A, Psarra A, Dimopoulou I, Sotiropoulou C, Augustatou K, et al. Neutrophil CD64 expression and serum IL-8: sensitive markers of severity and outcome in sepsis. Cytokine. 2006;36:283–90.
41. Gentile L, Cuenca A, Vanzant E, Efron P, McKinley B, Moore F, et al. Is there value in plasma cytokine measurements in patients with severe trauma and sepsis. Methods. 2013;61(1):3–9.
42. Hong T, Chang C, Ko W, Lin C, Liu H, Chow L, et al. Biomarkers of early sepsis may be correlated with outcome. J Transl Med. 2014;12:146.
43. Zhang J, She D, Feng D, Jia Y, Xie L. Dynamic changes of serum soluble triggering receptor expressed on myeloid cells-1 (sTREM-1) reflect severity and can predict prognosis: a prospective study. BMC Infect Dis. 2011;11:53.
44. Lvovschi V, Arnaud L, Parizot C, Freund Y, Juillien G, Ghillani-Dalbin P, et al. Cytokine profiles in sepsis have limited relevance for stratifying patients in the emergency department: a prospective observational study. PLoS One. 2011;6:e28870.
45. Bozza F, Salluh J, Japiassu A, Soares M, Assis E, Gomes R, et al. Cytokine profiles as markers of disease severity in sepsis: a multiplex analysis. Crit Care. 2007;11:R49.
46. Andaluz-Ojeda D, Bobillo F, Iglesias V, Almansa R, Rico L, Gandia F, et al. A combined score of pro- and anti- inflammatory interleukins improves mortality prediction in severe sepsis. Cytokine. 2012;57:332–6.
47. Tillett W, Francis T. Serological reactions in pneumonia with a non-protein somatic fraction of pneumococcus. J Exp Med. 1930;52:561–71.
48. Simon L, Gauvin F, Amre D, Saint-Louis P, Lacroix J. Serum procalcitonin and C-reactive protein levels as markers of bacterial infection: a systematic review and meta-analysis. Clin Infect Dis. 2004;39:206–17.
49. Povoa P, Coelho L, Almeida E, Fernandes A, Mealha R, Moreira P, et al. C-Reactive protein as a marker of infection in critically ill patients. Clin Microbiol Infect. 2005;11(2):101–8.
50. Schmit X, Vincent J. The time course of blood C-reactive protein concentrations in relation to the response to initial antimicrobial therapy in patients with sepsis. Infection. 2008;36:213–9.
51. O'Grady N, Barie P, Bartlett J, Bleck T, Carroll K, Kalil A, et al. Guidelines for evaluation of new fever in critically ill adult patients: 2008 update from the American College of Critical Care Medicine and the Infectious Diseases Society of America. Crit Care Med. 2008; 36(4):1330–49.
52. Harbarth S, Holeckova K, Froidevaux C, Pittet D, Ricou B, Grau G, et al. Geneva sepsis network diagnostic value of procalcitonin, interleukin-6 and interleukin-8 in critically ill patients admitted with suspected sepsis. Am J Respir Crit Care Med. 2001;164(3):396–402.
53. Muller B, Becker K, Schachinger H, Rickenbacher P, Huber P, Zimmerli W, et al. Calcitonin precursors are reliable markers of sepsis in a medical intensive care unit. Crit Care Med. 2000;28(4):977–83.
54. Schuetz P, Muller B, Christ-Crain M, Stolz D, Tamm M, Bouadma L, et al. Procalcitonin to initiate or discontinue antibiotics in acute respiratory tract infections. Cochrane Database Syst Rev. 2012;9:CD007498.
55. Schuetz P, Albrich W, Christ-Crain M, Chastre J, Mueller B. Procalcitonin for guidance of antibiotic therapy. Expert Rev Anti Infect Ther. 2010;8(5):575–87.

56. Wacker C, Prkno A, Brunkhorst F, Schlattmann P. Procalcitonin as a diagnostic marker for sepsis: a systematic reivew and meta-analysis. Lancet Infect Dis. 2013;13:426–35.
57. Yu C, Juan L, Hsu S, Chen C, Wu C, Lee C, et al. Role of procalcitonin in the diagnosis of infective endocarditis: a meta-analysis. Am J Emerg Med. 2013;31(6):935–41.
58. Tang B, Eslick G, Craig J, McLean A. Accuracy of procalcitonin for sepsis diagnosis in critically ill patients: systemic review and meta-analysis. Lancet Infect Dis. 2007;7(3):210–7.
59. Uzzan B, Cohen R, Nicolas P, Cucherat M, Perret G. Procalcitonin as a diagnostic test for sepsis in critically ill adults and after surgery or trauma: a systematic review and meta-analysis. Crit Care Med. 2006;34(7):1996–2003.
60. Mann E, Wood G, Wade C. Use of procalcitonin for the detection of sepsis in the critically ill burn patients: a systematic review of the literature. Burns. 2011;37:549–58.
61. Jensen J, Hein L, Lundgren B, Bestle M, Mohr T, Andersen M, et al. Procalcitonin guided interventions against infections to increase early appropriate antibiotics and improve survival in the intensive care unit; a randomized trial. Crit Care Med. 39(9):2048–58.
62. Sunden-Cullberg J, Norrby-Teglund A, Rouhiainen A, Rauvala H, Herman G, Tracey K, et al. Persistent elevation of high mobility group box-1 protein (HMGB-1) in patients with severe sepsis and septic shock. Crit Care Med. 2005;33:564–73.
63. Hatada T, Wada H, Nobori T, Okabayshi K, Maruyama K, Abe Y, et al. Plasma concentrations and importance of High Mobility Group Box protein in the prognosis of organ failure in patients with disseminated intravascular coagulation. Thromb Hemost. 2005;94:975–9.
64. Gibot S, Massin F, Cravoisy A, Barraud D, Nace L, Levy B, et al. High-mobility group box-1 protein plasma concentrations during septic shock. Intensive Care Med. 2007;33:1347–53.
65. Narvaez-Rivera R, Rendon A, Salinas-Carmona M, Rossa-Taraco A. Soluble RAGE as a severity marker in community acquired pneumonia associated sepsis. BMC Infect Dis. 2012;12:15.
66. Bouchon A, Dietrich J, Colonna M. Cutting edge: inflammatory responses can be triggered by TREM-1, a novel receptor expressed on neutrophils and monocytes. J Immunol. 2000;164:4991–5.
67. Gibot S. Clinical review: role of triggering receptor expressed on myeloid cells-1 during sepsis. Crit Care. 2005;9:485–9.
68. Jiyong J, Tiancha H, Wei C, Huahao S. Diagnostic value of the soluble triggering receptor expressed on myeloid cells-1 in bacterial infection: a meta-analysis. Intensive Care Med. 2009;35(4):587–95.
69. Jeong S, Song Y, Kim C, Kim H, Ku N, Han S, et al. Measurement of plasma sTREM-1 in patients with severe sepsis receiving early goal directed therapy and evaluation of its usefulness. Shock. 2012;37:574–8.
70. Looney R. Structure and function of human and mouse Fc gamma RII. Blood Cells. 1993;19(2):353–9.
71. Davis B, Olsen S, Ahmad E, Bigelow N. Neutrophil CD64 is an improved indicator of infection or sepsis in emergency department patients. Arch Pathol Lab Med. 2006;130(5):654–61.
72. Lewis S, Treacher D, Bergmeier L, Brain S, Chambers D, Pearson J, et al. Plasma from patients with sepsis up-regulates the expression of CD49d and CD64 on blood neutrophils. Am J Respir Cell Mol Biol. 2009;40(6):724–32.
73. Hsu K, Chan M, Wang J, Lin L, Wu C. Comparison of Fc-gamma receptor expression on neutrophils with procalcitonin for the diagnosis of sepsis in critically ill patients. Respirology. 2011;16(1):152–60.
74. Nuutila J, Hohenthal U, Laitinen I, Kotilainen P, Rajamaki A, Nikoskelainen J, et al. Simultaneous quantitative analysis of FcGammaRI (CD64) expression on neutrophils and monocytes: a new, improved way to detect infections. J Immunol Methods. 2007;328(1–2):189–200.
75. Jalava-Karvinen P, Hohenthal U, Laitinen I, Kotilainen P, Rajamaki A, Nikoskelainen J, et al. Simultaneous quantitative analysis of Fc gammaRI (CD64) and CR1 (CD35) on neutrophils in distinguishing between bacterial infections, viral infections and inflammatory diseases. Clin Immunol. 2009;133(3):314–23.

76. Muller Kobold A, Zijlastra J, Koene H. Levels of soluble Fc gamma RIII correlate with disease severity in sepsis. Clin Exp Immunol. 1998;227:220.
77. Christ-Crain M, Morgenthaler N, Struck J, Harbarth S, Bergmann A, Muller B. Mid-regional pro-adrenomedullin as a prognostic marker in sepsis: an observational study. Crit Care. 2009; 9:R816–24.
78. Angeletti S, Battistoni F, Fioravanti M, Bernardini S, Dicuonzo G. Procalcitonin and mid-regional pro-adrenomedullin test combination in sepsis diagnosis. Clin Chem Lab Med. 2013;51(5):1059–67.
79. Kofoed K, Andersen O, Kronborg G, Tvede M, Petersen J, Eugen-Olsen J, et al. Use of plasma C-reactive protein, procalcitonin, neutrophils, macrophage migration inhibitory factor, soluble urokinase-type plasminogen activator receptor, and soluble triggering receptor expressed on myeloid cells-1 in combination to diagnose infections. Crit Care. 2007;11:R38.
80. Haput T, Petersen J, Ellekilde G, Klausen H, Thorball C, Eugen-Olsen J, et al. Plasma suPAR levels are associated with mortality, admission time and Charlson comorbidity index in the acutely admitted medical patient: a prospective observational study. Crit Care. 2012;16:R130.
81. Ricciuto D, dos Santos C, Hawkes M, Toltl L, Conroy A, Rajwans N, et al. Angiopoietin-1 and angiopoietin-2 as clinically informative prognostic biomarkers of morbidity and mortality in severe sepsis. Crit Care Med. 2011;39:702–10.
82. Bozza F, Gomes R, Japiassu A, Soares M, Castro-Faria-Neto H, Bozza P, et al. Macrophage migration inhibitory factor levels correlate with fatal outcome in sepsis. Shock. 2004;22: 309–13.
83. Calandra T, Echtenacher B, Roy D, Pugin J, Metz C, Hultner L, et al. Protection from septic shock by neutralization of macrophage migration inhibitory factor. Nat Med. 2000;6:164–70.
84. Gibot S, Bene M, Noel R, Massin F, Guy J, Cravoisy A, et al. Combination biomarkers to diagnose sepsis in the critically ill patient. Am J Respir Crit Care Med. 2012;186(1):65–71.
85. Shapiro N, Trzeciak S, Hollander J, Birkhahn R, Otero R, Osborn T, et al. A prospective multicenter derivation of a biomarker panel to assess risk of organ dysfunction, shock and death in emergency department patients with suspected sepsis. Crit Care Med. 2009;37(1):96–104.

Chapter 12
Source Control in Sepsis

Michael Connolly and Charles Adams

Introduction

Source control is generally accepted to be a key component in the treatment and reversal of sepsis. It is comprised of the physical efforts to remove or contain a focus of invasive infection in order to restore normal function [1]. The principles of source control for sepsis have been known for centuries, but only recently have prioritizing and achieving source control in sepsis become more recognized due to the heightened awareness of sepsis as a result of the Surviving Sepsis Campaign [2]. The majority of research in sepsis has focused on early diagnosis, resuscitation, antibiotics, and other therapies, and despite source control being the cornerstone of therapy for sepsis for centuries, it has not been widely studied. Due to this lack of evidence, source control is often overlooked or underutilized much to the detriment of septic patients.

Definition

Source control is generally defined as an intervention designed to eradicate or limit a focus of infection and is achieved in one of three ways: drainage, debridement, or definitive control via resection or device removal [3]. Traditionally source control was achieved through surgical intervention, but due to technological advancements, source control is increasingly achieved via less invasive measures such as radiological-directed percutaneous drainage. Regardless of the method, source

M. Connolly, MD (✉) • C. Adams, MD
Department of Surgery, Alpert/Brown Medical School, 593 Eddy St, APL 453,
Providence, RI 02903, USA
e-mail: Connolly@brown.edu; MConnolly5@Lifespan.org

© Springer International Publishing AG 2017
N.S. Ward, M.M. Levy (eds.), *Sepsis*, Respiratory Medicine,
DOI 10.1007/978-3-319-48470-9_12

control must provide a prompt, effective means to allow egress of infection from the infected site or complete removal of the offending source (necrotic organ, dead tissue, or infected foreign body).

Diagnosis

Patients with evidence of infection should be thoroughly evaluated for the source of infection. The Surviving Sepsis Campaign urges routine screening of potentially infected seriously ill patients for severe sepsis in order to provide earlier therapeutic interventions [2]. Despite increases in technology, the key to detecting patients with severe infections remains a thorough history and physical exam. A majority of infections requiring source control can be identified early on with this simple evaluation alone. Laboratory testing should then be undertaken to narrow the differential diagnosis and alert the clinician to significant physiologic derangements requiring intervention. Finally, multiple radiographic modalities are available to aid in diagnosis with the choice of study determined by the clinical suspicion of the treating provider. Although modern radiographic techniques deliver exceptional quality images and frequently identify the source of infection, there are some disease processes in which obvious emergent source control should be undertaken and radiographic imaging omitted to avoid delays to definitive therapy. The best example of this is the patient with florid peritonitis who needs no further diagnostic imaging and should be taken to the operating room for exploration. In this setting, further diagnostic workup only delays source control and sets the stage for worsened outcomes.

Drainage

Drainage is the evacuation of infected fluid from a closed abscess space. Drainage may be achieved via a surgical incision, or for infections not requiring operative intervention, with placement of a percutaneous catheter. The goal of drainage procedures is to convert an uncontrolled, closed-space infection under pressure into a controlled sinus or fistula that freely drains the infection. Frequently, the systemic manifestations of sepsis are abrogated by draining the infection, and this serves as the physiological basis of the clinical axiom that "pus under pressure" kills patients.

Superficial abscesses that can be easily accessed should be opened surgically; however, deeper space infections frequently require an intervention using radiographic guidance. Using ultrasound or CT guidance, a catheter can be inserted into the abscess to achieve decompression and drainage of the abscess. Percutaneous drainage using radiographic imaging has been demonstrated to be a safe and effective method of controlling sepsis in both intra-abdominal and thoracic abscesses [4, 5]. Percutaneous drainage techniques are most effective when the abscess is uniloculated.

Cinat et al. demonstrated that a successful outcome following percutaneous drainage is most likely when abscesses are postoperative, not pancreatic, and not infected with yeast [6].

Despite significant advances in radiographic techniques and percutaneous catheters, deep-space infections, particularly those with a large burden of necrotic tissue, cannot always be treated with percutaneous drainage. In patients with multi-loculated abscesses, in patients with anatomically inaccessible abscesses, or in patients who have failed percutaneous drainage, open drainage is often required to achieve adequate drainage. The failure to recognize unsuccessful drainage or delays in operative drainage frequently lead to worsened outcomes in septic patients. It should be noted that a partially effective drainage procedure may be an effective temporizing maneuver that allows correction of severe physiologic derangements such that definitive, operative intervention may be performed in a more stable patient.

Debridement/Device Removal

Infected or necrotic tissue incites a vigorous inflammatory response in patients and should be excised when possible. Necrotizing soft tissue infections can spread rapidly and require early and extensive debridement to control the infection. Other necrotizing processes without infection, such as necrotizing pancreatitis, may be debrided after demarcation of the necrotizing tissue provided that the patient is stable enough to undergo surgical exploration. In fact, delayed debridement of necrotizing pancreatitis may lead to improved outcomes, but this remains controversial [7, 8].

Medical devices are frequently the source of infection in septic patients. Infections of these foreign bodies are difficult to eradicate due to the bacteria's ability to generate a biofilm that promotes adherence to the foreign body and prevents effective penetration of host defenses and antibiotics. Due to these factors, device removal is recommended whenever possible. Attempts to "eradicate" infection from an infected foreign body are rarely successful, and the infection typically flares as soon as the suppressive effect of antibiotics is removed.

Definitive Control

The ultimate source control frequently requires operative intervention to remove the focus of infection and repair the affected organ. This category includes resection for appendicitis or cholecystitis, repair of intestinal perforations, and resection of non-viable bowel or organs. Although these interventions frequently require the most invasive procedure, the operations result in the most definitive source control and frequently eliminate the need for any further interventions. For example, cholecystectomy for gangrenous cholecystitis completely removes the source of sepsis, unlike decompression with a cholecystostomy tube which only drains the infection, leaving the infected wall of the gallbladder to drive the host's septic response and may ultimately require future cholecystectomy for definitive restoration of normal function.

Indications for Source Control

Early goal-directed therapy increases survival in patients with severe sepsis or septic shock, but fluid resuscitation and antibiotics may not be sufficient therapy for patients with infections requiring source control [9]. As outlined in the Surviving Sepsis Guidelines [2], a specific anatomical diagnosis of infection should be sought as quickly as possible. In many cases, the identification of the infectious source of sepsis is frequently delayed or overlooked as the clinician focuses on the resuscitation of the critically ill patient. In fact, patients may be admitted to the intensive care unit with a diagnosis of sepsis, without a differential diagnosis of the source of sepsis and often without a clear-cut diagnosis other than "sepsis." All patients with severe sepsis or septic shock should have an attempt at identifying the source of infection because emergent source control is as important, if not more important, as the early recognition of sepsis and resuscitation in patients.

When source control is deemed necessary, interventions aimed to obtain it should be made as soon as possible. Invariably some procedures can be delayed for a limited period of time as the necessary institutional resources are mobilized and personnel become available, but it is imperative that patients are closely monitored during these inevitable delays. Additional therapies such as fluid and blood administration and antibiotics should be given during this period of preparation. Thus, the timing of source control depends on the severity of the patient's illness and can be broadly divided into emergent or urgent interventions.

Emergent source control is required in patients with severe, life-threatening infections or in those patients with poor premorbid physiological reserve who will not tolerate the sequelae of the septic response. These patients typically present with extensive physiologic derangements and organ failure. Patients in this group should be quickly identified, and immediate resuscitation and antibiotic therapy should be initiated. Source control should then be obtained, even if the patient has not been fully resuscitated, as the resuscitation can be continued in the operating room or interventional radiology suite. Although surgeons have classically performed emergent source control as part of their standard care of septic patients, there is a paucity of data on the effect of timing on patient outcomes. Nonetheless, some examples of infections requiring immediate source control include diffuse peritonitis, necrotizing soft tissue infections, and infections causing hemodynamic instability [10–12]. In patients requiring emergent source control, time is critical, and delays in obtaining source control in this patient group are associated with worsened outcomes [13].

For those patients whose physiological derangements are less severe or in those patients who have greater physiological reserve and less medical comorbidities, delayed source control may be desirable. In these patients, the risk of emergent intervention may be unnecessarily high and may be lessened by a brief period to allow adequate fluid resuscitation, correction of electrolyte abnormalities, reversal of coagulopathy, etc. A short delay in order to maximize surgical and anesthesiologist technical ability, operating room preparedness, and other resources may also be acceptable. Finally, image-guided drainage of an abscess is frequently the initial intervention of choice, but this may necessitate a delay until the interventional radiology team is available. While the concept of an "acceptable delay" seems counter to the expressed concept of emergent source control, this delay should only be undertaken if the cost in terms of time delay will be offset with a significant reduction in risk to the patient, or added benefit. In essence, a brief delay that favorably alters the risk to benefit ratio to the patient is worth undertaking, but any delay that does not yield reduced risk or added benefit must be avoided.

The appropriate delay to source control in non-emergent cases remains controversial because there is limited evidence. One consensus of experts accepts a delay of up to 24 h for patients with intra-abdominal sepsis in hemodynamically stable patients without peritonitis [14]. Appendicitis is the best-studied disease process looking at delays in source control. Although there is still some debate over delaying appendectomy, it appears that for most patients an in-hospital delay of less than 24 h is acceptable [15, 16]. However, in all cases of delayed source control, patients must be carefully monitored to ensure no deterioration in their clinical status. If they do worsen, immediate source control should be undertaken. Additionally, if there are no barriers to early source control, intervention should be undertaken as soon as possible to minimize complications.

Method of Source Control

The method used to obtain source control will vary depending on multiple factors, but ideally the method that results in adequate source control through the least invasive means is generally the most desirable. The clinician must weigh the risks and benefits of less or more invasive methods of source control to determine the appropriate modality. Integral to this decision process is an understanding of the natural history of each proposed therapy, as well as an understanding of limitations, common pitfalls, and complications since all of these factors must be considered in the decision analysis process. Often, the most invasive intervention must be performed in order to achieve rapid, effective source control.

Traditionally source control required surgical intervention to drain or remove the source of infection. The advent of advanced radiographic imaging and access techniques has allowed many infections to be controlled with less invasive procedures. Gerzoff et al. demonstrated that percutaneous drainage of intra-abdominal abscesses could be done safely and effectively using radiographic guidance [4]. The use of percutaneous drainage of both intra-abdominal and intra-thoracic infections is now commonplace [5, 17]. Successful percutaneous drainage of deep space infections controls the source of sepsis and delays or even eliminates the need for surgical intervention. Generally, percutaneous drainage procedures minimize the anatomic and physiologic derangements compared with surgical intervention, but the efficacy of drainage may be less definitive than surgical methods.

Despite significant advances in imaging and drainage techniques, treatment failures with percutaneous drainage still occur. Success rates for percutaneous drainage range from 70 to 90% depending on the source (location) of the infection [4, 6, 18, 19]. Multiple factors have been identified that predict failure of percutaneous drainage, including size of the abscess, poorly defined abscess, abscess that is not postoperative, abscess with yeast infection, residual collection after first drainage attempt, and increased number of drainage attempts [4, 17–19]. Patients being managed with percutaneous source control require frequent reassessment of the adequacy of source control, and if the patient clinically deteriorates, then more aggressive, and typically more invasive, source control is warranted.

Operative intervention is often required to obtain the best source control. Surgery facilitates drainage of abscesses and has the added benefit of removal of the offending source of the infection. Surgical therapy may employ resection (appendix, gallbladder, ischemic bowel, necrotizing soft tissue infection) or repair (duodenal ulcer, intestinal perforation). This intervention frequently controls the source of sepsis more completely, which may ultimately shorten the duration of physiological derangement and generally decreases the need for future interventions. It is notable though that once multisystem organ failure has occurred, surgical source control of the infection may not result in reversal of organ failure [20, 21].

Severe intra-abdominal infections resulting in sepsis are frequently complicated by postoperative abdominal compartment syndrome (ACS). ACS is defined as intra-abdominal hypertension resulting in multisystem organ failure driven by the accumulation of fluid within the abdomen and its contents restricted by the noncompliant abdominal fascia. The fluid may be tissue fluid or blood that exceeds the capacitance of the abdominal cavity leading to increased pressure. A planned open-abdomen approach, in which the abdomen is closed with a temporary abdominal dressing, is an accepted method of preventing ACS. Recurrent ACS may occur even in the setting of an open abdomen and portends a dismal prognosis. The open abdomen may facilitate repeat laparotomy and washout of intra-abdominal sepsis; however, there has been no convincing data that planned re-laparotomy improves outcomes in these patients [22]. The benefits of an open abdomen must be balanced against the complications since these patients have higher rates of anastomotic leak, entero-cutaneous fistula, and massive hernia [22–24]. Therefore, a planned open abdomen should be reserved for cases requiring a second look (bowel ischemia), to restore intestinal continuity after an abbreviated laparotomy in a critically ill patient or in patients with abdominal compartment syndrome. At present time there is insufficient data to recommend that the abdomen be left open in order to enhance source control [25].

Treatment of Selected Diseases

Gastrointestinal Tract

The gastrointestinal tract frequently is a source of severe sepsis and septic shock, with appendicitis ranking as the most common source of infection [26]. Although a short delay in appendectomy appears reasonable, patients with appendicitis should undergo appendectomy as soon as feasible in order to eliminate the infectious source. Like many surgical infectious diseases, the severity of the infection is on a continuum from mild physiological derangements extending all the way up to florid septic shock and multisystem organ failure. Accordingly, the optimal timing of intervention also spans a continuum, but it is critical that surgical source control not be deferred in patients manifesting clinical deterioration. In contrast to appendicitis, patients with intestinal perforations generally require emergent operative intervention to control the source of sepsis. The site of perforation will determine the extent of surgery required. The goals of therapy in these patients are to physically clear the infection as well as restore normal function if possible.

Sepsis from small and large bowel perforations requires an operation to control the perforation. Traditionally, control was obtained via resection of the diseased intestine, and in cases of severe sepsis and septic shock, bowel resection with a diverting ostomy remains the preferred method of source control. If the patient's physiology and comorbidities allow, lesser operations may suffice in obtaining some degree of source control without the additional burden of more invasive or definitive surgery. For example, in diverticulitis, an option may be laparoscopic drainage and lavage of the infection with definitive resection and anastomosis delayed until the sepsis and inflammation have resolved. A procedure such as this allows creation of a controlled fistula and avoidance of a colostomy while still draining the abscess in most patients [27].

Intestinal ischemia resulting in bowel compromise is a feared source of intra-abdominal sepsis. In some cases of intestinal ischemia, patients can be treated non-operatively with resuscitation and correction of the underlying cause of the ischemia; however intestinal infarction requires emergent operation to resect the segment of bowel affected. The diagnosis of intestinal ischemia can be challenging as physical exam, laboratory testing, and radiography can lack sensitivity; therefore, if suspected in a critically ill patient, operative exploration should be performed. Patients undergoing resection of necrotic bowel due to vascular catastrophe are best managed with a planned open abdomen and "second look" laparotomy to assure viable bowel prior to restoring bowel continuity [28].

Biliary Tract

The biliary tract is another frequent source of intra-abdominal sepsis, and the spectrum of illnesses ranges from simple non-complicated cholecystitis all the way up to ascending cholangitis and septic shock. Acute cholangitis is caused by biliary obstruction and systemic spread of the bacterial infection from the biliary tree into the liver and beyond. Obstruction of the biliary tree results in an increase in intraductal pressure leading quickly to translocation of bacteria into the bloodstream, resulting in severe sepsis and shock, with a high rate of mortality if not treated promptly. Acute cholangitis is often diagnosed based on the presence of three classic findings: right upper quadrant abdominal pain, fever, and jaundice. The mortality rate for this disease entity has traditionally been very high; prior to 1980, the mortality rate was 50 %, but this rate has dropped significantly in recent years with the rise of endoscopic decompression [29].

Treatment of acute cholangitis requires early diagnosis, prompt antibiotic therapy, and decompression of the biliary tree for source control. In severe cholangitis, antibiotics alone are insufficient, and emergent decompression must be performed. Decompression of the biliary tree can be accomplished via endoscopic, percutaneous, or surgical methods. The use of endoscopic retrograde cholangiopancreatography (ERCP) is effective in controlling sepsis and has been shown to have a lower morbidity and mortality than surgical approaches [30]. Delays in performing ERCP for cholangitis result in increased mortality, length of hospital stay, and readmission rates [31, 32].

Acute cholecystitis is a more common source of biliary sepsis, but usually causes less severe sepsis and shock than cholangitis. Laparoscopic cholecystectomy is the preferred method of source control when possible; however, in patients that are poor operative risk candidates, percutaneous drainage with a cholecystostomy tube is adequate to control the infection. A notable exception may be the previously noted condition of emphysematous cholecystitis in which bacterial invasion of the gallbladder wall by gas-forming organisms results in a gangrenous cholecystitis. In this setting, drainage procedures alone may be inadequate in controlling the source of infection, and extirpation of the infected organ may be necessary.

Pancreatitis

Pancreatitis, like many surgical infections, spans a range from chemical pancreatitis marked by mild elevations of laboratory tests to severe necrotizing pancreatic infections leading to death. Pancreatitis follows a variable and unpredictable course both in timing of disease progression and disease severity, making this a particularly dangerous and difficult disease to treat for clinicians. Patients with pancreatic infarction or necrosis are at risk of developing infected necrosis; however, the diagnosis is difficult to make on clinical grounds alone because the findings of fever, leukocytosis, and worsening organ failure are nonspecific and frequently occur in patients with severe pancreatitis with and without infection. Abdominal computed tomography is helpful in identifying pancreatic necrosis as well as the stigmata of infected pancreatic necrosis and is particularly helpful in guiding therapy. When infected pancreatic necrosis is identified, prompt drainage of the infection is required.

The timing and method of this drainage has been contested, but delayed surgical debridement appears to decrease the morbidity and mortality of pancreatic necrosectomy [7, 33, 34]. Therefore, initial control of infected pancreatic necrosis with percutaneous drainage should be considered in most patients with open necrosectomy reserved for only the sickest patients or those developing ACS. Percutaneous pancreatic drainage controls the liquid component of the infection and is a temporizing maneuver, but true source control requires surgical debridement of the solid, necrotic debris. Utilizing this "step-up" approach, true source control may be obtained in a way that has been shown to significantly reduce the mortality associated with operation for infected pancreatic necrosis [8].

Necrotizing Soft Tissue Infection

Necrotizing soft tissue infections have a mortality rate of 25–35% and an even higher rate of significant morbidity [35]. One of the most feared types of necrotizing soft tissue infections is necrotizing fasciitis. This rapidly progressive form of soft tissue infection can spread in a matter of hours, resulting in death of the patient. Source control via surgical debridement must be performed emergently if there is any hope of patient salvage, and the most important factor in preventing morbidity and mortality is time to surgical debridement. Indeed, multiple series have demonstrated that the only factor predictive of survival in the setting of necrotizing soft tissue infection is time to operative intervention [36, 37]. Patients with necrotizing soft tissue infections should be taken emergently to the operating room for wide excision and debridement. The extent of excision should extend beyond the obviously affected areas and frequently results in large open wounds. Although these wounds may result in significant morbidity, the risk of mortality increases substantially when debridement is incomplete [37]. After the initial debridement, wounds should be inspected within hours to ensure control of the infection, as many patients require serial debridement. In extreme cases, amputation of an extremity may be necessary because of rapidly spreading infection or worsening muscle necrosis due to bacterial invasion.

Infected Devices

The use of invasive medical devices is commonplace. Medical devices can range from simple devices used almost daily in the intensive care unit (urinary catheters, central venous catheters) to complex, life-saving devices (valve replacements, left ventricular assist devices). Unfortunately, medical devices frequently provide the nidus for infection in septic patients. Microbes are able to bind to these medical devices based upon the cell surface characteristics of the microorganisms and the type of foreign body material [38]. Once the device is colonized, the organisms produce a biofilm that protects the organisms from antibiotic therapy and results in persistent or difficult to eradicate infections [39].

The optimal treatment of an infected medical device is removal. Any patient with severe sepsis or septic shock related to a medical device should have prompt removal of the device and antibiotic therapy. Similarly to other infections, the urgency of removal depends on the clinical condition of the patient, but should be performed soon after identifying the device as the source.

Patients with implanted medical devices often have other potential sites for infection, making definitive diagnosis challenging. However, when possible or if a high degree of suspicion exists, the device should be removed. Additionally, the device should be removed if there is local skin infection, metastatic infective complications, or recurrence of infection after cessation of antibiotics [38]. Removal of the device can carry significant morbidity, such as in a patient with difficult vascular access or infected mesh from a hernia repair. Salvage therapy with antibiotics can be performed in stable patients in an attempt to avoid removal of the device; however, the presence of the foreign body and biofilm makes salvage attempts unsuccessful. Contingency plans should be arranged in the meantime in case of treatment failure, and salvage should not be attempted in patients with severe sepsis or shock.

Conclusion

Source control is a critical element in managing patients with sepsis, yet it is often overlooked by clinicians as they focus on fluid resuscitation, timing and selection of antibiotics, etc. In certain disease processes, such as necrotizing fasciitis or ascending cholangitis, source control is the most important step; therefore, early consideration of the source and prompt intervention are imperative. The timing of source control should be determined by the severity of the patient's condition, the expected course for that disease process, and the overall condition of the patient. The optimal method of source control is determined by evaluating the risks and benefits of the invasiveness of the therapy versus the need for partial or complete eradication of the source. In general, the method that provides the most complete control with the least disruption of anatomy is preferred.

References

1. Marshall JC, al Naqbi A. Principles of source control in the management of sepsis. Crit Care Clin. 2009;25:753–68.
2. Dellinger RP, Levy MM, Rhodes A, Annane D, Gerlach H, Opal SM, et al. Surviving sepsis campaign: international guidelines for management of severe sepsis and septic shock: 2012. Crit Care Med. 2013;41(2):580–637.
3. Jimenez MF, Marshall JC. Source control in the management of sepsis. Intensive Care Med. 2001;27:S49–62.

4. Gerzof SG, Robbins AH, Johnson WC, Birkett DH, Nabseth DC. Percutaneous catheter drainage of abdominal abscesses. A five-year experience. N Engl J Med. 1981;305:653–7.
5. Moulton JS, Benkert RE, Weisiger KH, Chambers JA. Treatment of complicated pleural fluid collections with image-guided drainage and intracavitary urokinase. Chest. 1995;108(5): 1252–9.
6. Cinat ME, Wilson SE, Din AM. Determinants for successful percutaneous image-guided drainage of intra-abdominal abscess. Arch Surg. 2002;137(7):845–9.
7. Fernandez-del Castillo C, Rattner DW, Makary MA, Mostafavi A, McGrath D, Warshaw AL. Debridement and closed packing for the treatment of necrotizing pancreatitis. Ann Surg. 1998;228(5):676–84.
8. van Santvoort HC, Besselink MG, Bakker OJ, Hofker HS, Boermeester MA, Dejong CH, et al. A setp-up approach or open necrosectomy for necrotizing pancreatitis. N Engl J Med. 2010;362:1491–502.
9. Rivers E, Nguyen B, Havstad S, Ressler J, Muzzin A, Knoblich B, et al. Early goal-directed therapy in the treatment of severe sepsis and septic shock. N Engl J Med. 2001;345:1368–77.
10. Gajic O, Urrutia LE, Sewani H, Schroeder DR, Cullinane DC, Peters SG. Acute abdomen in the medical intensive care unit. Crit Care Med. 2002;30(6):1187–90.
11. Boyer A, Vargas F, Coste F, Saubusse E, Castaing Y, Gbikpi-Benissan G, et al. Influence of surgical treatment timing on mortality from necrotizing soft tissue infections requiring intensive care management. Intensive Care Med. 2009;35(5):847–53.
12. Buck DL, Vester-Andersen M, Moller MH. Surgical delay is a critical determinant of survival in perforated peptic ulcer. Br J Surg. 2013;100(8):1045–9.
13. Wacha H, Hau T, Dittmer R, Ohmann C, The Peritonitis Study Group. Risk factors associated with intraabdominal infections: a prospective multicenter study. Langenbecks Arch Surg. 1999;384:24–32.
14. Solomkin JS, Mazuski JE, Bradley JS, Rodvold KA, Goldstein EJC, Baron EJ, et al. Diagnosis and management of complicated intra-abdominal infection in adults and children: guidelines by the surgical infection society and the infectious diseases society of America. Clin Infect Dis. 2010;50:133–64.
15. The United Kingdom National Surgical Research Collaborative. Safety of short, in-hospital delays before surgery for acute appendicitis. Ann Surg. 2014;259:894–903.
16. Drake FT, Mottey NE, Farrokhi ET, Florence MG, Johnson MG, Mock C, et al. Time to appendectomy and risk of perforation in acute appendicitis. JAMA Surg. 2014;149(8):837–44.
17. Kumar RR, Kim JT, Haukoos JS, Macias LH, Dixon MR, Stamos MJ, et al. Factors affecting the successful management of intra-abdominal abscesses with antibiotics and the need for percutaneous drainage. Dis Colon Rectum. 2005;49:183–9.
18. Kassi F, Dohan A, Soyer P, Vicaut E, Boudiaf M, Valleur P, et al. Predictive factors for failure of percutaneous drainage of postoperative abscess after abdominal surgery. Am J Surg. 2014;207:915–21.
19. Marin D, Ho LM, Barnhard H, Neville AM, White RR, Paulson EK. Percutaneous abscess drainage in patients with perforated acute appendicitis: effectiveness, safety, and prediction of outcome. Am J Roentgenol. 2010;194:422–9.
20. Eiseman B, Beart R, Norton L. Multiple organ failure. Surg Gynecol Obstet. 1977;144(3): 323–6.
21. Norton LW. Does drainage of intraabdominal pus reverse multiple organ failure. Am J Surg. 1985;149(3):347–50.
22. Hau T, Ohmann C, Wolmerhauser A, Wacha H, Yang Q. Planned relaparotomy vs relaparotomy on demand in the treatment of intra-abdominal infections. Arch Surg. 1995;130:1193–7.
23. van Ruler O, Mahler CW, Boer KR, Reuland EA, Gooszen HG, Opmeer BC, et al. Comparison of on-demand vs planned relaparotomy strategy in patients with severe peritonitis. JAMA. 2007;298(8):865–72.
24. Adkins AL, Robbins J, Villalba M, Bendick P, Shanley CJ. Open abdomen management of intra-abdominal sepsis. Am Surg. 2004;70(2):137–40.

25. Lamme B, Boermeester MA, Reitsma JB, Mahler CW, Obertop H, Gouma DJ. Meta-analysis of relaparotomy for secondary peritonitis. Br J Surg. 2002;89:1516–24.
26. Sartelli M, Catena F, Ansaloni L, Coccolini F, Corbella D, Moore EE, et al. Complicated intra-abdominal infections worldwide: the definitive data of the CIAOW study. World J Emerg Surg. 2014;9:37.
27. Toorenvliet BR, Swank H, Schoones JW, Hamming JF, Bemelman WA. Laparoscopic perito-neal lavage for perforated colonic diverticulitis: a systematic review. Colorectal Dis. 2010; 12(9):862–7.
28. Park WM, Glovicki P, Cherry KJ, Hallet JW, Bower TC, Panneton JM, et al. Contemporary management of acute mesenteric ischemia: factors associated with survival. J Vasc Surg. 2002;35(3):445–52.
29. Jamal MM, Yamini D, Singson Z, Samarasena J, Hashemzadeh M, Vega KJ. Decreasing hos-pitalization and the in-hospital mortality related to cholangitis in the united states. J Clin Gastroenterol. 2001;45:e92–6.
30. Lai E, Mok F, Tan E, Lo C, Fan S, You K, et al. Endoscopic biliary drainage for severe acute cholangitis. N Engl J Med. 1992;326:1582–6.
31. Kashab MA, Tariq A, Tariq U, Kim K, Ponor L, Lennon A, et al. Delayed and unsuccessful endoscopic retrograde cholangiopancreatography are associated with worse outcomes in patients with acute cholangitis. Clin Gastroenterol Hepatol. 2012;10:1157–61.
32. Navaneethan U, Gutierrez NG, Jegadeesan R, Venkatesh P, Butt M, Sanaka MR, et al. Delay in performing ERCP and adverse events increase the 30-day readmission risk in patients with acute cholangitis. Gastrointest Endosc. 2013;78:81–90.
33. Mier J, Luque-de Leon E, Castillo A, Robledo F, Blanco R. Early versus late necrosectomy in severe necrotizing pancreatitis. Am J Surg. 1997;173:71–5.
34. Hartwig W, Maksan SM, Foitzik T, Schmidt J, Herfarth C, Klar E. Reduction in mortality with delayed surgical therapy of severe pancreatitis. J Gastrointest Surg. 2002;6(3):481–7.
35. Anaya DA, McMahon K, Nathens AB, Sullivan SR, Foy H, Bulger E. Predictors of mortality and limb loss in necrotizing soft tissue infections. Arch Surg. 2005;140:151–8.
36. McHenry CR, Piotrowski JJ, Petrinic D, Malangoni MA. Determinants of mortality for necro-tizing soft-tissue infections. Ann Surg. 1995;221:558–63.
37. Bilton BD, Zibari GB, McMillan RW, Aultman DF, Dunn G, McDonald JC. Aggressive surgi-cal management of necrotizing fasciitis serves to decrease mortality: a retrospective study. Am Surg. 1998;64:397–400.
38. von Eiff C, Jansen B, Kohnen W, Becker K. Infections associated with medical devices. Drugs. 2005;65(2):179–214.
39. Costerton JW, Stewart PS, Greenberg EP. Bacterial Biofilms: a common cause of persistent infections. Science. 1999;284:1318–22.

Chapter 13
Hemodynamic Support in Sepsis

Jean-Louis Vincent

Introduction

Hemodynamic support in sepsis is more complex than it may seem at initial glance with multiple components thatneed to be considered, including choice of fluid and vasoactive agent, which variables to monitor and which targets to aimfor. Further complexity is added by the fact that the overall hemodynamic status of any patient is a reflection not only oftheir macro-hemodynamic situation but also of their micro-hemodynamics. Each patient must therefore be assessed andtreated on an individual basis to ensure that the most appropriate support is offered. Importantly, hemodynamic status is adynamic event, changing with the evolution of the disease and a patient's response to treatment so that interventions must berepeatedly adapted and reassessed.

Fluid Administration

The release of many inflammatory mediators in sepsis results in vasodilation and increased microvascular permeability, leading to increased extravascular losses associated with the need for a larger blood volume. There may also be fluid deficits due to lack of fluid intake, severe sweating, and sometimes gastrointestinal losses. All these elements contribute to the need for considerable volume administration in these patients. Moreover, fluid administration is required to achieve a hyperdynamic state, which is a typical feature of sepsis. A large cardiac preload is also required in the presence of myocardial depression associated with a decreased ventricular ejection fraction. Fig. 13.1 represents these elements.

J.-L. Vincent, MD (✉)
Department of Intensive Care, Erasme Hospital, Université Libre de Bruxelles,
Route de Lennik 808, Brussels 1070, Belgium
e-mail: jlvincent@intensive.org

© Springer International Publishing AG 2017
N.S. Ward, M.M. Levy (eds.), *Sepsis*, Respiratory Medicine,
DOI 10.1007/978-3-319-48470-9_13

Fig. 13.1 The reasons for
abundant fluid
requirements in sepsis

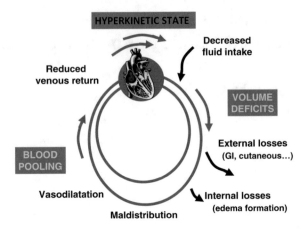

However, excessive fluid administration can result in increased morbidity and
mortality [3, 4] so that careful monitoring of fluid balance is required. The time factor is also very important, and fluid administration should be considered as a
dynamic process changing as the patient's status evolves, with initial, generous fluid
resuscitation if septic shock is present followed by later elimination of excess fluid.
The SOSD—salvage, optimization, stabilization, de-escalation—strategy should be
used to guide fluid administration according to the phase of the disease [5, 6]:

Salvage: During the early salvage phase, the most important consideration is to
  provide adequate, lifesaving fluid resuscitation. Fluids should therefore be given
  liberally, e.g., at 20–30 ml/kg, depending on the severity of the shock state; a
  slightly lower amount may be preferred in patients with profound hypoxemia
  from a pulmonary source. This initial phase should be quite short, before a monitor is in place to assess patient response.

Optimization: During the optimization phase, the patient is no longer in immediate
  danger, and fluid administration should be titrated according to patient needs, the
  aim being to optimize tissue perfusion and limit the development of organ dysfunction. Some monitoring is needed to assess the effects of the fluid administration
  while avoiding the development of pulmonary edema. A given level of cardiac filling pressures does not tell much about the potential response to fluids (except when
  it is very low), so that a dynamic approach is preferable. A fluid challenge technique
  [7] is the most obvious physiological approach, based on the Frank-Starling relation
  [8]. It is essential that the fluid challenge follows a strict protocol: too often, vague
  instructions are given making interpretation of the results difficult. The amount of
  fluid prescribed is also often too large ("give 500 mL of saline and we will see…"),
  so that the effects of the fluid challenge may become harmful.

The fluid challenge technique can be summarized by the four letters, TROL,
  signifying the type of fluid (see below), the rate (typically 150–250 mL in 10 min,
  depending on the weight of the patient), the objective (referring to an objective
  variable, such as arterial pressure or heart rate or cardiac output if measured), and
  the limit (a predefined maximal increase in a cardiac filling pressure, usually the
  central venous pressure (CVP)) [9]. The fluid challenge can be repeated as

necessary but must be discontinued if the limits are reached before the objective is achieved. Passive leg raising can be used as a sort of "internal" fluid challenge by shifting fluid from the legs to the thorax, but although at first glance the procedure seems simple, it is more complex than commonly thought [10]. Indeed, the response is very short-lasting and cannot be appreciated simply by a change in blood pressure, but requires continuous measurement of stroke volume (SV). In mechanically ventilated patients, one can also use the pulse pressure variation (PPV) if an arterial catheter is in place or the SV variation (SVV) if cardiac output is being monitored [11, 12], but this requires a fully controlled ventilator mode, with no triggering of the respirator by the patient. However, as sedative agents are now being used less because of their adverse effects on vascular tone and myocardial function, most ventilated patients will trigger the respirator at some point. Moreover, the use of relatively small tidal volumes, as recommended, decreases the amplitude of the signal and major arrhythmias also influence the measurements. Hence, PPV and SVV can be helpful signs, but only in very specific conditions, which are seldom present.

Stabilization: At this point, the patient is no longer in or at risk of shock and has reached a steady state so that only maintenance fluid therapy is required. Fluid infusion may still be required, but oral intake may be sufficient if this is possible.

De-escalation: In this phase, the patient is recovering and excess fluid must be removed, preferably by spontaneous diuresis. Furosemide is seldom needed, because if there is inadequate spontaneous diuresis, it is likely that kidney function is sufficiently impaired to necessitate the use of renal replacement therapy for fluid removal.

Choice of fluid is a complex issue and remains a matter of ongoing debate. The use of colloid solutions is associated with less fluid requirement and less edema formation, even in the presence of altered capillary permeability [13], but colloid choices are limited. The use of albumin may result in improved survival rates in sepsis, especially when shock is present [14, 15]. Hydroxyethyl starch (HES) solutions may be preferred because of their lower costs compared to albumin, but they may be associated with serious adverse effects in sepsis [16] and should therefore be avoided in these conditions. The place of gelatins is not well defined, largely because these solutions are not available in the USA. In the absence of a demonstrated benefit of colloid solutions, crystalloid solutions are usually recommended as first-line solutions, but they have their own problems. For example, large amounts of saline solution can induce hyperchloremic acidosis [17], which may have some adverse effects, including on renal function [18]. The so-called "balanced" fluids include other molecules (e.g., lactate, gluconate, malate) to act as buffers, but these may also have unwanted effects [19].

Vasoactive Agents

The presence of hypotension requires the use of vasopressor agents. Until recently, it was generally proposed that vasopressor therapy should be started only when the response to fluid was inadequate to restore an adequate perfusion pressure, but this approach is no longer recommended. Indeed, even when there is a good response to fluid, a patient may experience transient hypotension, and even short-lived episodes of hypotension can be deleterious to the organs [20]. It is, therefore, preferable to administer vasopressor agents, however briefly, in all cases of arterial hypotension. Norepinephrine is the vasopressor agent of choice as it has strong alpha-adrenergic properties but also some milder beta-adrenergic properties that help to maintain cardiac output. Dopamine is associated with higher mortality rates and it should not be used in these patients [21]. The use of epinephrine should be restricted to very severe cases, as it may affect the distribution of blood flow and alter cellular metabolism, as reflected by an increase in blood lactate levels [22]. Whether vasopressin analogs may be of use is still unclear, but it is possible that early use may protect the endothelial cell barrier and limit edema formation [23].

If there is evidence of myocardial depression, addition of dobutamine may be useful to increase blood flow and oxygen delivery (DO_2) to the organs. Although there are no prospective randomized controlled trials demonstrating the beneficial effects of dobutamine on outcomes in this setting, clinical experience shows that dobutamine administration can be associated with a rapid improvement in tissue perfusion [24]. The doses required are usually very limited (around 5 µg/kg/min). If the result is unsatisfactory, the dobutamine infusion can be discontinued, and the effect will rapidly disappear because of its short half-life. There may be a decrease in blood pressure when the dobutamine infusion is started, but this often reflects some underlying hypovolemia and should trigger another fluid challenge.

Monitoring

Monitoring of the central venous oxygen saturation ($ScvO_2$) can be useful in complex cases, when the adequacy of DO_2 is questioned. The typical hemodynamic pattern of sepsis is a high cardiac output associated with a normal or high $ScvO_2$, so that a low $ScvO_2$ suggests inadequate DO_2. A low $ScvO_2$ should, therefore, encourage administration of more intravenous fluids, including transfusions in patients with anemia, and the use of dobutamine. Large multicenter trials [25–27] did not confirm the improvement in survival reported in the study by Rivers et al. [28] on early goal-directed therapy, but many of the patients enrolled in these later studies had already been resuscitated and were not very ill [29]. Importantly, $ScvO_2$ measurements should not be used as the basis for a simple protocol [30], but integrated and interpreted with other variables so that the full picture of hemodynamic alterations can be appreciated and treatment oriented most effectively.

Measurements of blood lactate levels are essential to assess the severity of shock and, equally importantly, the response to treatment. Shock is associated with a blood lactate level >2 mmol/L [31]. Repeated lactate levels are very important to provide an indication of evolution and response to treatment; decreasing lactate levels are associated with a better prognosis [32–34]. Importantly, although the decrease in lactate concentrations has been referred to as lactate "clearance," this term is incorrect because the change in lactate concentrations reflects changes in both production and elimination of lactate [35].

Conclusion

The hemodynamic management of patients with sepsis is more complex than at first glance with multiple components that need to be considered in order to maintain organ function and prevent death. Importantly, each patient must be assessed and treated on an individual basis to ensure that the most appropriate support is offered. There is no optimal arterial pressure or cardiac output for all patients, and multiple variables should be assessed together to provide a full picture of each patient's hemodynamic status. Whether directing therapy at improving the microcirculation is beneficial remains a matter of ongoing research [36]. Analysis of trends in values over time is more useful than single measures and can help indicate whether or not a patient is responding to treatment.

References

1. De Backer D, Creteur J, Preiser JC, Dubois MJ, Vincent JL. Microvascular blood flow is altered in patients with sepsis. Am J Respir Crit Care Med. 2002;166:98–104.
2. Sakr Y, Dubois MJ, De Backer D, Creteur J, Vincent JL. Persistent microcirculatory alterations are associated with organ failure and death in patients with septic shock. Crit Care Med. 2004;32:1825–31.
3. Acheampong A, Vincent JL. A positive fluid balance is an independent prognostic factor in patients with sepsis. Crit Care. 2015;19:251.
4. Sirvent JM, Ferri C, Baro A, Murcia C, Lorencio C. Fluid balance in sepsis and septic shock as a determining factor of mortality. Am J Emerg Med. 2015;33:186–9.
5. Vincent JL, De Backer D. Circulatory shock. N Engl J Med. 2013;369:1726–34.
6. Hoste EA, Maitland K, Brudney CS, Mehta R, Vincent JL, Yates D, et al. Four phases of intravenous fluid therapy: a conceptual model. Br J Anaesth. 2014;113:740–7.
7. Vincent JL, Weil MH. Fluid challenge revisited. Crit Care Med. 2006;34:1333–7.
8. Katz AM. Ernest Henry Starling, his predecessors, and the "Law of the Heart". Circulation. 2002;106:2986–92.
9. Vincent JL. Let's give some fluid and see what happens" versus the "mini-fluid challenge. Anesthesiology. 2011;115:455–6.
10. Monnet X, Teboul JL. Passive leg raising: five rules, not a drop of fluid! Crit Care. 2015;19:18.
11. Marik PE, Cavallazzi R, Vasu T, Hirani A. Dynamic changes in arterial waveform derived variables and fluid responsiveness in mechanically ventilated patients: a systematic review of the literature. Crit Care Med. 2009;37:2642–7.
12. Vincent JL, Rhodes A, Perel A, Martin GS, Della Rocca G, Vallet B, et al. Clinical review: update on hemodynamic monitoring—a consensus of 16. Crit Care. 2011;15:229.
13. Orbegozo Cortes D, Gamarano Barros T, Njimi H, Vincent JL. Crystalloids versus colloids: exploring differences in fluid requirements by systematic review and meta-regression. Anesth Analg. 2015;120:389–402.

14. Finfer S, McEvoy S, Bellomo R, McArthur C, Myburgh J, Norton R. Impact of albumin compared to saline on organ function and mortality of patients with severe sepsis. Intensive Care Med. 2011;37:86–96.
15. Caironi P, Tognoni G, Masson S, Fumagalli R, Pesenti A, Romero M, et al. Albumin replacement in patients with severe sepsis or septic shock. N Engl J Med. 2014;370:1412–21.
16. Serpa Neto A, Veelo DP, Peireira VG, de Assuncao MS, Manetta JA, Esposito DC, et al. Fluid resuscitation with hydroxyethyl starches in patients with sepsis is associated with an increased incidence of acute kidney injury and use of renal replacement therapy: a systematic review and meta-analysis of the literature. J Crit Care. 2014;29:185–7.
17. Orbegozo Cortes D, Rayo Bonor A, Vincent JL. Isotonic crystalloid solutions: a structured review of the literature. Br J Anaesth. 2014;112:968–81.
18. Yunos NM, Bellomo R, Hegarty C, Story D, Ho L, Bailey M. Association between a chloride-liberal vs chloride-restrictive intravenous fluid administration strategy and kidney injury in critically ill adults. JAMA. 2012;308:1566–72.
19. Reddy S, Weinberg L, Young P. Crystalloid fluid therapy. Crit Care. 2016;20:59.
20. Bai X, Yu W, Ji W, Lin Z, Tan S, Duan K, et al. Early versus delayed administration of norepinephrine in patients with septic shock. Crit Care. 2014;18:532.
21. De Backer D, Aldecoa C, Njimi H, Vincent JL. Dopamine versus norepinephrine in the treatment of septic shock: a meta-analysis. Crit Care Med. 2012;40:725–30.
22. Levy B. Bench-to-bedside review: is there a place for epinephrine in septic shock? Crit Care. 2005;9:561–5.
23. He X, Su F, Taccone FS, Laporte R, Kjolbye AL, Zhang J, et al. A selective V1A receptor agonist, selepressin, is superior to arginine vasopressin and to norepinephrine in ovine septic shock. Crit Care Med. 2016;44(1):23–31.
24. Dellinger RP, Levy MM, Rhodes A, Annane D, Gerlach H, Opal SM, et al. Surviving sepsis campaign: international guidelines for management of severe sepsis and septic shock: 2012. Crit Care Med. 2013;41:580–637.
25. Yealy DM, Kellum JA, Huang DT, Barnato AE, Weissfeld LA, Pike F, et al. A randomized trial of protocol-based care for early septic shock. N Engl J Med. 2014;370:1683–93.
26. Peake SL, Delaney A, Bailey M, Bellomo R, Cameron PA, Cooper DJ, et al. Goal-directed resuscitation for patients with early septic shock. N Engl J Med. 2014;371:1496–506.
27. Mouncey PR, Osborn TM, Power GS, Harrison DA, Sadique MZ, Grieve RD, et al. Trial of early, goal-directed resuscitation for septic shock. N Engl J Med. 2015;372:1301–11.
28. Rivers E, Nguyen B, Havstad S, Ressler J, Muzzin A, Knoblich B, et al. Early goal-directed therapy in the treatment of severe sepsis and septic shock. N Engl J Med. 2001;345:1368–77.
29. De Backer D, Vincent JL. Early goal-directed therapy: do we have a definitive answer? Intensive Care Med. 2016;42:1048.
30. Vincent JL. The future of critical care medicine: integration and personalization. Crit Care Med. 2016;44:386–9.
31. Singer M, Deutschman CS, Seymour CW, Shankar-Hari M, Annane D, Bauer M, et al. The third international consensus definitions for sepsis and septic shock (Sepsis-3). JAMA. 2016;315:801–10.
32. Nguyen HB, Rivers EP, Knoblich BP, Jacobsen G, Muzzin A, Ressler JA, et al. Early lactate clearance is associated with improved outcome in severe sepsis and septic shock. Crit Care Med. 2004;32:1637–42.
33. Liu V, Morehouse JW, Soule J, Whippy A, Escobar GJ. Fluid volume, lactate values, and mortality in sepsis patients with intermediate lactate values. Ann Am Thorac Soc. 2013;10:466–73.
34. Dettmer M, Holthaus CV, Fuller BM. The impact of serial lactate monitoring on emergency department resuscitation interventions and clinical outcomes in severe sepsis and septic shock: an observational cohort study. Shock. 2015;43:55–61.
35. Vincent JL. Serial blood lactate levels reflect both lactate production and clearance. Crit Care Med. 2015;43:e209.
36. Shapiro NI, Angus DC. A review of therapeutic attempts to recruit the microcirculation in patients with sepsis. Minerva Anestesiol. 2014;80:225–35.

Chapter 14
Bundled Therapies in Sepsis

Laura Evans and William Bender

Introduction

In recent years, there has been an increased focus on delivering appropriate, efficient, and effective medical care. As a result of this, a number of tools and techniques have been developed and increasingly used to assist in this process. One such entity is that of care bundles or, more simply, bundles. These are a set of evidence-based interventions that, when implemented together, tend to result in significantly better outcomes than when implemented individually [1]. Bundles usually consistent of three to five elements and are targeted for a defined patient population or care setting. Their effectiveness is centered on bringing together independent practices and tying them into a package that needs to be completed for each encounter with these patients or care settings [2].

A variety of key factors are associated with the development of bundles. Each individual element within the bundle, when possible, should be based upon well-established evidence. If lower grade evidence including expert opinion is utilized, ongoing re-evaluation and periodic updating of the bundles and their associated elements should occur. As a general recommendation, the included elements should be between three and five in number and descriptive in manner rather than proscriptive, so as to aid in appropriate local customization [1]. In addition, a multidisciplinary approach should be used in their development and implementation. This not only ensures broad acceptance of the reasoning behind them but also allows for a consistent focus on how they should be utilized to deliver the most effective care possible. This broad, team-based approach to bundles also prevents them from devolving into simple checklists.

L. Evans (✉) • W. Bender
Pulmonary, Critical Care and Sleep Medicine, Bellevue Hospital/NYU School of Medicine, 550 First Ave, NBV 7N24, New York, NY 11201, USA
e-mail: laura.evans@nyumc.org

© Springer International Publishing AG 2017
N.S. Ward, M.M. Levy (eds.), *Sepsis*, Respiratory Medicine,
DOI 10.1007/978-3-319-48470-9_14

Checklists, while helpful, tend to contain a series of tasks and processes that often fall under either the "nice to do" or "have to do" categories [2]. They also have the potential to get overloaded with an increased number of elements while lacking a well-delineated owner. Their utilization also tends to be extremely broad and not targeted toward specific patients or care settings. As a result of all of this, omission of various elements within a checklist, or the entire list altogether, may not necessarily impact a patient to a large degree. This is in stark contrast to a bundle, however, given their focused usage and more scientifically robust construction. An omission of an element within a bundle, or a bundle altogether, is much more likely to result in a negative outcome for a patient.

This leads to arguably the most important factor associated with the development of care bundles: compliance with them is measured in an "all or none" approach. If all elements have been completed, or if an element was not completed but documented as contradicted for a specific reason, then the bundle is counted as complete for that specific patient or setting. If any element is absent in the documentation, then the bundle is incomplete. The "all or none" method limits variability and assures that evidenced-based care is being delivered consistently. In addition, it also promotes improvement methods to focus on processes of care so as to facilitate improved bundle usage, and ultimately patient outcomes [1].

History

Care bundles were initially developed around 20 years ago. They have been used within a number of different medical and surgical specialties and perhaps most prominently within cardiology [3]. In recent years, their use has been increasingly explored and utilized within the field of critical care. [4, 5]. Berenholtz et al. further advanced this idea with an article published in 2002. The authors reviewed 35 years' worth of critical care literature for interventions that could prevent avoidable morbidity and mortality in intensive care [6]. Six evidence-based interventions were ultimately identified that were felt to be able to improve intensive care outcomes: effective assessment of pain, appropriate use of blood transfusions, prevention of ventilator-associated pneumonia, appropriate sedation, appropriate peptic ulcer disease prophylaxis, and appropriate deep vein thrombosis prophylaxis [7]. The latter four of these interventions were subsequently clustered together to form a ventilator care bundle.

The Institute of Healthcare Improvement (IHI) then used these works to help develop two care bundles that ultimately were a key part of the "100,000 Lives Campaign" and the "5 Million Lives Campaign" [8]. The IHI Ventilator Bundle was the first of these and consisted of four elements: elevation of the head of the bed to between 30° and 45°, daily "sedation" vacations and assessment of readiness to extubate, peptic ulcer disease prophylaxis, and deep venous thrombosis prophylaxis. A fifth element, "daily oral care with chlorhexidine," was added a few years later [9]. The overall goal with this tool was to reliably provide care that prevented certain adverse events associated with patients receiving mechanical ventilation. The second bundle that was developed was the IHI Central Line Bundle. The five elements with this tool consisted of hand hygiene, maximal barrier precautions, chlorhexidine skin antisepsis, optimal catheter site selection, and daily review of line necessity with prompt removal of unnecessary lines [10]. Both these bundles were noted to have a positive effect with increasing rates of compliance resulting in decreased rates of ventilator adverse events and central line associated infections [11–13]. These successes subsequently allowed the bundle concept to be more easily applied to other areas within the field of critical care including severe sepsis and septic shock.

The Surviving Sepsis Campaign and Initial Care Bundles

The Surviving Sepsis Campaign was created in 2002 to increase awareness and improve care for patients with severe sepsis and septic shock. This movement represented a combined effort from multiple professional societies including the European Society of Intensive Care Medicine, and the Society of Critical Care Medicine with the overall goal of reducing mortality from sepsis by 25% by 2009, which represented the 5-year anniversary of its initial release of guidelines in 2004 [14]. The campaign has consisted of four phases. The first was undertaken in early 2002 and 2003 and consisted of an introduction to the campaign and along with a push to define the scope of the problem posed by sepsis and to also increase awareness [15]. The second phase consisted of the creation of evidence-based guidelines for the management of severe sepsis and septic shock via an international consensus committee and the initial set, as previously noted, was published in 2004. The third phase of the Surviving Sepsis Campaign was then undertaken with collaboration with the Institute of Healthcare Improvement. The goal of this step was to disseminate the guidelines into everyday clinical care while also gathering data on their implementation and effect [15].

This was accomplished using a variety of instruments including educational programs to continue to increase awareness and adherence with the guidelines as well as performance measures and quality improvement indicators deigned to provide feedback regarding how often patients were receiving guideline-based care [15, 16]. In addition, and arguably most importantly, two sepsis care bundles were created from elements within the Surviving Sepsis Guidelines. In keeping with the one of core mantras associated with care bundles, "the aim of the sepsis bundle is twofold: first, to eliminate the piecemeal application of guidelines that characterizes the majority of clinical environments today, and second, to make it easier for clinicians to bring the guidelines into practice" [16].

The initial bundles that were created from the Campaign's evidence-based guidelines were the Sepsis Resuscitation Bundle and the Sepsis Management Bundle. The Resuscitation Bundle consisted of six elements to be completed within the first 6 h of a patient's presentation. The elements included checking a serum lactate, obtaining blood cultures prior to the administration of antibiotics, administering broad spectrum antibiotics within 3 h of emergency department admission or within 1 h for non-emergency department intensive care unit admissions, delivering an initial fluid bolus of 20 mL/kg of crystalloid (or colloid equivalent) in the event of hypotension and/or a lactate level greater than 4 mmol/L followed by the administration of vasopressors for hypotension not responding to initial fluid resuscitation to maintain a mean arterial pressure (MAP) greater than or equal to 65, and lastly, in the event of persistent hypotension despite fluid resuscitation and/or a lactate level greater than 4 mmol/L achieving a central venous pressure (CVP) greater than 8 mmHg and/or a central venous oxygen saturation ($S_{cv}O_2$) of greater than 70% [17]. The Management Bundle consisted of four elements that recommended to be accomplished within the first 24 h of presentation. These included the administration of low-dose steroids for septic shock in accordance with standardized hospital policy, drotrecogin alfa (activated) administered in accordance with standardized hospital policy, glucose control maintained greater than the lower limit of normal but less than 150 mg/dL and inspiratory plateau pressures maintained less than 30 cmH_2O for mechanically ventilated patients (see Fig. 14.1) [17].

These two bundles were subsequently disseminated with the rest of the Campaign's educational materials and quality indicators. To fully facilitate the improvement of the delivery of care for sepsis, an international registry was also created as part of the Surviving Sepsis Campaign and a number of regional networks were established to facilitate data collection and assistance with performance improvement [15]. The first large-scale analysis of the Campaign and its participating sites was published in 2010. A total of 165 participating sites with 15,022 subjects between January 2005 and March 2008 were examined. Initial compliance at all sites in the first quarter with both bundles was noted to be low, at only 10.9% for the resuscitation bundle and 18.4% for the management bundle. These rates were noted to increase linearly with time, however, up to 31.3% ($p < 0.001$) by the end of 2 years for the resuscitation bundle and 36.1% ($p = 0.008$) for the management bundle (see Fig. 14.2). In addition, compliance with each indi-

Severe Sepsis Bundles:
Sepsis Resuscitation Bundle
(To be accomplished as soon as possible and scored over first 6 hours):
1. Serum lactate measured.
2. Blood cultures obtained prior to antibiotic administration.
3. From the time of presentation, broad-spectrum antibiotics administered within 3 hours for ED admissions and 1 hour for non-ED ICU admissions.
4. In the event of hypotension and/or lactate > 4 mmol/L (36 mg/dl): a) Deliver an initial minimum of 20 ml/kg of crystalloid (or colloid equivalent). b) Apply vasopressors for hypotension not responding to initial fluid resuscitation to maintain mean arterial pressure (MAP) > 65mm Hg.
5. In the event of persistent hypotension despite fluid resuscitation (septic shock) and/or lactate > 4 mmol/L (36 mg/dl):
a) Achieve central venous pressure (CVP) of >8mm Hg.
b) Achieve central venous oxygen saturation (ScvO2) of > 70%.*
Sepsis Management Bundle
(To be accomplished as soon as possible and scored over first 24 hours):
1 Low-dose steroids administered for septic shock in accordance with a standardized hospital policy.
2 Drotrecogin alfa (activated) administered in accordance with a standardized hospital policy.
3 Glucose control maintained > lower limit of normal. but < 150 mg/dl (8.3 mmol/L).
4 Inspiratory plateau pressures maintained < 30 cm H2O for mechanically ventilated patients.
*Achieving a mixed venous oxygen saturation (SvO2) of 65% is an acceptable alternative.

Fig. 14.1 Initial resuscitation and management bundles produced by the Surviving Sepsis Campaign in 2004. Reproduced from Levy MM, Dellinger RP, Townsend SR et al. The Surviving Sepsis Campaign: results of an international guideline-based performance improvement program targeting severe sepsis. Crit Care Med. 2010; 38:367–374

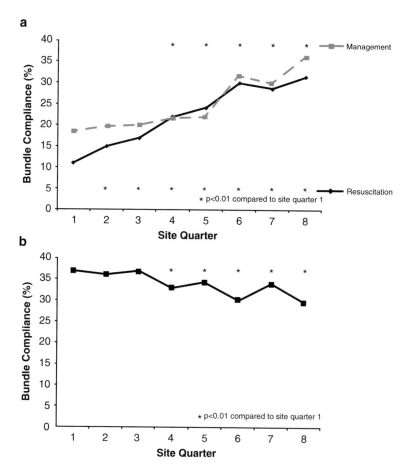

Fig. 14.2 Compliance and mortality change over time. (**a**) Change in the percentage of patients compliant with all elements of the resuscitation bundle (*dotted line*) and the management bundle (*solid line*) over 2 years of data collection (*$p < 0.01$ compared with the first quarter). Note that both Y axes are truncated at 40% to emphasize relative change over time as opposed to absolute change. (**b**) Change in hospital mortality over time (*$p < 0.01$ compared with first quarter). Reproduced from Levy MM, Dellinger RP, Townsend SR et al. The Surviving Sepsis Campaign: results of an international guideline-based performance improvement program targeting severe sepsis. Crit Care Med. 2010; 38:367–374

vidual bundle element was noted to increase significantly as well, with the exception of inspiratory plateau pressure, which was high at baseline [17]. Unadjusted hospital mortality was noted to decrease during this 2 year period from 37 to 30.8% ($p = 0.001$) and the adjusted odds ratio for mortality was noted to improve for each successive quarter that a site participated in the Campaign. This resulted in an adjusted absolute drop of 0.8% per quarter with an overall drop of 5.4% (95% confidence interval 2.5–8.4) over 2 years [17]. These results were interpreted as encouraging but a definitive relationship between increased compliance and mortality reduction could not be directly established given the overall study design. There was clear association, however, with participation in the Surviving Sepsis Campaign and continuous quality improvement in sepsis care as well as decreased hospital mortality [3, 17]. This relationship continued to be demonstrated in the most recent analysis of the Campaign as well. Over a period of now seven and a half years, increased compliance was noted to be associated with a 25% relative risk reduction in mortality [18].

A similar trend was also noted in studies performed outside the Surviving Sepsis Campaign but still utilizing both care bundles. In a prospective observational study published by Gao et al. in 2005, which was one of the first studies examining bundle compliance and hospital mortality, the impact of compliance with both the resuscitation and management bundles was examined in 101 consecutive critically ill patients with severe sepsis and septic shock at two teaching hospitals in England [19]. The rate of compliance with the resuscitation bundle was noted to be 52% and the management bundle was 30%. Noncompliance with the resuscitation bundle was associated with a relative risk of in-hospital mortality of 2.12 (95% confidence interval 1.20–3.76) while noncompliance with the management bundle was associated with a relative risk of in-hospital mortality of 1.76, although this did not achieve statistical significance [19].

A prospective observational study performed at a teaching hospital in Belgium examined not only bundle compliance and mortality but also the time to compliance [20]. Among 69 consecutive patients admitted to the intensive care unit with severe sepsis or septic shock, compliance with the resuscitation bundle was obtained in 72%. This cohort had a significant lower mortality rate of 16% as compared to a mortality rate of 44% among those patients whose care was not compliant with the resuscitation bundle [20]. No significant difference in mortality was noted in the patients whose care was compliant with the management bundle, but among patients whose care was compliant with the management bundle after only 12 h, a statistically significant lower mortality rate of 10% was noted as compared to 39% among whose who were compliant after 24 h [20].

A subsequent meta-analysis, which consisted of a total of 21 studies including the two highlighted above, examined the use of both the resuscitation and management bundles and their association with survival among patients with severe sepsis and septic shock. A total of 23,438 patients were pooled for analysis and the overall compliance rate with the bundles was noted to be around 50% [21]. Compliance with the resuscitation bundle was noted to be two times more likely to be associated with survival (odds ratio of 2.124, 95% confidence interval 1.701–2.651), while compliance with both bundles together demonstrated a slightly lower but still significant impact (odds ratio 1.744, 95% 1.421–2.141) [21].

More recently, significant improvements were noted in mortality in conjunction with an increase in bundle compliance among 4329 adults admitted with severe sepsis or septic shock among a group of 18 ICUs in both Utah and Idaho from 2004 through 2010 [22]. In this particular cohort, mortality was observed to decrease from 21.2% in 2004 to 8.7% in 2010 while all-or-none total bundle compliance simultaneously increased from 4.9 to 73.4%. Interestingly, and not overly surprising, increased compliance with the initial resuscitation bundle was noted to be associated with a lower probability of being eligible for further resuscitation and the need for management bundle elements [22].

Current Sepsis Bundle Practices

As the Surviving Sepsis Campaign moved through its third phase and into its fourth, which is focused on reinvigorating the campaign and recommitting to improving mortality from sepsis, two revised sets of guidelines were released, first in 2008 and then again most recently in 2012 [15]. With both updates, changes were made reflective of the most recent evidence available for the evaluation and treatment of sepsis [23]. As a result of the most recent guideline changes in 2012, along with continued evaluation of data from the international registry, two major changes were made to the care bundles.

The first of these was that the management bundle, which consisted of several elements targeted for completion within the first 24 h, was removed in its entirety [22]. After analyzing the series of well-designed randomized controlled trials examining the use of steroids in adult septic shock, no benefit was noted on outcome [23, 24]. A lack of definitive conclusiveness was also noted for the management of blood sugars [23, 25, 26]. At the same time, given the results of the PROWESS-SHOCK trial, which showed no benefit for droctrecogin alfa (recombinant human activated protein C) in patients with severe septic shock as well as its subsequent removal from the market by the FDA, its role in the guidelines and subsequent care bundles was negated [23, 27]. In the SSC dataset, compliance with the inspiratory plateau pressure target of less than 30 cmH_2O was consistently over 80% and thus it was dropped as a target for performance improvement.

The second major change was to the resuscitation bundle. The major impetus for this change was tied to one of the important premises associated with care bundles, that there should be constant reevaluation of the bundle elements with periodic updating so as to encourage continuous improvement of both care process and outcomes [1, 5]. A recent review of seven and a half year's worth of data consisting of nearly 30,000 patients in the Surviving Sepsis Campaign database revealed a 25% relative risk reduction in mortality associated with a statistically significant increase in bundle compliance and for every hour delay seen with antibiotic administration, a 5–7% increase in mortality was noted [18, 28, 29]. In addition, lactate, blood culture obtainment, antibiotic administration, intravenous fluid administration, central venous pressure, and central venous oxygen saturation ($ScvO_2$) were all noted to be statistically significant independently and significantly associated with a decreased odds ratio of mortality (see Table 14.1) [18, 29].

As a result of these findings, the resuscitation bundle was divided into two parts, with the goal of emphasizing early detection and early intervention. The first component, the initial resuscitation bundle, currently consists of four elements to be completed within the first 3 h of a patient's presentation: measure a lactate level,

Table 14.1 Hospital mortality adjusted odds ratio modeled individually for each element in bundle compliance using a generalized estimating equation population-averaged logistic regression

	Participation in SSC, year	Hospital mortality OR[a]	95% CI	p
Initial care bundle (first 6 h of presentation)				
Measured lactate	<2	0.80	0.73–0.89	<0.001
	2 to <3	0.67	0.59–0.76	<0.001
	≥3	069	0.63–0.75	<0.001
Blood cultures before antibiotics	Not applicable[b]	0.82	0.77–0.87	<0.001
Broad-spectrum antibiotics	Not applicable[b]	0.85	0.81–0.90	<0.0001
Fluids and vasopressors	<2	0.86	0.73–1.01	0.074
	2 to <3	0.63	0.48–0.81	<0.001
	≥3	0.74	0.62–0.88	0.001
CVP > 8mmHg	Not applicable[b]	0.84	0.78–0.91	<0.0001
Scvo₂ > 70%	Not applicable[b]	0.83	0.76–0.90	<0.001
All resuscitation measures	Not applicable[b]	0.79	0.73–0.85	<OɹO01
Management bundle (First 24 h after presentation)				
Steroid policy	<2	0.96	0.84–1.09	0.527
	2 to <3	0.76	0.64–0.89	0.001
	≥3	0.88	0.79–0.99	0.031
rhAPC policy	Not applicable	0.93	0.87–1.00	0.061
Glucose policy	Not applicable	0.71	0.68–0.75	< 0.001
Plateau pressure control	Not applicable	0.81	0.74–0.89	< 0.001
All management measures	Not applicable	0.74	0,69–0.79	< 0.001

Reproduced from Levy MM, Rhodes A, Phillips GS et al. Surviving Sepsis Campaign: Association between performance metrics and outcomes in a 7.5-year study. Crit Care Med. 2014; October 1. Epub ahead of print
SSC surviving sepsis campaign, *OR* odds ratio, *CVP* central venous pressure, *Scvo₂* central venous oxygen saturation, *rhA PC* recombinant human activated protein C
[a]Hospital mortality odds ratio for those patients where the bundle- element was achieved compared to when the bundle was not achieved, and the results are adjusted by sight quarter of participation and the Sepsis Severity Score
[b]No significant interaction ($p < 0.05$) between the bundle element and years of participation in the Surviving Sepsis Campaign. If the interaction was significant, then the odds-ratio is given for each level of participation

obtain blood cultures prior to administration of antibiotics, administer broad spectrum antibiotics, and administer 30 mL/kg of crystalloid fluid for hypotension or a lactate level greater than 4 mmol/L [23]. The second part, the septic shock bundle, currently consists of three elements to be completed within 6 h of a patient's presentation; apply vasopressors for hypotension that does not respond to initial fluid resuscitation to maintain a mean arterial pressure (MAP) greater than or equal to 65, in the event of persistent arterial hypotension despite volume resuscitation or an initial lactate greater than or equal to 4 mmol/L a central venous pressure (CVP) and/or central venous oxygen saturation (ScvO₂) should be measured, and lastly, to re-measure a lactate level if the initial lactate was elevated (see Fig. 14.3) [23].

SURVIVING SEPSIS CAMPAIGN BUNDLES

TO BE COMPLETED WITHIN 3 HOURS:
1) Measure lactate level
2) Obtain blood cultures prior to administration of antibiotics
3) Administer broad spectrum antibiotics
4) Administer 30 mL/kg cry stalloid for hypotension or lactate ≥4mmol/L

TO BE COMPLETED WITHIN 6 HOURS:
5) Apply vasopressors (for hypotension that does not respond to initial fluid resuscitation) to maintain a mean arterial pressure (MAP) ≥ 65 mm Hg
6) In the event of persistent arterial hypotension despite volume resuscitation (septic shock) or initial lactate ≥ 4 mmol/L (36 mg/dL):
   - Measure central venous pressure (CVP)*
   - Measure central venous oxygen saturation ($Scvo_2$)*
7) Remeasure lactate if initial lactate was elevated*

*Targets for quantitative resuscitation included in the guidelines are CVP of ≥8 mm Hg. $Scvo_2$ of ≥70%, and normalization of lactate.

Fig. 14.3 Current surviving sepsis campaign bundles. Reproduced from Dellinger RP, Levy MM, Rhodes A et al. Surviving Sepsis Campaign: International Guidelines for Management of Severe Sepsis and Septic Shock: 2012. Crit Care Med. 2013; 41:580–637

Controversies with Sepsis Bundle Practices

Despite the increased uptake of care bundles within the field of critical care, a number of criticisms of them exist along with criticisms regarding their usage in the evaluation and treatment of patients with severe sepsis and septic shock. These critiques are varied in their approach and reasoning and they often cite a number of reasons for opposition to the idea of using care bundles. These range from arguing that the bundles are used by industries as a marketing tool or that they are inefficient due to the inclusion of too many individual elements [30, 31].

One of the major and often repeated criticisms is that there is a lack of formal evidence supporting the process of bundling. Opponents note that the idea of bundle synergy has not been clearly examined. In addition, it is argued that results from before and after the implementation of bundles are not definitive "proof-of-concept" demonstrations or are appropriate substitutes for prospective randomized trials [32]. This point regarding a lack of robust scientific evaluation of the impact of bundles on clinical outcomes has been acknowledged by bundle proponents, including the Surviving Sepsis Campaign, and thus studies demonstrating their effectiveness should be interpreted with some degree of caution [17, 19]. At the same time, however, there has been no data demonstrating any degree of harm posited by the use of care bundles and their established trend of effectiveness has continued with their continued use [28, 33]. In addition, bundles are reflective of a method focused on overall performance improvement for the entire process of care associated with a particular patient or care setting [2, 11]. Thus, standardized controlled trials and their associated outcomes may be insensitive in their ability to capture all of the relevant results from this method.

A second major criticism of the use of care bundles in sepsis is that in adopting an "all or none" approach to bundle compliance, a lack of clinical autonomy and a failure to tailor therapy to each individual patient develops [32, 34]. An element that seems to get missed in this argument, however, is that all the elements within the sepsis care bundles have always been acknowledged to potentially not apply to every patient with severe sepsis or septic shock [33]. If a particular element is felt to not apply to a particular patient or care setting, as long as that reasoning is documented and acknowledged then the bundle may still be counted as complete [1, 33]. In recent years, this issue has centered on the use of central venous pressure for assistance with guiding volume resuscitation [32, 34, 35]. Given the presence of new data from both inside and outside the Campaign, the Surviving Sepsis Campaign's bundles have subsequently reflected this change and as previously noted, it is now part of the septic shock bundle to simply be checked within the first 6 h in the presence of persistent hypotension or hyperlactatemia [23, 33]. The simple act of transducing a central venous pressure in a patient with septic shock is unlikely to be harmful and the subsequent result can be added to the clinical data available to the clinician at the bedside to then make an informed decision regarding further therapy. At the same time, the majority of the critiques of this "all or none" approach are centered in tertiary or quaternary centers where more often than not, multiple advanced therapies and providers are available at the bedside in a moment's notice [30, 34, 35]. A large number of smaller institutions exist, however, and may not have these same resources and advanced capabilities. Thus, relying on an "all or none" approach with these care bundles in these settings limits potentially harmful variability and allows the delivery of consistent, performance improvement driven care [33, 36].

Conclusion

In closing, it is clear that care bundles seem to be effective instruments in delivering consistent care and improving patient outcomes across the field of medicine. Over the past few years, they seem to have been particularly effective in improving the processes of care and outcomes associated with sepsis, largely through the work of the Surviving Sepsis Campaign [18, 28]. One of key tenets of care bundles, however, is that they are reflective of an ongoing improvement process that is embraced by the entire environment around them [1, 6]. As the field of critical care continues to embrace this concept in increasing numbers, bundled care for sepsis as well as sepsis care overall, will undoubtedly continue to improve and the elements included in care bundles will change and evolve over time as the evidence base changes and the field moves forward [37].

References

1. Resar R, Griffin FA, Haraden C, Nolan TW. Using care bundles to improve health care quality. IHI innovation series white paper. Cambridge, MA: Institute for Healthcare Improvement; 2012. www.IHI.org. Accessed 2 Jun 2014
2. Haraden C. What is a bundle. Cambridge, MA: The Institute of Healthcare Improvement; 2014. www.IHI.org. Accessed 1 Jul 2014
3. Horner DL, Bellamy MC. Care bundles in intensive care. Contin Educ Anaesth Crit Care Pain. 2012;12:199–202.
4. Rivers E, Nguyen B, Havstad S, Ressler J, Muzzin A, Knoblich B, et al. Early goal-directed therapy in the treatment of severe sepsis and septic shock. N Engl J Med. 2001;345:1368–77.
5. Masterton RG. Sepsis care bundles and clinicians. Intensive Care Med. 2009;35:1149–51.
6. Fulbrook P, Mooney S. Care bundles in critical care: a practical approach to evidence-based practice. Nurs Crit Care. 2003;8(6):249–55.
7. Berenholtz SM, Dorman T, Ngo K, Provonost PJ. Qualitative review of intensive care unit quality indicators. J Crit Care. 2002;17:12–5.
8. McCannon CJ, Hackbarth AD, Griffin FA. Miles to go: an introduction to the 5 Million Lives Campaign. Jt Comm J Qual Patient Saf. 2007;33(8):477–84.
9. Institute for Healthcare Improvement. How-to guide: prevent ventilator-associated pneumonia. Cambridge, MA: Institute for Healthcare Improvement; 2012. www.IHI.org. Accessed 2 Jun 2014
10. Institute for Healthcare Improvement. How-to guide: prevent central line-associated blood-stream infections (CLABSI). Cambridge, MA: Institute for Healthcare Improvement; 2012. www.IHI.org. Accessed 2 Jun 2014
11. Resar R, Pronovost P, Haraden C, Simmonds T, Rainey T, Nolan T. Using a bundle approach to improve ventilator care processes and reduce ventilator-associated pneumonia. Jt Comm J Qual Patient Saf. 2005;31(5):243–8.
12. Furuya EY, Dick A, Perencevich EN, Pogorzelska M, Goldmann D, Stone PW. Central line bundle implementation in US intensive care units and impact on bloodstream infections. PLoS One. 2011;6(1):e15452.
13. Institute for Healthcare Improvement. IHI shares achievements of the 5 Million Lives Campaign. Cambridge, MA: Institute for Healthcare Improvement; 2008. http://www.ihi.org/about/news/Documents/IHIPressRelease_IHISharesAchievementsof5MillionLivesCampaign_Oct08.pdf. Accessed 2 Jun 2014.
14. Dellinger RP, Carlet JM, Masur H, Gerlach H, Calandra T, Cohen J, et al. Surviving sepsis campaign guidelines for management of severe sepsis and septic shock. Crit Care Med. 2004;32:858–73.
15. Surviving sepsis campaign history. http://www.survivingsepsis.org/About-SSC/Pages/History.aspx. Accessed 3 Jul 2014.
16. Levy MM, Pronovost PJ, Dellinger RP, Townsend S, Resar RK, Clemmer TP, et al. Sepsis change bundles: converting guidelines into meaningful change in behavior and clinical outcome. Crit Care Med. 2004;32:S595–7.
17. Levy MM, Dellinger RP, Townsend SR, Linde-Zwirble WT, Marshall JC, Bion J, Schorr C, et al. The surviving sepsis campaign: results of an international guideline-based performance improvement program targeting severe sepsis. Crit Care Med. 2010;38:367–74.
18. Levy MM, Rhodes A, Phillips GS, Townsend SR, Schorr CA, Beale R, et al. Surviving sepsis campaign: association between performance metrics and outcomes in a 7.5-year study. Crit Care Med. 2015;43(1):3–12.
19. Gao F, Melody T, Daniels DF, Giles S, Fox S. The impact of compliance with 6-hour and 24-hour sepsis bundles on hospital mortality in patients with severe sepsis-prospective observational study. Crit Care. 2005;9:R764–70.
20. Zambon M, Ceola M, Almeida-de-Castro R, Gullo A, Vincent JL. Implementation of the surviving sepsis campaign guidelines for severe sepsis and septic shock: we could go faster. J Crit Care. 2008;23:455–60.

21. Chamberlain DJ, Willis EM, Bersten AB. The severe sepsis bundles as processes of care: a meta-analysis. Aust Crit Care. 2011;24:229–43.
22. Miller III RR, Dong L, Nelson NC, Brown SM, Kuttler KG, Probst DR, et al. Multicenter Implementation of a severe sepsis and septic shock treatment bundle. Am J Respir Crit Care Med. 2013;188:77–82.
23. Dellinger RP, Levy MM, Rhodes A, Annane D, Gerlach H, Opal SM, et al. Surviving sepsis campaign: international guidelines for management of severe sepsis and septic shock: 2012. Crit Care Med. 2013;41:580–637.
24. Patel GP, Balk RA. Systemic steroids in severe sepsis and septic shock. Am J Respir Crit Care Med. 2012;185:133–9.
25. The NICE-SUGAR. Study Investigators (2009) intensive versus conventional glucose control in critically ill patients. N Engl J Med. 2009;360:1283–97.
26. Preiser JC, Devos P, Ruiz-Santana S, Mélot C, Annane D, Groeneveld J, et al. A prospective randomized multi-centre controlled trial on tight glucose control by intensive insulin therapy in adult intensive care units: the glucontrol study. Intensive Care Med. 2009;35:1738–48.
27. Ranieri VM, Thompson BT, Barie PS, Dhainaut JF, Douglas IS, Finfer S, et al. Drotrecogin alfa (activated) in adults with septic shock. N Engl J Med. 2012;366:2055–64.
28. Levy MM. The SSC improvement initiative: 2012 revised sepsis bundles. 42nd critical care congress review; 2013:9
29. Levy MM. The SSC improvement initiative: 2012 revised sepsis bundles. 42nd critical care congress review. 2013. https://www.youtube.com/watch?v=v08mYfxBJAE. Accessed 1 Sept 2014.
30. Amerling R, Winchester JF, Ronco C. Guidelines have done more harm than good. Blood Purif. 2008;26:73–6.
31. Camporota L, Brett S. Care bundles: implementing evidence or common sense. Crit Care. 2011;15:159–60.
32. Marik PE, Raghunathan K, Bloomstone J. Point/counterpoint: are the best patient outcomes achieved when ICU bundles are rigorously adhered to? No. Chest. 2013;144:374–8.
33. Dellinger RP, Townsend SR. Point/counterpoint: are the best patient outcomes achieved when ICU bundles are rigorously adhered to? Rebuttal. Chest. 2013;144:378–9.
34. Jones AE. Unbundling early sepsis resuscitation. Ann Emerg Med. 2014;63:654–5.
35. Marik PE, Cavallazzi R. Does the central venous pressure predict fluid responsiveness? An updated meta-analysis and a plea for some common sense. Crit Care Med. 2013;41:1774–81.
36. Dellinger RP, Townsend SR. Point/counterpoint: are the best patient outcomes achieved when ICU bundles are rigorously adhered to? Yes. Chest. 2013;144:372–4.
37. Surviving sepsis campaign statement regarding hemodynamic and oximetric monitoring in response to ProCESS and ARISE trials. http://www.survivingsepsis.org/Guidelines/Pages/default.aspx. Accessed 2 Oct 2014.

Chapter 15
Genetics in the Prevention and Treatment of Sepsis

John P. Reilly, Nuala J. Meyer, and Jason D. Christie

Introduction

Sepsis, the systemic response to acute infection, continues to be a leading cause of hospitalization, intensive care unit admission, and mortality in the United States despite significant advances in our understanding of sepsis pathogenesis and improvements in hospital-provided medical care [1, 2]. Modern hospital and intensive care unit practices, including early administration of antibiotics, fluid resuscitation, hemodynamic support, and mechanical ventilation, appear to be improving outcomes among patients with sepsis and septic shock [2, 3]. However, despite decades of research, the majority of clinic trials evaluating pharmacologic therapies targeting the host response to infection have demonstrated inconsistent or negative results [4–14]. The potential of genetics to improve the prevention and treatment of sepsis lies in furthering our understanding of the heterogeneity in host responses to

J.P. Reilly
Division of Pulmonary, Allergy, and Critical Care Medicine, Perelman School of Medicine, University of Pennsylvania, 5005 Gibson Building, 3400 Spruce Street, Philadelphia, PA 19104, USA
e-mail: john.reilly@uphs.upenn.edu

N.J. Meyer
Division of Pulmonary Allergy, and Critical Care Medicine, Perelman School of Medicine, University of Pennsylvania, 5039 West Gates Building, 3400 Spruce Street, Philadelphia, PA 19104, USA
e-mail: nuala.meyer@uphs.upenn.edu

J.D. Christie (✉)
Division of Pulmonary, Allergy, and Critical Care Medicine, Perelman School of Medicine, University of Pennsylvania, Blockley Hall, Room 719, 422 Guardian Drive, Philadelphia, PA 19104, USA
e-mail: jchristi@upenn.edu

© Springer International Publishing AG 2017
N.S. Ward, M.M. Levy (eds.), *Sepsis*, Respiratory Medicine,
DOI 10.1007/978-3-319-48470-9_15

infection, identifying those infected individuals at highest risk of incident sepsis, multi-organ system failure, or death, and selecting patients most likely to benefit from therapies targeted at sepsis pathogenesis.

The Heritability of Sepsis Susceptibility and Outcomes

An individuals' response to infection can vary greatly from mild symptoms that improve without intervention, to multi-organ system failure, septic shock, and death. Important clinical factors, including pathogen and host factors, are responsible for a large proportion of this heterogeneity. There is significant variability in each pathogen's virulence, invasiveness, and antibiotic resistance, which all contribute to the likelihood and severity of an infection [15]. Additionally, clinical factors of the host, including age, comorbidities, and site of infection, also contribute to the risk and prognosis of sepsis [16–19]. However, just as genetic variability in a given pathogen can determine virulence or antibiotic resistance, it has long been recognized that there is a strong heritable component to an individual's susceptibility and host response to infection [20].

Until recently, infectious diseases have been a leading cause of death in human populations and have exerted strong evolutionary pressures that have shaped the genetic diversity seen in today's human populations [21, 22]. In fact, genes involved in the immune system's response to infection are some of the most diverse in the human genome [23]. Classic examples of host-pathogen interactions resulting in genetic heterogeneity include several genotypes common in populations evolutionarily exposed to malaria. The hemoglobin S polymorphism of the β-globin (*HBB*) gene results in sickle cell disease in those with two copies of the polymorphism (i.e., hemoglobin S homozygotes), but also results in resistance from malarial infection in those with one copy (i.e., heterozygotes) [24]. Additionally, the Duffy null genotype results in the absence of the Duffy antigen receptor for chemokines on erythrocytes and is associated with protection from malarial infection [25]. These two functional genetic variants are very common in West African populations but are extremely rare in individuals of European or Asian ancestry. They likely persist at high frequencies due to selective pressures from historic host-pathogen interactions between African populations and malaria. Interestingly, the Duffy null genotype has recently been associated with increased risk of the acute respiratory distress syndrome, a common complication of sepsis, supporting the inference that evolutionary pressures result in genetic variability that alters risk of today's diseases [26].

The strongest evidence that the susceptibility and response to infectious disease is heritable comes from a landmark study of adopted children in Denmark in the pre-antibiotic era [20]. This study of the Danish Adoption Register found that adopted children had a nearly sixfold greater risk of premature death from infection if their biological parent also died prematurely from infection. However, if an adoptive parent died prematurely from infection, an increased risk of premature death from infection was not observed in his/her adopted children. Together, their findings support a strong genetic heritability contributing to risk and prognosis of infection and likely sepsis. In fact, in the Danish study, the heritability of premature death from infection was greater than that of vascular disease and cancer. Since Sorensen and colleagues' publication, several researchers have confirmed that susceptibility to and outcomes from infection are heritable [27–29]. Given this evidence, sepsis can be conceptualized as arising from the complex interaction of the environment, including pathogen exposure, and individual genetic factors important in the host response to infection.

With the completion of the Human Genome Project in 2003, investigators now have enhanced tools to not only estimate the heritability of infectious disease susceptibility and outcomes but also to determine the specific genetic variation that results in altered risk [30]. Over the last several decades, numerous associations between genetic variants and infectious disease risk and/or outcomes have been reported. While this chapter is by no means an exhaustive review of all reported genetic associations with infectious disease and/or sepsis, we will review the methods being implemented to study the genetics of sepsis, highlight several key reported and replicated genetic factors associated with sepsis, and discuss potential future applications of genetics to sepsis prevention and treatment.

Currently, the growing literature reporting genetic associations with acute infection and sepsis risk and/or outcomes has not yet translated to clinically applicable advancements. However, there is potential for genetic research to improve future patient care on many levels including (1) improved prediction of those at highest risk for sepsis allowing individuals to be targeted for preventative therapies or clinical trial enrollment, (2) improved evaluation of sepsis prognosis allowing for better triage to more or less intensive care, (3) development of new insight into sepsis pathogenesis by identifying unexpected genetic associations with sepsis risk or outcomes, and (4) identification of subgroups of patients most likely to respond to specific pharmacologic therapies targeted at specific sepsis mechanisms.

Approach to the Study of Sepsis Genetics

Sepsis is a clinical syndrome that results from an individual's physiologic response to an acute infection, a response that is at least in part genetically determined [20]. A large number of rare single gene disorders, exhibiting Mendelian inheritance, produce primary immunodeficiencies [31, 32]. These rare disorders often result in profound immunosuppression and can confer a dramatic increase risk of infection and sepsis. However, the majority of genetic factors that influence sepsis susceptibility and outcomes likely make modest contributions to altered risk. It is likely the interplay of multiple modest genetic factors and the environment that results in the complex and heterogeneous syndrome, sepsis. By identifying these genetic factors, we may begin to more accurately assess individual risk and develop therapies targeted at mechanisms uncovered by genetic investigation.

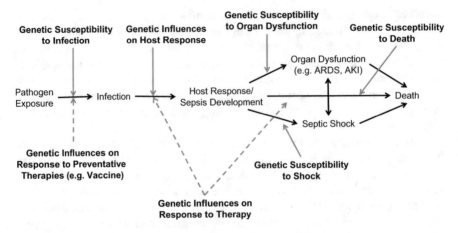

Fig. 15.1 Components of sepsis pathogenesis that are potentially influenced by an individual's genetics. A genotype may alter risk of infection once exposed to a pathogen; influence the host response to infection; alter risk of organ failure (e.g., acute respiratory distress syndrome, acute kidney injury), progression to septic shock, or death; or influence an individual's response to treatment and/or preventative therapies (e.g., vaccination)

In order to identify genetic variants altering the risk of sepsis or outcomes from sepsis, we must first develop a conceptual framework for the components of sepsis that may be influenced by an individual's genetics (Fig. 15.1). First, the likelihood of infection by a particular pathogen once an individual is exposed is potentially modified by genetics. In this light, specific genetic variants may alter risk of infection to all pathogens, a particular class of pathogen, or a very specific pathogen. Second, genetic variation in genes of the immune system may result in a host response to infection that varies across individuals, resulting in distinct genetic risk factors for the development of sepsis once an individual is infected. The pathophysiology of genetic variation and altered sepsis risk is likely complex. Whereas some genetic variants may result in a relative immunodeficiency enhancing a pathogen's invasiveness and therefore a host's severity of illness, other variants may result in an enhanced immune reaction to infection that promotes the physiology defining the sepsis syndrome. Third, among those patients who develop sepsis, genetic variation may alter risk of a specific organ system failure (e.g., acute kidney injury, acute respiratory distress syndrome), progression to septic shock, and/or mortality. Lastly, genetic variation may determine the likelihood of an individual to respond to particular sepsis therapies, such as fluid resuscitation, vasopressors, corticosteroids, or novel pharmacologic agents. Each of these components of sepsis susceptibility and outcomes may possess unique genetic risk factors, while there may be certain genetic variants that are common to multiple aspects of sepsis pathophysiology.

The complexity and heterogeneity of the immune response to infection and the subsequent development of sepsis present unique challenges to the study of sepsis genetics. The complexity of sepsis begins with an imperfect syndrome definition that relies on highly sensitive, but often not specific, clinical parameters [33, 34].

The importance of identifying the correct sepsis phenotype is paramount to conducting genetic association studies and may be enhanced in the future by the use of molecular biomarkers in sepsis diagnosis. Additionally, numerous and diverse environmental factors likely interact with an individual's genetics to determine the host response to infection, most importantly, the characteristics of the infecting pathogens. The study of sepsis genetics is also limited by the complexity of sepsis pathogenesis. The possible initial hyperimmune response followed by a relatively immunosuppressed state seen in sepsis pathogenesis may result in the identification of genes that have roles in altering risk specific to the early or late stages of sepsis. Additionally, patients enrolled in genetic association studies of sepsis are most often enrolled while hospitalized. Septic patients, who do not develop severe enough illness to present for medical care, have poor access to medical care or die prior to presenting to a hospital are often excluded from studies of sepsis genetics. Limiting the window of observation to the hospital has the potential to introduce ascertainment bias if a genetic variant is associated with the likelihood of presenting to the hospital. Despite these complexities, a significant number of genetic association studies have been conducted to date that provide insight into the genetic regulation of an individual's response to infection.

The focus of a genetic association study is to examine the association of one or many genetic polymorphisms with a phenotypic trait, such as sepsis. Genetic polymorphisms are inherited variations in human DNA sequence that occur in a least 1% of the population. The most common and well-studied genetic polymorphisms are single-base pair substitutions (i.e., single nucleotide polymorphisms, or SNPs), base pair deletions, and base pair insertions. With modern techniques, the detection of SNPs is straightforward and can be performed by an assay for an SNP or with the use of multiplexed DNA arrays whereby the genotype of multiple SNPs is determined simultaneously. Genetic polymorphisms can be present in portions of a gene that code for a protein, referred to as exons, and may therefore change the amino acid structure of a translated protein, potentially resulting in alterations of protein function. Alternatively, polymorphisms can exist in regions of a gene that do not specifically code for a protein, including the promoter, a region responsible for regulating gene transcription, and the introns, regions of the gene that are removed by RNA splicing prior to translation of RNA into proteins. Promoter and intronic polymorphisms often affect gene regulation and therefore dynamic levels of a protein at a given time. Importantly, specific combinations of genetic polymorphisms, often in close proximity to one another, tend to be inherited together in a haplotype block, referred to as linkage disequilibrium [35]. Therefore, the identification of a specific variant and disease association does not necessarily indicate that the specific polymorphism tested is the polymorphism responsible for the association. Further studies of the genetic locus identified, along with functional studies of the effects of a given polymorphism on protein level, structure, or function, are needed to determine the genetic variation responsible for altered disease risk.

Once the population of interest is defined, there are several approaches of identifying genetic associations. The genetic basis of classic Mendelian disorders is often studied using an approach referred to as linkage analysis [36]. In linkage analysis, genetic associations are identified by examining the inheritance of genetic markers relative to the inheritance of a disease in families with multiple affected individuals. The linkage-based approach is limited in complex diseases with a strong environmental component, such as infection and sepsis, because of the requirement for multiple affected family members. The most common approach used in studies of sepsis genetics has been the candidate gene association study [37]. In candidate gene studies, functional variants in a gene hypothesized to be important in sepsis are tested for an association with sepsis risk or outcomes in a case-control or cohort study design. To date, the candidate gene approach has most often focused on known genes involved in the innate immune system, cytokine responses, and coagulation pathways. The advantages of the candidate gene approach include a simple relatively inexpensive study design and the requirement for significantly smaller sample sizes than larger-scale approaches. Unfortunately, there are several disadvantages to the candidate gene approach and the quality of studies reported in the literature is highly variable [38]. The first main disadvantage is the requirement of a biologically plausible "candidate gene" and the "candidate" genetic variation within that gene. Therefore, the candidate gene approach limits the discovery of novel genetic factors [28, 39]. Additionally, findings of candidate gene studies often fail to replicate in other study populations, possibly reflecting limited study power, failure to correct for multiple hypothesis testing, or unidentified population stratification. Population stratification refers to the existence of subpopulations within a study population (e.g., ethnicities or racial groups) that differ in genetic characteristics and disease risk resulting in potential confounding of the genotype-phenotype relationship [40]. Despite these limitations, the candidate gene approach has identified several genetic variants that have replicated in multiple populations and likely represent true genetic risk factors for sepsis. Several of these variants are discussed below.

With the advent of microarray-based high-throughput genotyping technology, hundreds of thousands of polymorphisms across the genome can now be quickly assayed, and genome-wide association studies (GWAS) are increasingly being performed. The GWAS approach includes the genotype determination of >500,000 polymorphisms, capturing >80% of the variation in the genome. Each polymorphism is then tested for enrichment in the case or control population of a genetic association study. The advantages of GWAS include the assessment of the majority of individual's genetic variation, the ability to discover novel, previously unstudied associations, and the ability to adjust for genetic ancestry (i.e., population stratification). Given the huge amount of hypotheses tested in a GWAS, the current standard for determining statistical significance is p-value of $< 5 \times 10^{-8}$; therefore, the main limitation of GWAS is the requirement for huge sample sizes and/or large effect sizes to achieve stringent statistical thresholds [41]. Additionally, GWAS does not provide information regarding polymorphism function and focuses on common variants in the human genome potentially missing rare variant explaining a degree of sepsis heritability. GWAS has only very recently begun to be applied to sepsis research; however, future studies will certainly be conducted in increasingly large patient populations.

Other approaches to studying sepsis genetics have included the evaluation of gene expression (mRNA quantification in specific cell populations) during infection and sepsis and/or determining the association between genetic polymorphisms and the gene expression of certain components of the immune system important in sepsis. Additionally, future genetic association studies will include exome- or genome-wide sequencing, whereby the DNA sequence of all exons or the entire genome is performed. While this approach is currently expensive and computationally intense, whole exome or genome sequencing can identify rare variants that confer significant altered risk of sepsis. Furthermore, enhanced understanding of transcriptional regulation from the ENCODE project will likely lead to further understanding of genetic influences on disease risk and outcomes [42].

Candidate Gene Associations

As discussed above, a large number of candidate gene association studies have been conducted to identify genetic risk factors for sepsis and/or outcomes from sepsis [39, 43–46]. Table 15.1 provides a list of candidate genes that have been associated with sepsis risk or outcome to date. The findings of studies conducted thus far range from single-center studies in one population to associations that have been replicated in several independent populations. Importantly, as discussed above, candidate gene studies,

Table 15.1 Candidate genes associated with sepsis risk or mortality

Candidate gene/gene product	Hypothesized role in sepsis	References
Antigen/pathogen recognition		
Mannose-binding lectin (*MBL*)	Pattern recognition of carbohydrates	[51, 54–60, 63]
MBL-associated serine protease 2 (*MASP2*)	Activated by MBL and cleaves complement components	[191]
Toll-like receptor 1 (*TLR1*)	Pattern recognition of peptidoglycan and lipoproteins	[68, 69]
Toll-like receptor 2 (*TLR2*)	Pattern recognition of lipoteichoic acid and peptidoglycan	[60, 70, 71]
Toll-like receptor 4 (*TLR4*)	Pattern recognition of lipopolysaccharide (LPS)	[72–76]
Toll-like receptor 5 (*TLR5*)	Pattern recognition of flagellin	[71, 77]
CD14	Pattern recognition of LPS	[60, 93–96]
LPS binding protein (*LBP*)	Binding to LPS and presenting to macrophages	[100, 101]
Nucleotide-binding oligomerization domain-containing protein 2 (*NOD2*)	Pattern recognition of muramyl dipeptide moieties	[192]
IgG2 receptor (FγRIIa, *FCGR2A*)	Receptor for immunoglobulin G antibodies	[193–195]
Bacterial permeability-increasing protein (*BPI*)	Binding to LPS	[100, 196]

(continued)

Table 15.1 (continued)

Candidate gene/gene product	Hypothesized role in sepsis	References
Inflammatory response		
Tumor necrosis factor-α (*TNFα*)	Pro-inflammatory cytokine	[102, 107, 111–113]
Lymphotoxin α (*LTA*)	Pro-inflammatory cytokine	[111, 112]
Interleukin-1α (*IL1A*)	Pro-inflammatory cytokine	[118, 122, 124]
Interleukin-1β (*IL1B*)	Pro-inflammatory cytokine	[117–119, 122–124]
IL-1 receptor antagonist (*IL1RN*)	Competitive inhibitor of IL-1α and IL-1β	[120–125, 127, 128]
Interleukin-6 (*IL-6*)	Pro-inflammatory cytokine	[129–131, 133, 134]
Interleukin-18 (*IL-18*)	Pro-inflammatory cytokine	[197]
Interleukin-10 (*IL-10*)	Anti-inflammatory cytokine	[136–141]
Heat shock protein 70 (*HSP70*)	Multitude of immune-modulating effects	[115]
Myeloid differentiation factor 88 (*MYD88*)	Activated by TLRs resulting in pro-inflammatory signals	[78]
IL-1 receptor-associated kinase 1 (*IRAK-1*)	Downstream from TLRs, pro-inflammatory signaling	[86]
IL-1 receptor-associated kinase 4 (*IRAK-4*)	Downstream from TLRs, pro-inflammatory signaling	[79]
Macrophage migration inhibitory factor (*MIF*)	Pro-inflammatory cytokine	[198–201]
Interferon γ (*IFNG*)	Pro-inflammatory cytokine	[202]
CXCL2	Pro-inflammatory chemokine	[203]
Tissue inhibitor of matrix metalloproteinase-1 (*TIMP1*)	Inhibitor of matrix metalloproteinases	[204]
Apolipoprotein E (*APOE*)	Binds and traffic antigens, resulting in immune activation	[205]
SVEP1	Cell adhesion molecule	[206]
Coagulation		
Plasminogen activator inhibitor (*PAI1*)	Inhibits tissue plasminogen, procoagulant	[146–155]
Protein C (*PROC*)	Coagulation factor	[156–159]
Factor V (*F5*)	Coagulation factor activates thrombin	[161–163]
Regulators of cardiovascular response		
β₂ adrenergic receptor (*ADRB2*)	Blood pressure and cardiac output regulation	[167]
Vasopressinase (*LNPEP*)	Clearance of vasopressin	[168]
Angiotensin II type 1 receptor-associated protein (*AGTRAP*)	Vascular reactivity	[169]
Angiotensin converting enzyme (*ACE*)	Effects on vascular tone and inflammatory response	[207, 208]

to date, have been limited in many instances by small sample sizes, poor reproducibility, and possible false positive results. Therefore, many of these associations may not be confirmed as future studies are conducted in large cohorts of patients with the assessment of larger-scale genetic variation. Those genes representing promising avenues for future research are discussed below. They have been grouped into several common categories, antigen or pathogen recognition, cytokines, coagulation pathways, and regulators of cardiovascular response to sepsis.

Antigen/Pathogen Recognition

The innate immune system includes extensive processes whereby the host recognizes conserved structures of microbes called pathogen-associated molecular patterns [47, 48]. Genes that encode specific pattern recognition receptors exhibit significant variability possibly conferring altered susceptibility to infection, ranging from severe immunodeficiency to moderate increases in infection and/or sepsis risk [48].

Mannose-Binding Lectin (MBL)

The soluble serum protein MBL functions as a pattern recognition receptor by binding to carbohydrate structures of microorganisms, resulting in activation of compliment via the lectin pathway and phagocytosis by macrophages [49]. Relatively low levels of MBL are common in the population and have been associated with increased risk of sepsis and pneumonia in several independent studies [50–53]. Multiple SNPs within the *MBL* gene modulate levels and function of MBL and are therefore strong candidate variants for an association with sepsis risk or outcomes [54]. These SNPs include those located in the coding region resulting in altered protein structure and function, in addition to promoter polymorphisms that alter transcription and, therefore, serum levels of the MBL protein. A large number of candidate gene studies have examined associations between MBL polymorphisms and either sepsis risk, outcomes, or infection with particular pathogens [51, 55–60]. Many of these studies demonstrate a strong association between specific SNPs, known to alter MBL function or transcription, and sepsis or infection; however, replication of these associations has been inconsistent [61, 62]. A recent meta-analysis supports the conclusion that genetic variation in the MBL gene confers altered risk of sepsis; however, this conclusion was not true for all genetic variation reported in the literature, may be affected by publication bias, and requires larger confirmatory studies [63].

Toll-Like Receptors (TLR)

TLRs are a large family of pattern recognition receptors that are responsible for activating the innate immune system upon recognition of conserved microbial structures [64, 65]. Each member of the TLR family recognizes different microbial patterns; therefore, impairment of any particular TLR may result in increased susceptibility to particular classes of pathogens [66]. For example, TLR2 recognizes lipoteichoic acid and peptidoglycan, cell wall components of Gram-positive bacteria, whereas TLR4 recognizes lipopolysaccharide from Gram-negative bacteria, and TLR5 recognizes flagellin present on organisms such as *Legionella pneumophila* [67]. Genetic variation in the genes encoding TLR1, TLR2, TLR4, and TLR5, in addition to the downstream signaling molecules myeloid differentiation factor 88 (MyD88) and interleukin 1 receptor-associated kinase−1 and −4 (IRAK-1, IRAK-4), has been reported to confer altered risk of sepsis or sepsis outcomes [60, 68–79]. Again, these studies are all limited by small sample sizes and often conflicting results.

In one particular study, investigators evaluated the whole blood inflammatory response to pathogen-associated molecules in healthy volunteers based on genetic variation in 49 TLR related genes. They identified variants in *TLR1* gene that modify this inflammatory response and, subsequently, demonstrated an increased risk of organ dysfunction and death in septic patients possessing these variants [68]. TLR1 was the first human TLR identified and recognizes lipopeptides on bacterial cell walls [80]. Subsequent investigators have examined further genetic variation in *TLR1*, demonstrating further associations and partially replicated previous findings in populations of septic patients [69].

The receptor TLR2 recognizes Gram-positive bacteria and is coded for by the highly polymorphic *TLR2* gene. Studies have focused on several non-synonymous SNPs in the coding region of the *TLR2* gene. The first SNP results in a substitution of arginine for glutamine at amino acid 753 and was initially reported to increase risk of Gram-positive sepsis [70]; however, several subsequent studies have not replicated this association [81–83]. Other *TLR2* SNPs have been reported to alter sepsis risk or outcomes, but require further evaluation [60, 71].

Unlike TLR2, TLR4 recognizes components of Gram-negative bacteria and has genetic variation associated with decreased immune response to inhaled endotoxin in healthy volunteers [72, 73]. This same variation has been associated with Gram-negative infections and meningococcal disease is some reports [74–76], but not others [84, 85]. Additionally, studies have reported associations between *TLR5* genetic variation and infection and/or sepsis [71, 77]. Genetic variation in the downstream mediators, MyD88, IRAK-1, and IRAK-4, have also been reported to be association with infection and/or sepsis [78, 79, 86].

CD14 and Lipopolysaccharide Binding Protein (LBP)

CD14 is a receptor that recognizes LPS on Gram-negative bacteria in association with TLR4 and MD2, resulting in activation of the innate immune system and release of cytokines [87]. Levels of soluble serum CD14 are associated with infection, sepsis, and death [88–92]. A promoter polymorphism in the *CD14* gene (−159C/T) results in altered CD14 levels and has been associated with increased susceptibility and outcome from septic shock [60, 93, 94]. A second promoter polymorphism (−260C/T) has also been reported to alter *CD14* transcription and therefore risk of sepsis, septic shock, and mortality [94–96]; however, others have reported no association between −260C/T and sepsis [75, 97, 98]. Given CD14 is responsible for activating the innate immune response in the setting of infection with Gram-negative bacteria, it is possible that some of the different conclusions of prior studies result from the use populations with different amounts of Gram-positive and Gram-negative infections.

LBP is responsible for binding lipopolysaccharide from Gram-negative bacteria, presenting it to the TLR4-CD14-MD2 complex on macrophages, activating the innate immune response [99]. Studies of *LBP* genetic variation and Gram-negative sepsis demonstrate inconsistent results [100, 101]; therefore, more research is needed to determine the role of *LBP* variation in sepsis.

Cytokines

Examining variation in the genes encoding cytokines was a logical first step for candidate gene association studies in sepsis. Cytokines have long been recognized as an important component of the host response to infection and have been subject to many genetic association studies in sepsis.

Tumor Necrosis Factor-α (TNFα)

One of the first genetic associations with sepsis reported in the literature was the −308 G/A SNP in the *TNF* gene [102]. TNFα is an important pro-inflammatory cytokine recognized as a primary mediator of sepsis pathophysiology [103]. Animal studies have demonstrated the ability of anti-TNFα therapy to prevent the development of sepsis [104, 105]. However, several prior randomized controlled trials examined the effectiveness of anti-TNFα therapy in human sepsis, only to produce negative results [8, 10]. The −308G to A SNP is located in the promoter region of the *TNF* gene and is associated with increased production of TNFα [106]. The −308A allele has been associated with increased risk of septic shock and mortality from septic shock [102, 107]. Therefore, individuals possessing the high-risk allele possibly represent the ideal target population for future studies of anti-TNF therapies. Unfortunately, several more recent studies have failed to replicate these previous genetic associations [108, 109]. A particular challenging aspect of genetic association studies linking TNFα to sepsis is the presence of the *TNF* gene in a highly polymorphic region of the major histocompatibility complex on chromosome 6. Linkage disequilibrium between multiple inflammatory genes in the region makes identification of the causal variant conferring altered risk challenging and may explain some of the inconsistent results seen in the literature.

Lymphotoxin Alpha (LTA)

LTA, formerly referred to as TNFβ, is a cytokine produced by lymphocytes that results in induction of the inflammatory response [110]. Several early genetic association studies reported an association between the +252G/A SNP in the first intron of the *LTA* gene [111, 112]; however, more recent studies have not supported these findings [113, 114]. The *LTA* gene is located on chromosome 6 in the same major histocompatibility complex region as *TNF*, in addition to heat shock protein 70 (*HSP70*) among other inflammatory genes. Polymorphisms in *HSP70* have also been reported to be associated with risk of septic shock [115]; therefore, associations in the LTA gene may be the result of linkage disequilibrium with other genes located in the same region.

Interleukin-1 (IL-1) Family

The IL-1 family consists of two pro-inflammatory cytokines, IL-1α and IL-1β, which are important mediators of the sepsis immune response, in addition to the anti-inflammatory cytokine, IL-1 receptor antagonist (IL-1RA) [116]. IL-1RA binds to the IL-1 receptor but does not produce an inflammatory response, competitively inhibiting IL-1α and IL-1β. The *IL1A*, *IL1B*, and *IL1RN* genes encode for IL-1α, IL-1β, and IL-1RA, respectively, and are located close together on human chromosome 2. A clinical trial of a recombinant form of IL-1RA in the treatment of sepsis failed to demonstrate positive results; however, investigations of genetic heterogeneity in the IL-1 family of genes may identify patients more likely to respond to anti-IL-1 therapy [11]. Five polymorphisms in IL-1 genes have been reported to be associated with sepsis risk [117–126]. These polymorphisms include the SNPs −889 in the promoter region of the *IL1A* gene, −511 and −31 in the promoter region of *IL1B* gene, +3954 in exon 5 of the *IL1B* gene, and a variable number of tandem repeats in intron 2 of the *IL1RN* gene. A recent meta-analysis supports the association of the *IL1A* −889, *IL1B* +3954, and the *IL1RN* variable number of tandem repeats with sepsis susceptibility, but not the other two reported variants [124]. However, the meta-analysis may be limited by publication bias and study heterogeneity and requires further replication in larger populations. Additionally, a synonymous coding variant in *IL1RN* not included in the meta-analysis has also been associated with increased LPS-evoked IL-1RA plasma protein and improved survival during septic shock [127]. While this association has not been replicated as a sepsis mortality factor, the same variant has consistently been associated with reduced risk of acute respiratory distress syndrome [128].

Interleukin-6 (IL-6)

IL-6 is an important pro-inflammatory cytokine secreted in the setting of infection. Several genetic association studies of the *IL-6* gene and sepsis have been conducted only to produce conflicting results. Specifically, several studies have focused on the

−174G/C promoter SNP, which has been associated with IL-6 levels and improved survival among septic patients [129–131]. Other studies have not confirmed these associations [132, 133]. Taking an alternative approach, haplotypes made up of several SNPs in the *IL-6* gene have also been reported to be strongly associated with mortality and organ dysfunction among the septic [133, 134]. However, future research is needed in order to understand the functional significance of these haplotypes and how they translate to altered sepsis outcomes.

Interleukin-10 (IL-10)

IL-10 is an anti-inflammatory cytokine that is responsible for suppression of antigen presenting cells and downregulation of pro-inflammatory cytokines [135]. The most extensively studied genetic variants of *IL-10* in sepsis include three promoter polymorphisms (−1082G/A, −819T/C, and −592C/A) [136–140]. Specifically, the −1082G/A is associated with altered levels of IL-10 and altered Gram-positive sepsis risk and outcomes [137]. Additionally, a haplotype of three SNPs was found to be associated with mortality in pulmonary sepsis but not extrapulmonary sepsis [141].

Coagulation Pathways

A hallmark of the sepsis syndrome is activation of coagulation pathways, which may contribute to multi-organ system failure during sepsis. Interest in coagulation in sepsis peaked with the development of recombinant human activated protein C (rhAPC) or drotrecogin alfa. This therapy promotes fibrinolysis and inhibits thrombosis and was initially demonstrated to improve 28-day mortality in sepsis [5]. However confirmatory studies failed to demonstrate improved mortality and rhAPC was withdrawn from the marked in 2011 [7]. Several investigators have examined candidate genes important in coagulation as risk factors for sepsis. These investigations have the potential to identify particular subgroups of sepsis that may be most likely to respond to future therapies targeting coagulation.

Plasminogen Activator Inhibitor-1 (PAI-1)

PAI-1 inhibits tissue plasminogen activator and urokinase, functioning as a procoagulant factor that inhibits fibrinolysis [142]. Elevation in PAI-1 levels in plasma and bronchoalveolar lavage fluid is associated with worse outcomes in sepsis, pneumonia, and acute respiratory distress syndrome [143–145]. An insertion/deletion polymorphism in the promoter of the *PAI1* gene, −675 5G/4G, results in altered transcription and therefore altered levels of PAI-1 [146]. The 4G allele results in higher PAI-1 levels and has been reported to confer higher risk of mortality from meningococcal sepsis and severe pneumonia [147–155]. Supporting the biological plausibility of a *PAI1* variant and sepsis associations, the 4G allele also confers an exaggerated response in PAI-1 levels following ex vivo whole blood stimulation with LPS [154]. These findings elegantly demonstrate how a genetic risk factor for sepsis can have minimal effects of an individual in steady state, but can result in significant impacts after exposure to an environmental pathogen.

Protein C and Factor V Leiden

Protein C is an important coagulation factor with significant genetic variation. Two promoter SNPs in the protein C gene (*PROC*), −1654C/T and −1641G/A, have been reported to alter blood levels of protein C and sepsis outcomes [156–159]. Further research is needed to confirm these findings.

Factor V is a protein important in the coagulation cascade that serves to activate thrombin and generate fibrin deposition. A coding SNP with the factor V gene (*F5*) is responsible for the Factor V Leiden polymorphism, the most common inherited thrombophilia in European ancestry populations [160]. Several studies have reported an association between the Factor V Leiden polymorphism and sepsis susceptibility and/or outcomes [161–163]; however, other studies have not confirmed these findings [164, 165]. In a recent meta-analysis of eight studies, the Factor V Leiden polymorphism was not associated with sepsis risk or outcomes [166], highlighting the challenges of interpreting small candidate gene studies and the need for larger studies.

Regulators of Cardiovascular Response

In patients with septic shock, exogenous vasopressors are often used to augment the body's own mechanisms to maintain blood pressure. The most common vasopressors used to treat septic shock include the adrenergic vasopressors, norepinephrine and epinephrine, in addition to vasopressin. Therefore, genetic polymorphisms in genes involved in vascular reactivity or response to vasopressors are potential candidate risk factors for mortality among patients with sepsis and/or septic shock. Additionally, these genetic polymorphisms also represent candidate polymorphisms that may predict an individual's response to vasopressor therapy. Several studies have examined the associations of genetic variants in the β_2 adrenergic receptor, vasopressin pathway genes, and angiotensin pathway genes with sepsis outcomes in multiple populations [167–169]. Nakada and colleagues identified a haplotype of three SNPs in the β_2 adrenergic receptor gene (*ADRB2*), known to be associated with response to adrenergic agonists in asthmatics, and tested the association between this haplotype and mortality in sepsis [167]. In two independent cohorts, the risk haplotype was associated with increased norepinephrine dose and ultimately mortality. In another study, the same authors examined 17 SNPs in five vasopressin pathway genes and identified an SNP in the vasopressinase gene (*LNPEP*) that conferred a higher plasma vasopressin clearance and increased 28-day mortality [168].

In addition, an association between an SNP in the angiotensin II type 1 receptor-associated protein and increased protein expression, decreased blood pressure, and increased mortality was detected in a study of angiotensin pathway genes [169]. These associations require further validation; however, they represent promising avenues of research that could provide prognostic information for patients with sepsis or lead to future studies of determining genotype to guide vasopressor management.

Genome-Wide Association Studies

Only recently have patient cohorts been large enough to perform GWAS in infection and/or sepsis; therefore, large-scale data continues to be limited. However, several large GWAS relevant to sepsis are currently being performed, including a GWAS of bacteremia by the Wellcome Trust and of sepsis by the UK Critical Care Genomics Group. While limited, the GWAS in infection and/or sepsis, published to date, provide insight into the power of GWAS to identify novel variants associated with disease, assess treatment affects by genotype, and implicate novel pathways in disease susceptibility and/or outcomes. The first published GWAS studying a heterogeneous population of patients with severe sepsis was performed in those patient enrolled in the PROWESS randomized controlled trial of rhAPC [170]. These authors conducted several GWA analyses in the PROWESS population. In the first analysis, the authors sought to determine a population with improved response to rhAPC therapy based on genetic variants. Using a gene-environment interaction analysis, in this case SNP-by-treatment group interaction, the authors identified an SNP in the 5′ untranslated region of LOC222052 near to the insulin-like growth factor I (IGF1)—binding protein gene associated with improved treatment effect on mortality. Additionally, in a multimarker analysis where the authors considered gene-gene interactions, they identified combinations of three variants, rs7725278 in the intergenic region near the dopamine receptor D1, rs2256527 in the intergenic region near LOC391273, and rs10910651 in an intron of pecanex-like 2, associated with improved response to rhAPC. The functional significance of these variants is unknown, and rhAPC is no longer available in the United States; however, this study demonstrates how novel genetic associations between genetic variants and treatment effects can be identified in the future. In addition to the gene-treatment interaction analyses, the authors also tested whether any single SNPs could identify a subgroup with a 20% difference in mortality in the placebo group. In this population of approximately 700 subjects, no genetic variant reached statistical significance, possibly reflecting the small sample size and heterogeneous population.

While not specifically performed in septic populations, several GWA studies have been performed examining the association of genetic variants with severity of specific infections. These studies demonstrate how some genetic variants may alter the host response to specific infectious pathogens, while others may alter host response to all infections or particular categories of infections. The largest published GWA studies that have some relevance to sepsis are those performed in meningococcemia, malaria, and acute viral infections [171–175]. *Neisseria meningitidis* is a Gram-negative, polysaccharide-encapsulated bacterium that is responsible for meningococcal meningitis and sepsis and is associated with high mortality and morbidity. In a recent case-control GWAS in European discovery and validation populations, variants in the Factor H (*CFH*) and CFH-related genes (*CFHR3, CFHR1*) were associated with decreased susceptibility to meningococcal disease [171]. Complement deficiency is a known risk factor for *Neisseria* infection [176]; however, specific components of the complement pathway have not been identified to be associated with meningococcemia risk. The proteins coded for by the *CFH* and related genes are important negative regulators of complement signaling and therefore may be novel therapeutic targets for preventing meningococcal sepsis. Importantly, genes in the CFH pathway have not been previously studied in the candidate gene approach, demonstrating the power of GWAS to identify novel genetic variants in sepsis and infection.

Several GWA studies have examined the association of genetic variants and risk of severe malaria resulting from infection with *Plasmodium falciparum* [172–174]. These studies have demonstrated consistent signals in two genes, *HBB* and *ABO*, confirming previous epidemiologic studies demonstrating these associations, in addition to identifying two novel loci in the *ATP2B4* gene and in an intergenic region near the tight-junction protein gene *MARVELD3*. The hemoglobin S polymorphism responsible for sickle cell disease and malaria resistance is located in the *HBB* gene, so it is not surprising this polymorphism was identified in the GWAS. Additionally, polymorphisms in the *ABO* gene are responsible for determining ABO blood type. Blood type O has previously been reported to confer resistance to severe malarial infection [177], a finding that is now confirmed by GWAS. ABO blood type has also been reported to be associated with altered risk of the acute respiratory distress syndrome in patients with severe sepsis, possibly indicating overlapping genetically influenced mechanisms for severe malarial infection and sepsis outcomes [178]. In addition to studies of host genetics, a GWAS of *Plasmodium falciparum* genetic variation exhibited a strong association between variation in the pathogen's drug transporter genes and resistance to antimalarial agents, suggesting the need for future studies of host-pathogen genetic interactions [179].

Other approaches to identifying genetic associations with sepsis include conducting GWAS of levels of inflammatory mediators or of an individual's response to an inflammation-inducing agent. In a large population of individuals from Sardinia, researchers conducted a GWAS examining the association of genetic variation with blood levels of several inflammatory biomarkers, specifically, interleukin-6 (IL-6), erythrocyte sedimentation rate (ESR), monocyte chemotactic protein-1 (MCP-1), and C-reactive protein (CRP) [180]. They identified several variants associated with each biomarker, many of which were novel. Another study identified genome-wide variation associated with whole blood responses of IL-6, IL-1β, and TNF-α production to a TLR1/2 lipopeptide agonist in healthy individuals [181]. Genetic variation within the *TLR10/1/6* locus on chromosome 4 was noted to be associated with the cytokine response. Future studies of human models of sepsis could focus on genetic predictors of response to various pro-inflammatory agents, possibly identifying pathways unique to individual infections or classes of infection.

Gene Expression Studies

The objective of gene expression profiling is to quantify mRNA expression of thousands of genes simultaneously in a particular setting, such as sepsis. By linking gene expression to a sepsis phenotype, the approach has the potential to lead to discovery of novel mechanistic pathways or therapeutic targets for sepsis, biomarkers to aid in outcome prediction, or gene-expression-based subclasses of sepsis that may require unique therapeutic approaches. Gene expression profiling also provides a molecular signature of sepsis made up of hundreds to thousands of changes in gene expression from the baseline resting state. Beyond the complexity of the data produced, a limitation of gene expression studies is that they provide a single snapshot of time within a very dynamic process, such as sepsis. In addition, the mRNA expression pattern is often cell type specific, and the target cell in sepsis is far from clear. Despite these challenges, several genome-wide expression studies of whole blood or circulating white blood cells have been performed in adult and pediatric populations with sepsis or human volunteers challenged with endotoxin [182–189]. These studies have focused on several aspects of sepsis including predicting mortality, differentiating Gram-negative and Gram-positive responses, and examining the effects of corticosteroids on gene expression in pediatric septic shock. Regardless of the study focus, gene expression studies have consistently demonstrated a considerable upregulation of inflammation and innate immunity related genes in sepsis.

Future Directions

Despite a tremendous amount of research and advancement, investigations of genetics in sepsis have not yet translated into improved prediction, prevention, or treatment of the over one million Americans who develop sepsis each year [190]. However, the potential of genetic investigation to transform sepsis care remains, particularly given the evidence that sepsis risk and outcomes are genetically determined and that mortality from infection is a major evolutionary pressure. Future research should include investigations in larger cohorts of patients utilizing increasingly advanced analytic techniques. These future investigations will likely include larger population genome-wide association, gene expression, and sequencing studies; studies of gene-gene, gene-environment, and epigenetic interactions; identification of genetic predictors of response to therapy (pharmacogenomics); and analysis of the complicated interactions of host and pathogen genetics. With the future research these approaches may produce, the potential impact of genetic investigation on sepsis care may include enhanced risk stratification, discovery of novel therapies, and identification of subgroups of patients most likely to respond to targeted and personalized therapies.

References

1. Walkey AJ, Wiener RS, Lindenauer PK. Utilization patterns and outcomes associated with central venous catheter in septic shock: a population-based study. Crit Care Med. 2013;41(6):1450–7.
2. Kaukonen KM, Bailey M, Suzuki S, Pilcher D, Bellomo R. Mortality related to severe sepsis and septic shock among critically ill patients in Australia and New Zealand, 2000–2012. JAMA. 2014;311(13):1308–16.
3. Miller III RR, Dong L, Nelson NC, Brown SM, Kuttler KG, Probst DR, et al. Multicenter implementation of a severe sepsis and septic shock treatment bundle. Am J Respir Crit Care Med. 2013;188(1):77–82.
4. Annane D, Sebille V, Charpentier C, Bollaert PE, Francois B, Korach JM, et al. Effect of treatment with low doses of hydrocortisone and fludrocortisone on mortality in patients with septic shock. JAMA. 2002;288(7):862–71.
5. Bernard GR, Vincent JL, Laterre PF, LaRosa SP, Dhainaut JF, Lopez-Rodriguez A, et al. Efficacy and safety of recombinant human activated protein C for severe sepsis. N Engl J Med. 2001;344(10):699–709.
6. Sprung CL, Annane D, Keh D, Moreno R, Singer M, Freivogel K, et al. Hydrocortisone therapy for patients with septic shock. N Engl J Med. 2008;358(2):111–24.
7. Ranieri VM, Thompson BT, Barie PS, Dhainaut JF, Douglas IS, Finfer S, et al. Drotrecogin alfa (activated) in adults with septic shock. N Engl J Med. 2012;366(22):2055–64.
8. Abraham E, Anzueto A, Gutierrez G, Tessler S, San Pedro G, Wunderink R, et al. Double-blind randomised controlled trial of monoclonal antibody to human tumour necrosis factor in treatment of septic shock. NORASEPT II Study Group. Lancet. 1998;351(9107):929–33.
9. Abraham E, Laterre PF, Garbino J, Pingleton S, Butler T, Dugernier T, et al. Lenercept (p55 tumor necrosis factor receptor fusion protein) in severe sepsis and early septic shock: a randomized, double-blind, placebo-controlled, multicenter phase III trial with 1,342 patients. Crit Care Med. 2001;29(3):503–10.
10. Abraham E, Wunderink R, Silverman H, Perl TM, Nasraway S, Levy H, et al. Efficacy and safety of monoclonal antibody to human tumor necrosis factor alpha in patients with sepsis syndrome. A randomized, controlled, double-blind, multicenter clinical trial. TNF-alpha MAb Sepsis Study Group. JAMA. 1995;273(12):934–41.
11. Opal SM, Fisher Jr CJ, Dhainaut JF, Vincent JL, Brase R, Lowry SF, et al. Confirmatory interleukin-1 receptor antagonist trial in severe sepsis: a phase III, randomized, double-blind, placebo-controlled, multicenter trial. The Interleukin-1 Receptor Antagonist Sepsis Investigator Group. Crit Care Med. 1997;25(7):1115–24.
12. Szakmany T, Hauser B, Radermacher P. N-Acetylcysteine for sepsis and systemic inflammatory response in adults. Cochrane Database Syst Rev. 2012;9:CD006616.
13. Abraham E, Reinhart K, Opal S, Demeyer I, Doig C, Rodriguez AL, et al. Efficacy and safety of tifacogin (recombinant tissue factor pathway inhibitor) in severe sepsis: a randomized controlled trial. JAMA. 2003;290(2):238–47.
14. Rice TW, Wheeler AP, Bernard GR, Vincent JL, Angus DC, Aikawa N, et al. A randomized, double-blind, placebo-controlled trial of TAK-242 for the treatment of severe sepsis. Crit Care Med. 2010;38(8):1685–94.
15. Shorr AF, Tabak YP, Killian AD, Gupta V, Liu LZ, Kollef MH. Healthcare-associated bloodstream infection: a distinct entity? Insights from a large U.S. database. Crit Care Med. 2006;34(10):2588–95.
16. Martin GS, Mannino DM, Moss M. The effect of age on the development and outcome of adult sepsis. Crit Care Med. 2006;34(1):15–21.
17. Sands KE, Bates DW, Lanken PN, Graman PS, Hibberd PL, Kahn KL, et al. Epidemiology of sepsis syndrome in 8 academic medical centers. JAMA. 1997;278(3):234–40.
18. Girard TD, Opal SM, Ely EW. Insights into severe sepsis in older patients: from epidemiology to evidence-based management. Clin Infect Dis. 2005;40(5):719–27.

19. Krieger JN, Kaiser DL, Wenzel RP. Urinary tract etiology of bloodstream infections in hospitalized patients. J Infect Dis. 1983;148(1):57–62.
20. Sorensen TI, Nielsen GG, Andersen PK, Teasdale TW. Genetic and environmental influences on premature death in adult adoptees. N Engl J Med. 1988;318(12):727–32.
21. Finch CE. Evolution in health and medicine Sackler colloquium: evolution of the human lifespan and diseases of aging: roles of infection, inflammation, and nutrition. Proc Natl Acad Sci U S A. 2010;107(Suppl 1):1718–24.
22. Akey JM. Constructing genomic maps of positive selection in humans: where do we go from here? Genome Res. 2009;19(5):711–22.
23. Murphy PM. Molecular mimicry and the generation of host defense protein diversity. Cell. 1993;72(6):823–6.
24. Aidoo M, Terlouw DJ, Kolczak MS, McElroy PD, ter Kuile FO, Kariuki S, et al. Protective effects of the sickle cell gene against malaria morbidity and mortality. Lancet. 2002;359(9314):1311–2.
25. Miller LH, Mason SJ, Clyde DF, McGinniss MH. The resistance factor to Plasmodium vivax in blacks. The Duffy-blood-group genotype, FyFy. N Engl J Med. 1976;295(6):302–4.
26. Kangelaris KN, Sapru A, Calfee CS, Liu KD, Pawlikowska L, Witte JS, et al. The association between a Darc gene polymorphism and clinical outcomes in African American patients with acute lung injury. Chest. 2012;141(5):1160–9.
27. Westendorp RG, Langermans JA, Huizinga TW, Elouali AH, Verweij CL, Boomsma DI, et al. Genetic influence on cytokine production and fatal meningococcal disease. Lancet. 1997;349(9046):170–3.
28. Burgner D, Jamieson SE, Blackwell JM. Genetic susceptibility to infectious diseases: big is beautiful, but will bigger be even better? Lancet Infect Dis. 2006;6(10):653–63.
29. Bellamy R, Hill AV. Genetic susceptibility to mycobacteria and other infectious pathogens in humans. Curr Opin Immunol. 1998;10(4):483–7.
30. Hattori M. Finishing the euchromatic sequence of the human genome. Nature. 2004;431(7011):931–45.
31. Casanova JL, Fieschi C, Bustamante J, Reichenbach J, Remus N, von Bernuth H, et al. From idiopathic infectious diseases to novel primary immunodeficiencies. J Allergy Clin Immunol. 2005;116(2):426–30.
32. Casanova JL, Abel L. Inborn errors of immunity to infection: the rule rather than the exception. J Exp Med. 2005;202(2):197–201.
33. Bone RC, Balk RA, Cerra FB, Dellinger RP, Fein AM, Knaus WA, et al. Definitions for sepsis and organ failure and guidelines for the use of innovative therapies in sepsis. The ACCP/SCCM Consensus Conference Committee. American College of Chest Physicians/Society of Critical Care Medicine. Chest. 1992;101(6):1644–55.
34. Vincent JL, Opal SM, Marshall JC, Tracey KJ. Sepsis definitions: time for change. Lancet. 2013;381(9868):774–5.
35. Gabriel SB, Schaffner SF, Nguyen H, Moore JM, Roy J, Blumenstiel B, et al. The structure of haplotype blocks in the human genome. Science. 2002;296(5576):2225–9.
36. Risch N, Merikangas K. The future of genetic studies of complex human diseases. Science. 1996;273(5281):1516–7.
37. Vink JM, Boomsma DI. Gene finding strategies. Biol Psychol. 2002;61(1–2):53–71.
38. Clark MF, Baudouin SV. A systematic review of the quality of genetic association studies in human sepsis. Intensive Care Med. 2006;32(11):1706–12.
39. Chapman SJ, Hill AV. Human genetic susceptibility to infectious disease. Nat Rev Genet. 2012;13(3):175–88.
40. Marchini J, Cardon LR, Phillips MS, Donnelly P. The effects of human population structure on large genetic association studies. Nat Genet. 2004;36(5):512–7.
41. McCarthy MI, Abecasis GR, Cardon LR, Goldstein DB, Little J, Ioannidis JP, et al. Genome-wide association studies for complex traits: consensus, uncertainty and challenges. Nat Rev Genet. 2008;9(5):356–69.

42. ENCODE Project Consortium. An integrated encyclopedia of DNA elements in the human genome. Nature. 2012;489(7414):57–74.
43. Chung LP, Waterer GW. Genetic predisposition to respiratory infection and sepsis. Crit Rev Clin Lab Sci. 2011;48(5–6):250–68.
44. Sutherland AM, Walley KR. Bench-to-bedside review: association of genetic variation with sepsis. Crit Care. 2009;13(2):210.
45. Wong HR. Genetics and genomics in pediatric septic shock. Crit Care Med. 2012;40(5):1618–26.
46. Namath A, Patterson AJ. Genetic polymorphisms in sepsis. Crit Care Clin. 2009;25(4):835–56. x
47. Akira S, Uematsu S, Takeuchi O. Pathogen recognition and innate immunity. Cell. 2006;124(4):783–801.
48. Netea MG, van der Meer JW. Immunodeficiency and genetic defects of pattern-recognition receptors. N Engl J Med. 2011;364(1):60–70.
49. Jack DL, Turner MW. Anti-microbial activities of mannose-binding lectin. Biochem Soc Trans. 2003;31(Pt 4):753–7.
50. Rantala A, Lajunen T, Juvonen R, Bloigu A, Silvennoinen-Kassinen S, Peitso A, et al. Mannose-binding lectin concentrations, MBL2 polymorphisms, and susceptibility to respiratory tract infections in young men. J Infect Dis. 2008;198(8):1247–53.
51. Huh JW, Song K, Yum JS, Hong SB, Lim CM, Koh Y. Association of mannose-binding lectin-2 genotype and serum levels with prognosis of sepsis. Crit Care. 2009;13(6):R176.
52. Eisen DP, Dean MM, Boermeester MA, Fidler KJ, Gordon AC, Kronborg G, et al. Low serum mannose-binding lectin level increases the risk of death due to pneumococcal infection. Clin Infect Dis. 2008;47(4):510–6.
53. Eisen DP, Minchinton RM. Impact of mannose-binding lectin on susceptibility to infectious diseases. Clin Infect Dis. 2003;37(11):1496–505.
54. Garred P, Larsen F, Seyfarth J, Fujita R, Madsen HO. Mannose-binding lectin and its genetic variants. Genes Immun. 2006;7(2):85–94.
55. Gordon AC, Waheed U, Hansen TK, Hitman GA, Garrard CS, Turner MW, et al. Mannose-binding lectin polymorphisms in severe sepsis: relationship to levels, incidence, and outcome. Shock. 2006;25(1):88–93.
56. Horiuchi T, Gondo H, Miyagawa H, Otsuka J, Inaba S, Nagafuji K, et al. Association of MBL gene polymorphisms with major bacterial infection in patients treated with high-dose chemotherapy and autologous PBSCT. Genes Immun. 2005;6(2):162–6.
57. Summerfield JA, Ryder S, Sumiya M, Thursz M, Gorchein A, Monteil MA, et al. Mannose binding protein gene mutations associated with unusual and severe infections in adults. Lancet. 1995;345(8954):886–9.
58. Garnacho-Montero J, Garcia-Cabrera E, Jimenez-Alvarez R, Diaz-Martin A, Revuelto-Rey J, Aznar-Martin J, et al. Genetic variants of the MBL2 gene are associated with mortality in pneumococcal sepsis. Diagn Microbiol Infect Dis. 2012;73(1):39–44.
59. Garred P, Strom JJ, Quist L, Taaning E, Madsen HO: Association of mannose-binding lectin polymorphisms with sepsis and fatal outcome, in patients with systemic inflammatory response syndrome. J Infect Dis 2003, 188(9):1394–1403.
60. Sutherland AM, Walley KR, Russell JA. Polymorphisms in CD14, mannose-binding lectin, and Toll-like receptor-2 are associated with increased prevalence of infection in critically ill adults. Crit Care Med. 2005;33(3):638–44.
61. Klostergaard A, Steffensen R, Moller JK, Peterslund N, Juhl-Christensen C, Molle I. Sepsis in acute myeloid leukaemia patients receiving high-dose chemotherapy: no impact of chitotriosidase and mannose-binding lectin polymorphisms. Eur J Haematol. 2010;85(1):58–64.
62. Kronborg G, Weis N, Madsen HO, Pedersen SS, Wejse C, Nielsen H, et al. Variant mannose-binding lectin alleles are not associated with susceptibility to or outcome of invasive pneumococcal infection in randomly included patients. J Infect Dis. 2002;185(10):1517–20.
63. Zhang AQ, Yue CL, Pan W, Gao JW, Zeng L, Gu W, et al. Mannose-binding lectin polymorphisms and the risk of sepsis: evidence from a meta-analysis. Epidemiol Infect. 2014;1-12

64. Beutler B. Inferences, questions and possibilities in Toll-like receptor signalling. Nature. 2004;430(6996):257–63.
65. Casanova JL, Abel L, Quintana-Murci L. Human TLRs and IL-1Rs in host defense: natural insights from evolutionary, epidemiological, and clinical genetics. Annu Rev Immunol. 2011;29:447–91.
66. Misch EA, Hawn TR. Toll-like receptor polymorphisms and susceptibility to human disease. Clin Sci (Lond). 2008;114(5):347–60.
67. Hayashi F, Smith KD, Ozinsky A, Hawn TR, Yi EC, Goodlett DR, et al. The innate immune response to bacterial flagellin is mediated by Toll-like receptor 5. Nature. 2001;410(6832):1099–103.
68. Wurfel MM, Gordon AC, Holden TD, Radella F, Strout J, Kajikawa O, et al. Toll-like receptor 1 polymorphisms affect innate immune responses and outcomes in sepsis. Am J Respir Crit Care Med. 2008;178(7):710–20.
69. Pino-Yanes M, Corrales A, Casula M, Blanco J, Muriel A, Espinosa E, et al. Common variants of TLR1 associate with organ dysfunction and sustained pro-inflammatory responses during sepsis. PLoS One. 2010;5(10):e13759.
70. Lorenz E, Mira JP, Cornish KL, Arbour NC, Schwartz DA. A novel polymorphism in the toll-like receptor 2 gene and its potential association with staphylococcal infection. Infect Immun. 2000;68(11):6398–401.
71. Abu-Maziad A, Schaa K, Bell EF, Dagle JM, Cooper M, Marazita ML, et al. Role of polymorphic variants as genetic modulators of infection in neonatal sepsis. Pediatr Res. 2010;68(4):323–9.
72. Arbour NC, Lorenz E, Schutte BC, Zabner J, Kline JN, Jones M, et al. TLR4 mutations are associated with endotoxin hyporesponsiveness in humans. Nat Genet. 2000;25(2):187–91.
73. Michel O, LeVan TD, Stern D, Dentener M, Thorn J, Gnat D, et al. Systemic responsiveness to lipopolysaccharide and polymorphisms in the toll-like receptor 4 gene in human beings. J Allergy Clin Immunol. 2003;112(5):923–9.
74. Lorenz E, Mira JP, Frees KL, Schwartz DA. Relevance of mutations in the TLR4 receptor in patients with gram-negative septic shock. Arch Intern Med. 2002;162(9):1028–32.
75. Agnese DM, Calvano JE, Hahm SJ, Coyle SM, Corbett SA, Calvano SE, et al. Human toll-like receptor 4 mutations but not CD14 polymorphisms are associated with an increased risk of gram-negative infections. J Infect Dis. 2002;186(10):1522–5.
76. Faber J, Henninger N, Finn A, Zenz W, Zepp F, Knuf M. A toll-like receptor 4 variant is associated with fatal outcome in children with invasive meningococcal disease. Acta Paediatr. 2009;98(3):548–52.
77. Hawn TR, Verbon A, Lettinga KD, Zhao LP, Li SS, Laws RJ, et al. A common dominant TLR5 stop codon polymorphism abolishes flagellin signaling and is associated with susceptibility to legionnaires' disease. J Exp Med. 2003;198(10):1563–72.
78. von Bernuth H, Picard C, Jin Z, Pankla R, Xiao H, Ku CL, et al. Pyogenic bacterial infections in humans with MyD88 deficiency. Science. 2008;321(5889):691–6.
79. Ku CL, von Bernuth H, Picard C, Zhang SY, Chang HH, Yang K, et al. Selective predisposition to bacterial infections in IRAK-4-deficient children: IRAK-4-dependent TLRs are otherwise redundant in protective immunity. J Exp Med. 2007;204(10):2407–22.
80. Rock FL, Hardiman G, Timans JC, Kastelein RA, Bazan JF. A family of human receptors structurally related to Drosophila Toll. Proc Natl Acad Sci U S A. 1998;95(2):588–93.
81. Moore CE, Segal S, Berendt AR, Hill AV, Day NP. Lack of association between Toll-like receptor 2 polymorphisms and susceptibility to severe disease caused by *Staphylococcus aureus*. Clin Diagn Lab Immunol. 2004;11(6):1194–7.
82. von Aulock S, Schroder NW, Traub S, Gueinzius K, Lorenz E, Hartung T, et al. Heterozygous toll-like receptor 2 polymorphism does not affect lipoteichoic acid-induced chemokine and inflammatory responses. Infect Immun. 2004;72(3):1828–31.
83. Everett B, Cameron B, Li H, Vollmer-Conna U, Davenport T, Hickie I, et al. Polymorphisms in Toll-like receptors-2 and -4 are not associated with disease manifestations in acute Q fever. Genes Immun. 2007;8(8):699–702.

84. Read RC, Pullin J, Gregory S, Borrow R, Kaczmarski EB, di Giovine FS, et al. A functional polymorphism of toll-like receptor 4 is not associated with likelihood or severity of meningococcal disease. J Infect Dis. 2001;184(5):640–2.

85. Allen A, Obaro S, Bojang K, Awomoyi AA, Greenwood BM, Whittle H, et al. Variation in Toll-like receptor 4 and susceptibility to group A meningococcal meningitis in Gambian children. Pediatr Infect Dis J. 2003;22(11):1018–9.

86. Arcaroli J, Silva E, Maloney JP, He Q, Svetkauskaite D, Murphy JR, et al. Variant IRAK-1 haplotype is associated with increased nuclear factor-kappaB activation and worse outcomes in sepsis. Am J Respir Crit Care Med. 2006;173(12):1335–41.

87. Schutt C. Cd14. Int J Biochem Cell Biol. 1999;31(5):545–9.

88. Landmann R, Reber AM, Sansano S, Zimmerli W. Function of soluble CD14 in serum from patients with septic shock. J Infect Dis. 1996;173(3):661–8.

89. Brunialti MK, Martins PS, de Barbosa Carvalho H, Machado FR, Barbosa LM, et al. TLR2, TLR4, CD14, CD11B, and CD11C expressions on monocytes surface and cytokine production in patients with sepsis, severe sepsis, and septic shock. Shock. 2006;25(4):351–7.

90. Burgmann H, Winkler S, Locker GJ, Presterl E, Laczika K, Staudinger T, et al. Increased serum concentration of soluble CD14 is a prognostic marker in gram-positive sepsis. Clin Immunol Immunopathol. 1996;80(3 Pt 1):307–10.

91. Carrillo EH, Gordon L, Goode E, Davis E, Polk Jr HC. Early elevation of soluble CD14 may help identify trauma patients at high risk for infection. J Trauma. 2001;50(5):810–6.

92. Landmann R, Zimmerli W, Sansano S, Link S, Hahn A, Glauser MP, et al. Increased circulating soluble CD14 is associated with high mortality in gram-negative septic shock. J Infect Dis. 1995;171(3):639–44.

93. Gibot S, Cariou A, Drouet L, Rossignol M, Ripoll L. Association between a genomic polymorphism within the CD14 locus and septic shock susceptibility and mortality rate. Crit Care Med. 2002;30(5):969–73.

94. de Aguiar BB, Girardi I, Paskulin DD, de Franca E, Dornelles C, Dias FS, et al. CD14 expression in the first 24 h of sepsis: effect of -260C>T CD14 SNP. Immunol Invest. 2008;37(8):752–69.

95. Barber RC, Aragaki CC, Chang LY, Purdue GF, Hunt JL, Arnoldo BD, et al. CD14-159 C allele is associated with increased risk of mortality after burn injury. Shock. 2007;27(3):232–7.

96. Barber RC, Chang LY, Arnoldo BD, Purdue GF, Hunt JL, Horton JW, et al. Innate immunity SNPs are associated with risk for severe sepsis after burn injury. Clin Med Res. 2006;4(4):250–5.

97. Heesen M, Bloemeke B, Schade U, Obertacke U, Majetschak M. The −260 C−>T promoter polymorphism of the lipopolysaccharide receptor CD14 and severe sepsis in trauma patients. Intensive Care Med. 2002;28(8):1161–3.

98. Hubacek JA, Stuber F, Frohlich D, Book M, Wetegrove S, Rothe G, et al. The common functional C(−159)T polymorphism within the promoter region of the lipopolysaccharide receptor CD14 is not associated with sepsis development or mortality. Genes Immun. 2000;1(6):405–7.

99. Weiss J. Bactericidal/permeability-increasing protein (BPI) and lipopolysaccharide-binding protein (LBP): structure, function and regulation in host defence against Gram-negative bacteria. Biochem Soc Trans. 2003;31(Pt 4):785–90.

100. Hubacek JA, Stuber F, Frohlich D, Book M, Wetegrove S, Ritter M, et al. Gene variants of the bactericidal/permeability increasing protein and lipopolysaccharide binding protein in sepsis patients: gender-specific genetic predisposition to sepsis. Crit Care Med. 2001;29(3):557–61.

101. Barber RC, O'Keefe GE. Characterization of a single nucleotide polymorphism in the lipopolysaccharide binding protein and its association with sepsis. Am J Respir Crit Care Med. 2003;167(10):1316–20.

102. Mira JP, Cariou A, Grall F, Delclaux C, Losser MR, Heshmati F, et al. Association of TNF2, a TNF-alpha promoter polymorphism, with septic shock susceptibility and mortality: a multicenter study. JAMA. 1999;282(6):561–8.

103. Beutler B. TNF, immunity and inflammatory disease: lessons of the past decade. J Invest Med. 1995;43(3):227–35.
104. Tracey KJ, Fong Y, Hesse DG, Manogue KR, Lee AT, Kuo GC, et al. Anti-cachectin/TNF monoclonal antibodies prevent septic shock during lethal bacteraemia. Nature. 1987;330(6149):662–4.
105. Opal SM, Cross AS, Kelly NM, Sadoff JC, Bodmer MW, Palardy JE, et al. Efficacy of a monoclonal antibody directed against tumor necrosis factor in protecting neutropenic rats from lethal infection with Pseudomonas aeruginosa. J Infect Dis. 1990;161(6):1148–52.
106. Wilson AG, Symons JA, McDowell TL, McDevitt HO, Duff GW. Effects of a polymorphism in the human tumor necrosis factor alpha promoter on transcriptional activation. Proc Natl Acad Sci U S A. 1997;94(7):3195–9.
107. Nadel S, Newport MJ, Booy R, Levin M. Variation in the tumor necrosis factor-alpha gene promoter region may be associated with death from meningococcal disease. J Infect Dis. 1996;174(4):878–80.
108. Stuber F, Udalova IA, Book M, Drutskaya LN, Kuprash DV, Turetskaya RL, et al. 308 tumor necrosis factor (TNF) polymorphism is not associated with survival in severe sepsis and is unrelated to lipopolysaccharide inducibility of the human TNF promoter. J Inflamm. 1995;46(1):42–50.
109. Read RC, Teare DM, Pridmore AC, Naylor SC, Timms JM, Kaczmarski EB, et al. The tumor necrosis factor polymorphism TNF (−308) is associated with susceptibility to meningococcal sepsis, but not with lethality. Crit Care Med. 2009;37(4):1237–43.
110. Pfeffer K. Biological functions of tumor necrosis factor cytokines and their receptors. Cytokine Growth Factor Rev. 2003;14(3–4):185–91.
111. Waterer GW, Quasney MW, Cantor RM, Wunderink RG. Septic shock and respiratory failure in community-acquired pneumonia have different TNF polymorphism associations. Am J Respir Crit Care Med. 2001;163(7):1599–604.
112. Majetschak M, Flohe S, Obertacke U, Schroder J, Staubach K, Nast-Kolb D, et al. Relation of a TNF gene polymorphism to severe sepsis in trauma patients. Ann Surg. 1999;230(2):207–14.
113. Henckaerts L, Nielsen KR, Steffensen R, Van Steen K, Mathieu C, Giulietti A, et al. Polymorphisms in innate immunity genes predispose to bacteremia and death in the medical intensive care unit. Crit Care Med. 2009;37(1):192–201. e191-193
114. Sole-Violan J, de Castro F, Garcia-Laorden MI, Blanquer J, Aspa J, Borderias L, et al. Genetic variability in the severity and outcome of community-acquired pneumonia. Respir Med. 2010;104(3):440–7.
115. Temple SE, Cheong KY, Ardlie KG, Sayer D, Waterer GW. The septic shock associated HSPA1B1267 polymorphism influences production of HSPA1A and HSPA1B. Intensive Care Med. 2004;30(9):1761–7.
116. Pruitt JH, Copeland III EM, Moldawer LL. Interleukin-1 and interleukin-1 antagonism in sepsis, systemic inflammatory response syndrome, and septic shock. Shock. 1995;3(4):235–51.
117. Emonts M, Vermont CL, Houwing-Duistermaat JJ, Haralambous E, Gaast-de Jongh CE, Hazelzet JA, et al. Polymorphisms in PARP, IL1B, IL4, IL10, C1INH, DEFB1, and DEFA4 in meningococcal disease in three populations. Shock. 2010;34(1):17–22.
118. Gu W, Zeng L, Zhou J, Jiang DP, Zhang L, Du DY, et al. Clinical relevance of 13 cytokine gene polymorphisms in Chinese major trauma patients. Intensive Care Med. 2010;36(7):1261–5.
119. Shimada T, Oda S, Sadahiro T, Nakamura M, Hirayama Y, Watanabe E, et al. Outcome prediction in sepsis combined use of genetic polymorphisms – a study in Japanese population. Cytokine. 2011;54(1):79–84.
120. Arnalich F, Lopez-Maderuelo D, Codoceo R, Lopez J, Solis-Garrido LM, Capiscol C, et al. Interleukin-1 receptor antagonist gene polymorphism and mortality in patients with severe sepsis. Clin Exp Immunol. 2002;127(2):331–6.
121. Fang XM, Schroder S, Hoeft A, Stuber F. Comparison of two polymorphisms of the interleukin-1 gene family: interleukin-1 receptor antagonist polymorphism contributes to susceptibility to severe sepsis. Crit Care Med. 1999;27(7):1330–4.

122. Ma P, Chen D, Pan J, Du B. Genomic polymorphism within interleukin-1 family cytokines influences the outcome of septic patients. Crit Care Med. 2002;30(5):1046–50.
123. Wan QQ, Ye QF, Ma Y, Zhou JD. Genetic association of interleukin-1beta (−511C/T) and its receptor antagonist (86-bpVNTR) gene polymorphism with susceptibility to bacteremia in kidney transplant recipients. Transplant Proc. 2012;44(10):3026–8.
124. Zhang AQ, Pan W, Gao JW, Yue CL, Zeng L, Gu W, et al. Associations between interleukin-1 gene polymorphisms and sepsis risk: a meta-analysis. BMC Med Genet. 2014;15:8.
125. Zapata-Tarres M, Arredondo-Garcia JL, Rivera-Luna R, Klunder-Klunder M, Mancilla-Ramirez J, Sanchez-Urbina R, et al. Interleukin-1 receptor antagonist gene polymorphism increases susceptibility to septic shock in children with acute lymphoblastic leukemia. Pediatr Infect Dis J. 2013;32(2):136–9.
126. Zhang DL, Zheng HM, Yu BJ, Jiang ZW, Li JS. Association of polymorphisms of IL and CD14 genes with acute severe pancreatitis and septic shock. World J Gastroenterol. 2005;11(28):4409–13.
127. Meyer NJ, Ferguson JF, Feng R, Wang F, Patel PN, Li M, et al. A functional synonymous coding variant in the IL1RN gene is associated with survival in septic shock. Am J Respir Crit Care Med. 2014;190(6):656–64.
128. Meyer NJ, Feng R, Li M, Zhao Y, Sheu CC, Tejera P, et al. IL1RN coding variant is associated with lower risk of acute respiratory distress syndrome and increased plasma IL-1 receptor antagonist. Am J Respir Crit Care Med. 2013;187(9):950–9.
129. Fishman D, Faulds G, Jeffery R, Mohamed-Ali V, Yudkin JS, Humphries S, et al. The effect of novel polymorphisms in the interleukin-6 (IL-6) gene on IL-6 transcription and plasma IL-6 levels, and an association with systemic-onset juvenile chronic arthritis. J Clin Invest. 1998;102(7):1369–76.
130. Gaudino M, Andreotti F, Zamparelli R, Di Castelnuovo A, Nasso G, Burzotta F, et al. The -174G/C interleukin-6 polymorphism influences postoperative interleukin-6 levels and postoperative atrial fibrillation. Is atrial fibrillation an inflammatory complication? Circulation. 2003;108(Suppl 1):II195–9.
131. Schluter B, Raufhake C, Erren M, Schotte H, Kipp F, Rust S, et al. Effect of the interleukin-6 promoter polymorphism (−174G/C) on the incidence and outcome of sepsis. Crit Care Med. 2002;30(1):32–7.
132. Roth-Isigkeit A, Hasselbach L, Ocklitz E, Bruckner S, Ros A, Gehring H, et al. Inter-individual differences in cytokine release in patients undergoing cardiac surgery with cardio-pulmonary bypass. Clin Exp Immunol. 2001;125(1):80–8.
133. Sutherland AM, Walley KR, Manocha S, Russell JA. The association of interleukin 6 haplo-type clades with mortality in critically ill adults. Arch Intern Med. 2005;165(1):75–82.
134. Flores C, Ma SF, Maresso K, Wade MS, Villar J, Garcia JG. IL6 gene-wide haplotype is associated with susceptibility to acute lung injury. Transl Res. 2008;152(1):11–7.
135. Moore KW, de Waal MR, Coffman RL, O'Garra A. Interleukin-10 and the interleukin-10 receptor. Annu Rev Immunol. 2001;19:683–765.
136. Surbatovic M, Grujic K, Cikota B, Jevtic M, Filipovic N, Romic P, et al. Polymorphisms of genes encoding tumor necrosis factor-alpha, interleukin-10, cluster of differentiation-14 and interleukin-1ra in critically ill patients. J Crit Care. 2010;25(3):542. e541–548
137. Stanilova SA, Miteva LD, Karakolev ZT, Stefanov CS. Interleukin-10-1082 promoter poly-morphism in association with cytokine production and sepsis susceptibility. Intensive Care Med. 2006;32(2):260–6.
138. Gallagher PM, Lowe G, Fitzgerald T, Bella A, Greene CM, McElvaney NG, et al. Association of IL-10 polymorphism with severity of illness in community acquired pneumonia. Thorax. 2003;58(2):154–6.
139. Schaaf BM, Boehmke F, Esnaashari H, Seitzer U, Kothe H, Maass M, et al. Pneumococcal septic shock is associated with the interleukin-10-1082 gene promoter polymorphism. Am J Respir Crit Care Med. 2003;168(4):476–80.
140. Carregaro F, Carta A, Cordeiro JA, Lobo SM, Silva EH, Leopoldino AM. Polymorphisms IL10-819 and TLR-2 are potentially associated with sepsis in Brazilian patients. Mem Inst Oswaldo Cruz. 2010;105(5):649–56.

141. Wattanathum A, Manocha S, Groshaus H, Russell JA, Walley KR. Interleukin-10 haplotype associated with increased mortality in critically ill patients with sepsis from pneumonia but not in patients with extrapulmonary sepsis. Chest. 2005;128(3):1690–8.
142. Aso Y. Plasminogen activator inhibitor (PAI)-1 in vascular inflammation and thrombosis. Front Biosci. 2007;12:2957–66.
143. Song Y, Lynch SV, Flanagan J, Zhuo H, Tom W, Dotson RH, et al. Increased plasminogen activator inhibitor-1 concentrations in bronchoalveolar lavage fluids are associated with increased mortality in a cohort of patients with Pseudomonas aeruginosa. Anesthesiology. 2007;106(2):252–61.
144. Ware LB, Matthay MA, Parsons PE, Thompson BT, Januzzi JL, Eisner MD. Pathogenetic and prognostic significance of altered coagulation and fibrinolysis in acute lung injury/acute respiratory distress syndrome. Crit Care Med. 2007;35(8):1821–8.
145. Hermans PW, Hazelzet JA. Plasminogen activator inhibitor type 1 gene polymorphism and sepsis. Clin Infect Dis. 2005;41(Suppl 7):S453–8.
146. Dawson SJ, Wiman B, Hamsten A, Green F, Humphries S, Henney AM. The two allele sequences of a common polymorphism in the promoter of the plasminogen activator inhibitor-1 (PAI-1) gene respond differently to interleukin-1 in HepG2 cells. J Biol Chem. 1993;268(15):10739–45.
147. Westendorp RG, Hottenga JJ, Slagboom PE. Variation in plasminogen-activator-inhibitor-1 gene and risk of meningococcal septic shock. Lancet. 1999;354(9178):561–3.
148. Menges T, Hermans PW, Little SG, Langefeld T, Boning O, Engel J, et al. Plasminogen-activator-inhibitor-1 4G/5G promoter polymorphism and prognosis of severely injured patients. Lancet. 2001;357(9262):1096–7.
149. Haralambous E, Hibberd ML, Hermans PW, Ninis N, Nadel S, Levin M. Role of functional plasminogen-activator-inhibitor-1 4G/5G promoter polymorphism in susceptibility, severity, and outcome of meningococcal disease in Caucasian children. Crit Care Med. 2003;31(12):2788–93.
150. Binder A, Endler G, Muller M, Mannhalter C, Zenz W. 4G4G genotype of the plasminogen activator inhibitor-1 promoter polymorphism associates with disseminated intravascular coagulation in children with systemic meningococcemia. J Thromb Haemost. 2007;5(10):2049–54.
151. Garcia-Segarra G, Espinosa G, Tassies D, Oriola J, Aibar J, Bove A, et al. Increased mortality in septic shock with the 4G/4G genotype of plasminogen activator inhibitor 1 in patients of white descent. Intensive Care Med. 2007;33(8):1354–62.
152. Sapru A, Hansen H, Ajayi T, Brown R, Garcia O, Zhuo H, et al. 4G/5G polymorphism of plasminogen activator inhibitor-1 gene is associated with mortality in intensive care unit patients with severe pneumonia. Anesthesiology. 2009;110(5):1086–91.
153. Madach K, Aladzsity I, Szilagyi A, Fust G, Gal J, Penzes I, et al. 4G/5G polymorphism of PAI-1 gene is associated with multiple organ dysfunction and septic shock in pneumonia induced severe sepsis: prospective, observational, genetic study. Crit Care. 2010;14(2):R79.
154. Yende S, Angus DC, Ding J, Newman AB, Kellum JA, Li R, et al. 4G/5G plasminogen activator inhibitor-1 polymorphisms and haplotypes are associated with pneumonia. Am J Respir Crit Care Med. 2007;176(11):1129–37.
155. Li L, Nie W, Zhou H, Yuan W, Li W, Huang W. Association between plasminogen activator inhibitor-1-675 4G/5G polymorphism and sepsis: a meta-analysis. PLoS One. 2013;8(1):e54883.
156. Chen QX, Wu SJ, Wang HH, Lv C, Cheng BL, Xie GH, et al. Protein C -1641A/−1654C haplotype is associated with organ dysfunction and the fatal outcome of severe sepsis in Chinese Han population. Hum Genet. 2008;123(3):281–7.
157. Spek CA, Koster T, Rosendaal FR, Bertina RM, Reitsma PH. Genotypic variation in the promoter region of the protein C gene is associated with plasma protein C levels and thrombotic risk. Arterioscler Thromb Vasc Biol. 1995;15(2):214–8.
158. Walley KR, Russell JA. Protein C -1641 AA is associated with decreased survival and more organ dysfunction in severe sepsis. Crit Care Med. 2007;35(1):12–7.

159. Russell JA, Wellman H, Walley KR. Protein C rs2069912 C allele is associated with increased mortality from severe sepsis in North Americans of East Asian ancestry. Hum Genet. 2008;123(6):661–3.

160. Ridker PM, Miletich JP, Hennekens CH, Buring JE. Ethnic distribution of factor V Leiden in 4047 men and women. Implications for venous thromboembolism screening. JAMA. 1997;277(16):1305–7.

161. Kerlin BA, Yan SB, Isermann BH, Brandt JT, Sood R, Basson BR, et al. Survival advantage associated with heterozygous factor V Leiden mutation in patients with severe sepsis and in mouse endotoxemia. Blood. 2003;102(9):3085–92.

162. Benfield TL, Dahl M, Nordestgaard BG, Tybjaerg-Hansen A. Influence of the factor V Leiden mutation on infectious disease susceptibility and outcome: a population-based study. J Infect Dis. 2005;192(10):1851–7.

163. Benfield T, Ejrnaes K, Juul K, Ostergaard C, Helweg-Larsen J, Weis N, et al. Influence of Factor V Leiden on susceptibility to and outcome from critical illness: a genetic association study. Crit Care. 2010;14(2):R28.

164. Bernard GR, Margolis BD, Shanies HM, Ely EW, Wheeler AP, Levy H, et al. Extended evaluation of recombinant human activated protein C United States Trial (ENHANCE US): a single-arm, phase 3B, multicenter study of drotrecogin alfa (activated) in severe sepsis. Chest. 2004;125(6):2206–16.

165. Tsantes AE, Tsangaris I, Bonovas S, Kopterides P, Rapti E, Dimopoulou I, et al. The effect of four hemostatic gene polymorphisms on the outcome of septic critically ill patients. Blood Coagul Fibrinolysis. 2010;21(2):175–81.

166. Zhang J, He Y, Song W, Lu Y, Li P, Zou L, et al. Lack of association between factor V leiden and sepsis: a meta-analysis. Clin Appl Thromb Hemost. 2015;21(3):204–10.

167. Nakada TA, Russell JA, Boyd JH, Aguirre-Hernandez R, Thain KR, Thair SA, et al. Beta2-adrenergic receptor gene polymorphism is associated with mortality in septic shock. Am J Respir Crit Care Med. 2010;181(2):143–9.

168. Nakada TA, Russell JA, Wellman H, Boyd JH, Nakada E, Thain KR, et al. Leucyl/cystinyl aminopeptidase gene variants in septic shock. Chest. 2011;139(5):1042–9.

169. Nakada TA, Russell JA, Boyd JH, McLaughlin L, Nakada E, Thair SA, et al. Association of angiotensin II type 1 receptor-associated protein gene polymorphism with increased mortality in septic shock. Crit Care Med. 2011;39(7):1641–8.

170. Man M, Close SL, Shaw AD, Bernard GR, Douglas IS, Kaner RJ, et al. Beyond single-marker analyses: mining whole genome scans for insights into treatment responses in severe sepsis. Pharmacogenomics J. 2013;13(3):218–26.

171. Davila S, Wright VJ, Khor CC, Sim KS, Binder A, Breunis WB, et al. Genome-wide association study identifies variants in the CFH region associated with host susceptibility to meningococcal disease. Nat Genet. 2010;42(9):772–6.

172. Band G, Le QS, Jostins L, Pirinen M, Kivinen K, Jallow M, et al. Imputation-based meta-analysis of severe malaria in three African populations. PLoS Genet. 2013;9(5):e1003509.

173. Jallow M, Teo YY, Small KS, Rockett KA, Deloukas P, Clark TG, et al. Genome-wide and fine-resolution association analysis of malaria in West Africa. Nat Genet. 2009;41(6):657–65.

174. Timmann C, Thye T, Vens M, Evans J, May J, Ehmen C, et al. Genome-wide association study indicates two novel resistance loci for severe malaria. Nature. 2012;489(7416):443–6.

175. Fumagalli M, Pozzoli U, Cagliani R, Comi GP, Bresolin N, Clerici M, et al. Genome-wide identification of susceptibility alleles for viral infections through a population genetics approach. PLoS Genet. 2010;6(2):e1000849.

176. Fijen CA, Kuijper EJ, te Bulte MT, Daha MR, Dankert J. Assessment of complement deficiency in patients with meningococcal disease in The Netherlands. Clin Infect Dis. 1999;28(1):98–105.

177. Fry AE, Griffiths MJ, Auburn S, Diakite M, Forton JT, Green A, et al. Common variation in the ABO glycosyltransferase is associated with susceptibility to severe Plasmodium falciparum malaria. Hum Mol Genet. 2008;17(4):567–76.

178. Reilly JP, Meyer NJ, Shashaty MG, Feng R, Lanken PN, Gallop R, et al. ABO blood type A is associated with increased risk of ARDS in whites following both major trauma and severe sepsis. Chest. 2014;145(4):753–61.
179. Mu J, Myers RA, Jiang H, Liu S, Ricklefs S, Waisberg M, et al. Plasmodium falciparum genome-wide scans for positive selection, recombination hot spots and resistance to antimalarial drugs. Nat Genet. 2010;42(3):268–71.
180. Naitza S, Porcu E, Steri M, Taub DD, Mulas A, Xiao X, et al. A genome-wide association scan on the levels of markers of inflammation in Sardinians reveals associations that underpin its complex regulation. PLoS Genet. 2012;8(1):e1002480.
181. Mikacenic C, Reiner AP, Holden TD, Nickerson DA, Wurfel MM. Variation in the TLR10/TLR1/TLR6 locus is the major genetic determinant of interindividual difference in TLR1/2-mediated responses. Genes Immun. 2013;14(1):52–7.
182. Calvano SE, Xiao W, Richards DR, Felciano RM, Baker HV, Cho RJ, et al. A network-based analysis of systemic inflammation in humans. Nature. 2005;437(7061):1032–7.
183. Johnson SB, Lissauer M, Bochicchio GV, Moore R, Cross AS, Scalea TM. Gene expression profiles differentiate between sterile SIRS and early sepsis. Ann Surg. 2007;245(4):611–21.
184. Payen D, Lukaszewicz AC, Belikova I, Faivre V, Gelin C, Russwurm S, et al. Gene profiling in human blood leucocytes during recovery from septic shock. Intensive Care Med. 2008;34(8):1371–6.
185. Tang BM, Huang SJ, McLean AS. Genome-wide transcription profiling of human sepsis: a systematic review. Crit Care. 2010;14(6):R237.
186. Tang BM, McLean AS, Dawes IW, Huang SJ, Lin RC. The use of gene-expression profiling to identify candidate genes in human sepsis. Am J Respir Crit Care Med. 2007;176(7):676–84.
187. Tang BM, McLean AS, Dawes IW, Huang SJ, Cowley MJ, Lin RC. Gene-expression profiling of gram-positive and gram-negative sepsis in critically ill patients. Crit Care Med. 2008;36(4):1125–8.
188. Wong HR, Cvijanovich NZ, Allen GL, Thomas NJ, Freishtat RJ, Anas N, et al. Corticosteroids are associated with repression of adaptive immunity gene programs in pediatric septic shock. Am J Respir Crit Care Med. 2014;189(8):940–6.
189. Wong HR, Cvijanovich N, Allen GL, Lin R, Anas N, Meyer K, et al. Genomic expression profiling across the pediatric systemic inflammatory response syndrome, sepsis, and septic shock spectrum. Crit Care Med. 2009;37(5):1558–66.
190. Martin GS. Sepsis, severe sepsis and septic shock: changes in incidence, pathogens and outcomes. Expert Rev Anti Infect Ther. 2012;10(6):701–6.
191. Stengaard-Pedersen K, Thiel S, Gadjeva M, Moller-Kristensen M, Sorensen R, Jensen LT, et al. Inherited deficiency of mannan-binding lectin-associated serine protease 2. N Engl J Med. 2003;349(6):554–60.
192. Brenmoehl J, Herfarth H, Gluck T, Audebert F, Barlage S, Schmitz G, et al. Genetic variants in the NOD2/CARD15 gene are associated with early mortality in sepsis patients. Intensive Care Med. 2007;33(9):1541–8.
193. Yuan FF, Wong M, Pererva N, Keating J, Davis AR, Bryant JA, et al. FcgammaRIIA polymorphisms in Streptococcus pneumoniae infection. Immunol Cell Biol. 2003;81(3):192–5.
194. Moens L, Van Hoeyveld E, Verhaegen J, De Boeck K, Peetermans WE, Bossuyt X. Fcgamma-receptor IIA genotype and invasive pneumococcal infection. Clin Immunol. 2006;118(1):20–3.
195. Khor CC, Chapman SJ, Vannberg FO, Dunne A, Murphy C, Ling EY, et al. A mal functional variant is associated with protection against invasive pneumococcal disease, bacteremia, malaria and tuberculosis. Nat Genet. 2007;39(4):523–8.
196. Michalek J, Svetlikova P, Fedora M, Klimovic M, Klapacova L, Bartosova D, et al. Bactericidal permeability increasing protein gene variants in children with sepsis. Intensive Care Med. 2007;33(12):2158–64.
197. Stassen NA, Breit CM, Norfleet LA, Polk Jr HC. IL-18 promoter polymorphisms correlate with the development of post-injury sepsis. Surgery. 2003;134(2):351–6.
198. Yende S, Angus DC, Kong L, Kellum JA, Weissfeld L, Ferrell R, et al. The influence of macrophage migration inhibitory factor gene polymorphisms on outcome from community-acquired pneumonia. FASEB J. 2009;23(8):2403–11.

199. Das R, Subrahmanyan L, Yang IV, van Duin D, Levy R, Piecychna M, et al. Functional polymorphisms in the gene encoding macrophage migration inhibitory factor are associated with Gram-negative bacteremia in older adults. J Infect Dis. 2014;209(5):764–8.
200. Renner P, Roger T, Bochud PY, Sprong T, Sweep FC, Bochud M, et al. A functional microsatellite of the macrophage migration inhibitory factor gene associated with meningococcal disease. FASEB J. 2012;26(2):907–16.
201. Lehmann LE, Book M, Hartmann W, Weber SU, Schewe JC, Klaschik S, et al. A MIF haplotype is associated with the outcome of patients with severe sepsis: a case control study. J Transl Med. 2009;7:100.
202. Stassen NA, Leslie-Norfleet LA, Robertson AM, Eichenberger MR, Polk Jr HC. Interferon-gamma gene polymorphisms and the development of sepsis in patients with trauma. Surgery. 2002;132(2):289–92.
203. Flores C, Maca-Meyer N, Perez-Mendez L, Sanguesa R, Espinosa E, Muriel A, et al. A CXCL2 tandem repeat promoter polymorphism is associated with susceptibility to severe sepsis in the Spanish population. Genes Immun. 2006;7(2):141–9.
204. Lorente L, Martin M, Plasencia F, Sole-Violan J, Blanquer J, Labarta L, et al. The 372 T/C genetic polymorphism of TIMP-1 is associated with serum levels of TIMP-1 and survival in patients with severe sepsis. Crit Care. 2013;17(3):R94.
205. Moretti EW, Morris RW, Podgoreanu M, Schwinn DA, Newman MF, Bennett E, et al. APOE polymorphism is associated with risk of severe sepsis in surgical patients. Crit Care Med. 2005;33(11):2521–6.
206. Nakada TA, Russell JA, Boyd JH, Thair SA, Walley KR. Identification of a nonsynonymous polymorphism in the SVEP1 gene associated with altered clinical outcomes in septic shock. Crit Care Med. 2015;43(1):101–8.
207. Marshall RP, Webb S, Bellingan GJ, Montgomery HE, Chaudhari B, McAnulty RJ, et al. Angiotensin converting enzyme insertion/deletion polymorphism is associated with susceptibility and outcome in acute respiratory distress syndrome. Am J Respir Crit Care Med. 2002;166(5):646–50.
208. Harding D, Baines PB, Brull D, Vassiliou V, Ellis I, Hart A, et al. Severity of meningococcal disease in children and the angiotensin-converting enzyme insertion/deletion polymorphism. Am J Respir Crit Care Med. 2002;165(8):1103–6.

Index

© Springer International Publishing AG 2017
N.S. Ward, M.M. Levy (eds.), *Sepsis*, Respiratory Medicine,
DOI 10.1007/978-3-319-48470-9

Printed in the United States
By Bookmasters